CONCEPTUAL MODELS OF NURSING

Analysis and Application

FOURTH EDITION

Joyce J. Fitzpatrick, RN, PhD, FAAN
Elizabeth Brooks Ford Professor and Dean
Frances Payne Bolton School of Nursing
Case Western Reserve University
Cleveland, Ohio

Ann L. Whall, RN, PhD, FAAN
Professor, School of Nursing
Associate Director, The Geriatrics Center
The University of Michigan
Ann Arbor, Michigan

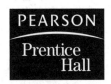

PEARSON
Prentice
Hall

Upper Saddle River, New Jersey

Library of Congress Cataloging-in-Publication Data

Conceptual models of nursing : analysis and application / [edited by] Joyce J. Fitzpatrick, Ann L. Whall.— 4th ed.
  p. ; cm.
  ISBN 0-13-048060-6
  1. Nursing—Philosophy. 2. Nursing models.
  [DNLM: 1. Models, Nursing. 2. Philosophy, Nursing. WY 20.5 C744 2005] I.
Fitzpatrick, Joyce J., (date) II. Whall, Ann L.
  RT84. 5. C664 2005
  610.73'01—dc22   2004001577

Publisher: Julie Levin Alexander
Publisher's Assistant: Regina Bruno
Editor-in-Chief: Maura Connor
Assistant Editor: Sladjana Repic
Editorial Assistant: Malgorzata Jaros-White
Director of Manufacturing & Production: Bruce Johnson
Managing Production Editor: Patrick Walsh
Production Liaison: Cathy O'Connell
Production Editor: Robin Reed, Carlisle Communications
Manufacturing Manager: Ilene Sanford
Manufacturing Buyer: Pat Brown
Design Director: Cheryl Asherman
Cover Designer: Amy Rosen
Senior Design Coordinator: Maria Guglielmo Walsh
Director of Marketing: Karen Allman
Executive Marketing Manager: Nicole Benson
Channel Marketing Manager: Rachele Strober
Marketing Coordinator: Janet Ryerson
Composition: Carlisle Communications
Printer/Binder: Phoenix Color Book Tech Park
Cover Printer: Phoenix Color

This book was set in Times by Carlisle Communications, Ltd. and was printed and bound by Phoenix Color Company. The cover was printed by Phoenix Color.

Notice: Care has been taken to confirm the accuracy of information presented in this book. The authors, editors, and the publisher, however, cannot accept any responsibility for errors or omissions or for consequences from application of the information in this book and make no warranty, express or implied, with respect to its contents.

The authors and publisher have exerted every effort to ensure that drug selections and dosages set forth in this text are in accord with current recommendations and practice at time of publication. However, in view of ongoing research, changes in government regulations, and the constant flow of information relating to drug therapy and drug reactions, the reader is urged to check the package inserts of all drugs for any change in indications of dosage and for added warnings and precautions. This is particularly important when the recommended agent is a new and/or infrequently employed drug.

Pearson Education Ltd.
Pearson Education Singapore, Pte. Ltd.
Pearson Education Canada, Ltd.
Pearson Education—Japan

Pearson Education Australia Pty., Limited
Pearson Education North Asia Ltd.
Pearson Educación de Mexico, S.A. de C.V.
Pearson Education Malaysia, Pte. Ltd.
Pearson Education, Inc., Upper Saddle River, NJ

10 9 8 7 6 5 4 3 2 1

ISBN: 0-13-048060-6

We dedicate this book to Martha E. Rogers,
an inspiration, a constant friend,
and an enduring motivation to achieve excellence.

CONTENTS

PREFACE

The 1st edition of this text was published in 1983. At that time our intent was to familiarize students with nursing models and to present a scholarly analysis of the models using a consistent format across models. In addition, our goal was to excite and challenge students to use these grand theories in research and practice. By the 2nd edition in 1989, most students were familiar with the nursing conceptual models, and we focused on presenting a historical panorama of models, again using the most current and best sources for explanation and analysis. The 3rd edition, published in 1996, was focused on synthesis and extension of our previous work. In that edition, we focused on the application of the nursing models to nursing practice, with specific attention to the relationship of the nursing models to nursing diagnoses guiding nursing interventions. This 4th edition comes at a time when there is significant integration of nursing conceptual models with both middle-range nursing theories and practice level theories throughout the discipline.

As nursing models have come to be understood as the embodiment of nursing philosophies, presenting the beliefs, understandings, and purposes of the discipline of nursing, it is most appropriate that they guide research, education, and practice. According to Ellis (1983), nursing models articulate the essence of nursing and serve as tangible sources of the perspective of nursing across time. Many of these conceptual models serve as sources for extensive programs of research, as curricular organizers, and as templates for practice. All of the models embody the nursing perspective and therefore may be used to guide knowledge development within nursing.

Within this 4th edition, the authors explore how nursing models might guide newer elements within nursing, such as the standardized nursing languages. Some models lend themselves to this application and some do not. The first two chapters present nursing conceptual models within the context of theory development within the discipline of nursing. We explore how nursing models may be used, along with other methods, to guide middle-range and prescriptive/practice theory development. Because there has been a shift toward emphasis on the development of practice theories for nursing, we have suggested analysis and evaluation guidelines that nursing might use to address such practice level theory. In this analysis we suggest that the perspective of nursing from conceptualization at the broadest levels, along with other criteria, be used to analyze and evaluate these theories. Likewise, as middle-range theory in nursing is used to guide nursing research, it too has become an important element within the knowledge base of the nursing discipline. Therefore, we also suggest middle-range theory be examined with nursing models as perspective and with the addition of related criteria. Examination of the full range of nursing theory in light of the perspective of nursing has long been advocated. If this examination is completed with nursing models as exemplars, the nursing discipline will be enhanced with a logically developed, coherent body of knowledge.

We believe that the analyses and evaluation methods presented in this text are an important way to develop a coherent knowledge base within nursing. Faculty and students in graduate programs in nursing will find this text most helpful in the development and evaluation of the theoretical base for advanced nursing practice, research, and education. Undergraduate faculty and students may also find this text valuable as a method by which to evaluate their theoretical base and apply the concepts to professional nursing practice.

REFERENCE

Ellis, R. (1983). Philosophical inquiry. In H. H. Werley & J. J. Fitzpatrick (Eds.), *Annual Review of Nursing Research, 1,* 211–228.

CONTRIBUTORS

Cynthia Cameron, PhD, RN
Associate Dean and Associate Professor
Graduate Program
University of Manitoba
Winnipeg, Manitoba
Canada

Veronica F. Engle, PhD, RN, FAAN
Professor
College of Nursing
University of Tennessee Health Science
Center
Memphis, TN

Joyce J. Fitzpatrick, PhD, RN, FAAN, FNAP
Elizabeth Brooks Ford Professor of
Nursing
Frances Payne Bolton School of Nursing
Case Western Reserve University
Cleveland, OH

Emily J. Fox-Hill, PhD, RN
Assistant Professor
College of Nursing
University of Tennessee Health Science
Center
Memphis, TN

Maureen A. Frey, PhD, RN
Director, Center for Excellence in
Pediatric Nursing
Children's Hospital of Michigan
Detroit, MI

Hertha L. Gast, PhD, RN
Assistant Professor
College of Nursing
Wayne State University
Detroit, MI

Ann C. Glasgow, MSN, ND(c), RN
Family Nurse Practitioner
Family Medicine Clinic
Oxford, MS

Edward J. Halloran, PhD, RN, FAAN
Associate Professor
School of Nursing
University of North Carolina
Chapel Hill, NC

Jean Croce Hemphill, PhD, RN
Family Nurse Practitioner
James H. Quillen VA Medical Center
Mountain Home, TN

Diane R. Lancaster, PhD, RN
Director, Nursing Research
Boston University Medical Center
Boston, MA

Carol J. Loveland-Cherry, PhD, RN, FAAN
Professor
School of Nursing
University of Michigan
Ann Arbor, MI

Linda Luna, PhD, RN
King Faisel Specialist Hospital and
Research Center
Rijadh, Kingdom of Saudi Arabia

Kristen S. Montgomery, PhD, RN
Assistant Professor
College of Nursing
University of South Carolina
Columbia, SC

ix

Diana L. Morris, PhD, RN, FAAN
Associate Professor
Frances Payne Bolton School of Nursing
Case Western Reserve University
Cleveland, OH

Jana L. Pressler, PhD, RN
Associate Professor
School of Nursing
University of Missouri–Kansas City
Kansas City, MO

Stephanie I. Muth Quillin, PhD, RN
Associate Professor
Department of Family & Community
Nursing
College of Nursing
East Tennessee State University
Johnson City, TN

Pamela G. Reed, PhD, RN, FAAN
Professor
College of Nursing
University of Arizona
Tucson, AZ

Mary J. Thorson, PhD, RN
Assistant Professor
College of Pharmacy, Nursing and Allied
Health
Howard University
Washington, DC

Mary E. Tiedeman, PhD, RN
Associate Professor
College of Nursing
Brigham Young University
Provo, UT

**Patricia Hinton Walker, PhD, RN,
FAAN, FNAP**
Professor and Dean of Nursing
Graduate School of Nursing
Uniformed Services University of the
Health Sciences
Bethesda, MD

Ann L. Whall, PhD, RN FAAN
Professor
School of Nursing
Associate Director, The Geriatrics Center
University of Michigan
Ann Arbor, MI

Sharon A. Wilkerson, PhD, RN
Associate Professor
School of Nursing
Purdue University
West Lafayette, IN

**Tamara L. Zurakowski, PhD, RN,
CRNP**
Assistant Professor
School of Nursing
La Salle University
Philadelphia, PA

Carolyn L. Blue, PhD
Associate Professor
Purdue University, School of Nursing
West Lafayette, IN

Nancy Kramer, EdD, CPNP, ARNP
Professor and BSN Program Chair
Allen College
Waterloo, IA

Elizabeth Lenz, PhD, RN, FAAN
Dean and Professor
College of Nursing
Ohio State University
Columbus, OH

Kathleen M. Neill, DNSc, RN
Ethics Liaison
Center for Clinical Bioethics
Adjunct Associate Professor
Georgetown University
Washington, DC

Nursing Knowledge Development: Relationship to Science and Professional Practice

Joyce J. Fitzpatrick

Nursing is an evolving discipline, both in its science development (theory and research) and in its professional practice. At the same time, we have a rich history of thought from Florence Nightingale to the present-day nurse theorists, researchers, and clinicians. In addition, today much of nursing science and professional practice includes integration of nursing knowledge, from the broad conceptualizations of the nursing models to the level of practice theory.

Nursing conceptual models often are understood as the embodiment of nursing philosophies, presenting its beliefs, understandings, and purposes. Flowing from these grand theories are the middle range and practice theories that are more closely associated both conceptually and practically to the everyday activities of nurse educators, researchers, and clinicians. This deductive process of knowledge development leads nurses to discover new ideas and potential applications of knowledge. Scientists also can engage in inductive processes of building knowledge from their data. Both processes have relevance in the discipline of nursing.

In addition, nursing conceptual models provide the overall direction for practice, education, and research. Components of basic and applied research, ethics, and knowledge from philosophical and historical inquiry can be derived from these broad conceptualizations. The research and professional practice of the discipline also include integration of knowledge from other disciplines, particularly the health sciences.

Although it is imperative to address the process of our knowledge development in nursing, the content component of our knowledge development is as critical. Both process and content components of the knowledge within the nursing discipline are embedded in nursing conceptual models and the middle range and practice theories that flow from these models.

This chapter addresses the following questions: What is science? What is the nature of knowing in a science and a professional practice? How do the patterns of knowing of the scientist and professional practitioner complement each other?

Science represents one means of understanding ourselves and our world. In Kuhn's (1977) revolutionary view of science, the development of disciplines is based on the convergence of scientific thought. Kuhn proposes that the predominant model within a discipline is subject to the sociological development of the discipline, and that the processes for knowledge development are as important as the content that is being developed. Kuhn's view includes attention to both the theory and the research components of science; both are necessary for scientific development.

In a clinical discipline such as nursing, there are two distinct ways of knowing, requiring different sets of skills (Fitzpatrick, 2002, 2003). Clinicians develop knowledge through a process of synthesizing information quickly. They make clinical judgments based on this rapid synthesis of information. The more expert the clinician, the more quickly the information can be synthesized, and presumably the more accurate the clinical judgment. Clinical scholars use knowledge developed through evidence-based practice to further advance their clinical understandings. Best practices inform current clinical practice, and the clinical scholar relies on evidence from a variety of sources to guide clinical judgments.

One of the ways in which we develop knowledge in nursing as a discipline is through science. The scientific process provides the means for this knowledge development. Researchers view the world by examining each component in great depth. They are much more likely to spend time cautiously, viewing each detail from many different perspectives and gathering much data before reaching conclusions. The research process takes things apart, and only after considerable data collection and analyses does the research arrive at the interpretations and conclusions.

It is not common for the expert researcher also to be an expert clinician. Rather, because a different set of skills is required of each, the most effective teams for development of clinical nursing knowledge would include both clinicians and researchers, each bringing their different perspectives and their different skills to the knowledge development process.

Both research and clinical practice are guided by general and specific understandings of the world. At times, the broad understandings are referred to as "world views." Within the nursing discipline, as these models have become more deliberate and more systematically developed they have been understood as nursing conceptual models. As models and frameworks, these structures provide the foundation for development of both clinical and scientific knowledge. These models provide both the form (or the structures) and the content on which we base our science and professional practice. The more specific understandings are referred to as theories. Both the broad conceptualizations and the specific theories guide both research and professional practice in nursing.

Nursing as a discipline must attend to both the process of knowledge development and the content of nursing knowledge. The nurse scientist and the nurse clinician must have the tools with which to develop their knowledge, at the same time knowing the content parameters of the knowledge that is to be developed. Multiple modes of inquiry within both research and clinical practice are warranted, especially given that nursing has staked a knowledge claim to understandings of the holistic persons and their health. Nurse scientists and clinicians together can develop knowledge that builds the holistic framework, thus adding a dimension of knowledge that is not developed through other disciplines, or through the application of knowledge from these other disciplines to professional nursing practice.

Quality research is rather simple to identify from a general scientific standard. Peer-reviewed evaluation of the merit of research serves as the basic criteria, including use of the peer review process in judging both the award of research funds and the acceptance of manuscripts in scientific journals. Quality theory is also possible to evaluate, although a different set of criteria is used. There exists a basic set of evaluation criteria that is consistent across levels of theory. There also exists a set of standards upon which clinical knowledge can be judged. Thus, each component of knowledge development has its own parameters for judging the quality of the work.

Some characteristics are desirable in both clinical scholarship and research. Knowledge development from either approach would be enhanced by attention to excellence and creativity. At the same time it is important to attend to the desired outcomes and anticipated products of the knowledge development processes, whether developed through clinical scholarship or research. Outcome-driven models are most valued in contemporary professional work. Thus, both the clinical and the scientific way of knowing in nursing are built on a strong foundation of inquiry, with attention to both the process and content of the inquiry.

Both clinical scholarship and research are likely to flourish in environments where there is support for knowledge development, including attention to nurturing of innovation and creativity. Attention to the outcomes of knowledge development also is an important factor. Improvements in clinical outcomes now serve as important criteria by which we judge our professional nursing practice. The use of clinical knowledge also is important in anticipating trends, predicting needs for services, and designing and managing health services. As clinical scholars become more experienced, it is important for them to assume an active role in creating the environments in which knowledge development can advance. In addition, as scientists become more tuned in to the clinical phenomena uncovered by partners in professional nursing practice, they can engage in scholarship that is directly relevant to health outcomes of the individuals, families, and communities they serve.

In summary, it can best be understood that clinical scholarship and research together provide the core knowledge on which expert professional nursing practice is developed. One without the other is not sufficient to inform a clinical discipline such as nursing. Rather, clinical scholarship and research are intertwined and interdependent. Both professional practice and science benefit from the strengths inherent in a knowledge development approach that incorporates attention to these interrelated ways of knowing.

REFERENCES

Fitzpatrick, J. J. (2002). The balance in nursing: Clinical and scientific ways of knowing and being. *Nursing Education Perspectives, 23,* 57.

Fitzpatrick, J. J. (2003). The case for the clinical doctorate. *Reflections in Nursing Leadership, 29,* 8, 9, 13.

Kuhn, T. S. (1977). *The essential tension: Selected studies in scientific tradition and change.* Chicago: University of Chicago Press.

2

The Structure of Nursing Knowledge: Analysis and Evaluation of Practice, Middle Range, and Grand Theory

Ann L. Whall

The structure of knowledge in the discipline of nursing holds within it explanations that clarify the present and hold promise for the future. This chapter explores the structure of nursing knowledge and the interrelationships of nursing models, middle range, and nursing practice level theory. Ways in which each of these three levels of theory might be analyzed and evaluated are also presented.

Throughout this chapter, the term *theory* is defined in a structural manner; that is, as a group of concepts, interrelated via propositional statements, which is based upon a group of underlying assumptions. Within nursing there are usually three levels of theory discussed that are based upon their characteristic levels of abstraction. These three levels of theory are termed *grand* (the most abstract or not readily operationalized), through the *middle range* (more readily operationalized), to the more concrete or *micro/practice* level.

PHILOSOPHIC ISSUES

An important paradigm shift has taken place in the last few decades of the 20th century that affects the nature of nursing theory; little notice, however, has been taken of this change or is discussed in nursing within the

5

United States (Whall & Hicks, 2002). Lack of attention to the implications related to such change may forestall many opportunities both internal and external to nursing. The shift referred to is a unification of aspects of positivism and postmodernism into a neomodernist movement. Neomodernism takes into account the metanarratives or historic themes and patterns (often from nursing conceptual models) found within both empiricism and postmodernism.

Positivism

Positivism, one variation of which was logical positivism, dominated scientific thought from the mid-19th century (Whall & Hicks, 2002). One of logical positivism's major tenets that had great impact upon both nursing theory and research was the verification principle, which posited that phenomena were scientifically meaningful only if they were empirically verifiable via sense experience and/or via logical proofs (Phillips, 1987). Although empirics within nursing can take many forms (and generally are not reflective of a strict verificationist perspective), positivism's influence affects segments of nursing practice, education, and research (Whall, 1989). Positivism supports a "context stripping" approach in which various aspects of situations are seen as unimportant—especially contextual aspects that are not directly operationalizable. This viewpoint is contrary to nursing's historic perspective, as nursing has historically dealt with patient values and meanings (e.g., spiritual desires and cultural beliefs) which arguably affect virtually all nursing situations. The verificationist perspective of positivism was thus seen by many in nursing as greatly restrictive and, therefore, was not fully or generally embraced in nursing education and practice.

Postmodernism

Postmodern thinking in large part was a reaction to the restrictive views of science found within positivism, but also was a result of multiple other societal and philosophical influences. Postmodernism made its appearance within scientific discussions sometime around the beginning of the 20th century, although it was not recognized or seen as influential within U.S. nursing until approximately the last decade of the 20th century (Whall & Hicks, 2002).

Postmodernists criticized the universal claims of the positivists regarding scientific truth (Abbey, 2000; Schrag, 1997). Postmodernists characterized positivists as "context strippers," denoting inattention to the reciprocal relationships between individuals and their many environments, as well as objectifying those observed. The context of persons cannot, however, be ignored by nursing, as clinical situations are often chaotic, and characterized by multiple, diverse, and simultaneous interactions that are virtually uncontrollable.

Many characteristics of postmodernism were/are very congruent with traditional nursing values and experiences. Likewise, nurse theorists for the most part deviated in both educational background and research training from that of scientists holding strict positivist views. When the postmodernist movement expanded the possibilities for science, and newly accepted topics for theory and research afforded the discipline both interesting and fuller possibilities not available within a positivistic world. A great criticism of postmodernism, however, is the tendency to overanalyze, overevaluate, and deconstruct, and provide little alternative for reconstruction via synthesis of such findings. This has led some within nursing and other disciplines to accept all viewpoints as having equal merit, leading to much confusion.

Multiple nursing conceptual models were developed during an era of great postmodern influence; the models are reflective of postmodern views, but are also sometimes reflective of certain positivistic views. Although this text focuses upon both analysis and evaluation of three levels of nursing theory, the focus also is upon the synthesis of these outcomes for nursing practice; such an effort might be seen as most reflective of a neomodernist position.

Neomodernism

Exterior to nursing (and often European in origin), a shift within the scientific worldview (from positivism to postmodernism and now to neomodernism) has been a major topic of discussion for several years. These discussions by Laudan (1977) and Lakatos (1977) view science in a newer manner (Whall & Hicks, 2002). Laudan saw science as progressing, with a collection of assumptions, tools, methods, and axioms/principles guiding science. Within this view, many theories could reside but commonalities remained that were sometimes grounded in the past. Laudan's views are now more descriptive of the state of the discipline of nursing. Reed (1995) and others use the term neomodernism to describe the state of science that goes beyond both positivism and postmodernism. This "above and beyond" characteristic of neomodernism is an approach to science in which a deliberative effort is made to utilize important traditional metanarratives (such as found in grand theories/nursing conceptual models) to address current problems within science.

In Reed's view, this neomodernist approach includes the freedom to explore and propose alternative ways and methods for nursing science, while taking into account important historic values and traditions. Neomodernism, therefore, offers a more inclusive and a seemingly more liberated path than even postmodernism, and suggests an important role for nursing conceptual models as excellent sources of nursing metanarratives within this "new science." The metanarratives within neomoderism are defined as important enduring themes found within disciplinary products such as the nursing conceptual models.

Other Philosophic Issues

Philosophy in large part is concerned with what is termed ontological and epistemological questions. Ontology is a branch of philosophy addressing the nature of reality (Reed, 1997). Theory within a discipline is influenced by ontological assumptions about what exists and "how we know what we know." Ontology, for example, may deal with the questions of "reality."

Within nursing, ontological issues have been played out many times. For example, during the 1960s, nursing assumed the validity of a then-popular theory that schizophrenia was caused by "cold and rejecting" mothers. Later, however, when it was possible to visualize brain function, nursing came to accept that schizophrenia most likely existed due to impaired neurologic mechanisms. Data incongruent with the theory of the "schizophrenic mother" was then used to modify the understanding of schizophrenia and how nursing might work with persons or families with a member so afflicted.

Within nursing the discussion of the "ways of knowing" (e.g., empiric, esthetic, personal, and ethical) are discussions of an epistemological nature (Carper, 1978); epistemology in this sense is concerned with the structure of knowledge. Debates within the discipline as to the value of such products as Nursing Diagnoses, Nursing Intervention Classification Systems (NICs), and Nursing Outcomes Classification Systems (NOCs), are similar issues. Likewise, whether nursing theory could/should be deductively structured from nursing grand theories, or inductively derived from practice, or both, were/are discussions of an epistemologic nature. Therefore, discussions within nursing about the value of disciplinary products will continue, are epistemologic in nature, and based upon philosophic positions within nursing.

Within the neomodernist position currently influencing nursing, many somewhat conflictual viewpoints are seen as useful. Within such a view, nurse practitioners need to remain aware of multiple understandings of various phenomena held and this knowledge used to structure their practice. Within neomodernism, the usefulness and uses of such scholarly products of the discipline, such as research findings, could and would be guided by nursing metanarratives (or the historic beliefs and themes). It is thus essential that this neomodernist position be better understood and its influence within nursing be examined more closely.

In a neomodernist position there is also an understanding that reality is likely and potentially flawed, and that examining multiple ways of knowing is one way of attempting to establish an acceptable "reality" for nursing (for a time). Discussions within nursing about the nature of certain products such as evidence-based practice (EBP) are, therefore, important. For example, the nature of the role that experiential knowledge plays in EBP is an important issue (Whall, Sinclair, & Paraboo, 2004).

THE PERSPECTIVE, DOMAINS, PERSISTENT QUESTIONS, AND TRUTH CRITERIA OF NURSING

Ellis was a clear-thinking, futuristic scholar who concerned herself with major questions regarding the structure of nursing knowledge. The editors of this text, as members of a Nursing Theory Think Tank, noted Ellis' belief that by addressing structural questions first, one might better understand current issues within the discipline. Nursing science, according to Ellis, is composed of both processes and products; thus debates (e.g., a scientific process) about products (e.g., nursing models) are needed within the discipline. Both of these scientific elements (products and processes) are important within a neomodernist view.

According to Ellis, the major components of the structure of the discipline of nursing are *perspective, domains, persistent questions, truth criteria,* and *the community of scholars* (Algase & Whall, 1993, 1995). There are other elements, as outlined by Phoenix (1964), but Ellis often focused on these five components.

The *domains* of the discipline are the subjects or content areas upon which nursing practice is focused. One might conceptualize this content using older terms (e.g., medical surgical nursing or pediatrics) or using more contemporary terms (e.g., long-term care and critical care). It is very important to realize that no one discipline "owns" any particular area of knowledge; in the marketplace of ideas, any area may be claimed by a given discipline. Knowledge across disciplines is gradually modified and then becomes accepted within other disciplines. For example, blood pressure monitoring and electrocardiography were at first part of medical knowledge and then later became part of nursing. Nursing focuses upon caregiving, but so do other disciplines such as social work and other professions. Thus the domains or components of knowledge found within any one discipline have a history, fluctuate, may be shared with other disciplines, and can only be relatively identified as specific to a particular discipline at a point in time.

The *perspective* of a discipline is perhaps the most fascinating structural element that Ellis discussed, for it is composed in large part of historical and traditional precedents, philosophical and ethical components, visionary ideals, and commonly accepted practices. This perspective is very important because it can be used to identify and sanction what can be considered "nursing" theory, "nursing" research, and "nursing" practice. In other words, the way in which given domains of a science are addressed (and their distinction from other disciplines), is due largely to its perspective.

The perspective is also used to evaluate the content of the domains. An example of this evaluative function is the debate over advanced-practice knowledge within nursing. In-depth physical assessment knowledge, which was once the preserve or domain of physicians alone, has gradually became part of the primary assessment of advanced-practice nursing. A debate within nursing between traditionalists/nontraditionalists has stimulated opposing views with regard to such assessment. One group sees in-depth physical assessment as a normal extension of the domain of nursing, believing that as technology advances, domains are modified. This "avant-garde" group argues that although this assessment procedure is used in many disciplines, the perspective of a given discipline determines how and why it is applied. The perspectives of all disciplines are somewhat and relatively in a state of flux, but also contain stable elements, such as identifiable metanarratives across time.

The *persistent questions* within the discipline may be found in its practice, education, and research discussions, and clearly involve the products of nursing science: "Was the action ethical?" or "Was the holistic perspective of nursing evident?" are examples of such questions. These questions also currently address trends in research over time; questions regarding cost-benefit analysis are one such example.

The *truth criteria* used to evaluate nursing products are traditional as well as evolving. The analysis and evaluation guidelines used in this text and in its prior editions are in essence one type of truth criteria. Questions used by national accrediting bodies, state boards, institutional review boards, and human subjects review groups also represent nursing's institutionalized truth criteria.

The *community of scholars* are members of the discipline who aim to develop the discipline by broadening nursing's knowledge base through such endeavors as research and scholarly discussions and debates. The community of scholars, in Ellis' view, should be involved in questions that address issues at the "cutting edge" of the discipline.

Ellis believed one threat to the community of scholars was that their "scholarly" pursuits and debates might become so esoteric that they would become estranged from nursing practice and nursing practitioners. For example, the debate regarding logical positivism (Whall, 1989) was unheard and unknown by most practicing nurses, who never considered rejecting the spiritual aspect of care as "unscientific." Nursing scholars, therefore, must continually check the relevance of their scholarly pursuits and debates; at times they will lead nursing and at times they may follow, but in Ellis' view these scholars need to maintain their relevancy to nursing practice.

ANALYSIS AND EVALUATION OF THREE LEVELS OF KNOWLEDGE IN NURSING

This text derives its evaluation (or truth) criteria in part from nursing conceptual models, as well as from other early sources and meta-theoretic discussion within nursing. The analysis and evaluation criteria used for the three levels of theory (micro/practice, middle range, and grand nursing model levels) were modified so as to be relevant to the theoretic characteristics of each level of theory.

Practice or Micro Theory

Practice level theory, also called micro theory and/or prescriptive theory, is more specific or concrete than the other two levels of theory and addresses specific directions/prescriptions for practice. Research on decubitus ulcers, nasal gastric suction, or urinary catheterization, for example, can be readily identified as practice level theory. Practice level theory is also produced by other methods, including induction from practice and deduction from middle-range theory (MRT), as well as from research on nursing conceptual models. Many of nursing's early guidelines for care, which are found in hospital procedure books, were/are practice theory generated inductively and primarily from practice experience, using trial-and-error methods.

Benner, Hooper-Kytiakidis, and Stannard's work (1999) addresses an interesting manner in which expert practice knowledge may be produced. They describe an interpretive process in which nurses keep records of exemplar cases concerning clinical patterns. By (in part) reflecting on these narratives, nurses may produce practice level knowledge, suggesting a "thinking-in-action" approach to practice level theory/knowledge development. This thinking-in-action is based, however, upon an in-depth understanding of the situation, as opposed to strictly a rule-bound approach.

Johnson and Ratner's work (1997) suggests a similar developmental process for practice level theory or knowledge. They support the idea that one may "theorize" about praxis knowledge and/or capture this knowledge in theory, and that this "thinking-in-action" is an ongoing process.

The guidelines for analysis and evaluation of practice theory are in the form of questions that will lead to practice actions (Table 2–1). These guidelines do not address the analysis of the four metaparadigm concepts of person, environment, health, and nursing (such as used for evaluation of nursing conceptual models), rather these concepts are seen as implicit to

TABLE 2-1   Criteria for the Analysis and Evaluation of Practice Theory

Basic considerations

1. Definitional adequacy: Can the concepts be readily operationalized?
2. Empirical adequacy: Are the operationalized concepts congruent with empirical data?
3. Statement/propositional adequacy: Do the statements lead to clear directives for nursing care? Are the statements sufficient to the practice task at hand and not contradictory in nature?

Internal analysis and evaluation

1. Consideration of completeness and consistency: Are there gaps or inconsistencies within the theory that may lead to prescriptive conflicts and difficulties?
2. Assumptions of theory: Are these beliefs congruent with nursing's historical perspective? Are these assumptions congruent with existing ethical standards and social policy? Are these assumptions in conflict with given cultural groups?

External analysis and evaluation

1. Analysis of existing standards: Is the practice theory produced congruent with existing nursing standards? Is the practice theory produced congruent with care standards produced external to nursing (e.g., Agency for Health Care Policy Research guidelines)?
2. Analysis of nursing practice and education: Is the practice theory produced consistent with existing standards of education within nursing? Is the theory produced related to nursing diagnoses and nursing intervention practices?
3. Analysis of research: Is the practice theory supported by existing research internal and external to nursing?

the questions. Because practice theory is designed for immediate application to practice, questions regarding the match or fit with existing empirical data are most important. Likewise, the relevance and adequacy for immediate application to practice of concept definitions are important. Operational definitions, which are descriptors of how to apply practice theory, are very important for practice theory. Thus the adequacy of operational definitions is addressed.

The interrelationships of statements or propositions found within practice theory should also be addressed, perhaps using theoretical substruction (Dulock & Holzemer, 1991). Gaps and inconsistencies in the theory would thus become understood and problems with the adequacy of the theory become evident.

The internal analysis of practice theory may be approached by diagramming the sign (i.e., positive, negative, or unknown) of the interrelationship of all concepts found within the theory, as described very early by Hardy (1974). In this way, lapses and inconsistencies in the completeness of the concept structure are addressed. Propositional adequacy of the overall theory is important, and at the practice level it may be argued that more explicit statements, such as those that are necessary, sufficient, and directional in nature, are most important. Associational statements are also needed, but if these predominate, practice directions may not be specific enough.

The internal analysis and evaluation of practice theory considers gaps and inconsistencies within the theory. In part, this is answered via the diagramming of concepts and the analysis of propositions identified above. In addition, the overall theory is considered for problems involving completeness of thought and inconsistent conclusions.

The assumptions of the theory are also considered in light of the historical and current perspectives of nursing. The current perspective may be deduced from nursing models, which are of prime importance in determining whether nursing's historical perspective is evident. If there are conflicts with the practice theory and nursing's historical perspective, then an assessment of the outcomes of the theory is needed. As with middle-range theory, practice theory may fit within nursing models that are themselves incongruent with each other; if this occurs, the choices made should be evident. Assumptions of practice theory are also relevant to ethical and cultural implications of the theory. Application of practice theory that is in conflict with given cultural standards is arguably unethical. This assessment thus has practice application implications in nursing.

The external analysis and evaluation of all levels of theory is currently a "hot topic" because its support by EBP discussions and by discussion of experiential knowledge must be assessed. In this regard, comparison of theory with the standards of practice, produced both externally or internally to nursing, is an effort in this direction and is very important to practice theory. Nursing and other research is also examined and the question of its support for the theory, its neutrality, or its opposition to the theory is evaluated.

In summary, the body of nursing knowledge is so extensive today that analysis and evaluation of all levels of theory is necessary. Because a more interlocking body of knowledge in nursing may for the first time in history be possible to attain, assessment of the fit between the levels of theory found within nursing needs to be addressed. With such assessment, nursing knowledge may be greatly expanded and clarified. At the least, such assessment will lead to better understanding of the strengths and weaknesses of nursing's knowledge base, as well as the portions of theory that need to be better developed. Analysis of each theoretical level should also lead to more knowledgeable "consumers" of nursing theory.

Middle-Range Theory

MRT is particularly useful in research—it is sufficiently concrete to facilitate operationalization, and yet at the same time is broad or abstract enough to facilitate general application. Merton (1977) discussed MRT at length and defined it as lying somewhere between the most abstract ideas (e.g., grand theory/nursing models) and more circumscribed concrete ideas (e.g., care procedures). Intervention research in nursing often produces MRT.

Merton (1977) stated that MRT may fall within or be congruent with several more abstract grand theories that are themselves incongruent with each other; thus, too many practice theories fit within a given MRT that are themselves incongruent with each other. For example, decubitus ulcer care/practice theory might be congruent with two MRTs of elder care, which individually exhibit conflicting propositions and assumptions. There are many methods, therefore, by which MRT may be produced (Walker & Avant, 1995). For example, there is "armchair" theorizing, theorizing from practice situations or more general phenomena, and developing an MRT more by deductively generating statements from several existing theories (Whall, 1986).

The analysis and evaluation of MRT (Table 2–2) in this text uses guidelines (or truth criteria) similar to that for analysis and evaluation of the nursing conceptual models. However, the metaparadigm concepts (person, environment, health, and nursing), although inherent within this level of theory, have been eliminated from this analysis. Questions of more immediate relevance, such as the fit of the MRT with the existing nursing perspective and domains, are asked. The more global metaparadigm concepts found in the models are not always implicit in MRT, although they may be inferred. Likewise, middle-range concepts have more specific empirical referents (or can be understood through human sense data) than the more abstract models.

TABLE 2–2   Criteria for the Analysis and Evaluation of Middle-Range Theory

Basic considerations
1. What are the definitions and relative importance of major concepts?
2. What is the type and relative importance of major theoretical statements and/or propositions?

Internal analysis and evaluation
1. What are the assumptions underlying the theory? What is the relationship to philosophy of science positions?
2. Are concepts related/not interrelated via statements? Is there any resulting loss of information?
3. Is there internal consistency and congruency of all component parts of the theory?
4. What is the empirical adequacy of theory? Has it been examined in practice and research and has it held up to this scrutiny?

External analysis and evaluation
1. What is the congruence with related theory and research internal and external to nursing?
2. What is the congruence with the perspective of nursing, the domains, and the persistent questions?
3. What ethical, cultural, and social policy issues are related to the theory?

Theoretical statements found in MRT may be categorized in part using the system of Hardy (1974) or identified as ranging from casual to associative in nature. Theoretical statements or propositions of MRT should be assessed for their relative importance as well as for missing linkages between concepts. Theoretical substruction (Dulock & Holzemer, 1991), or the diagramming of all relationships found in a theory, may be used for this purpose. Missing relationships between concepts are also identified. For this purpose, a matrix is made of the sign of all the concepts; that is, one asks whether the relationship is positive, negative, or unknown. A decision is made about the relative importance of any missing concepts (i.e., whether missing data make the theory unclear).

Assumptions derived from the MRT are also analyzed by asking what is assumed to exist as a basis for the theory, and what situation exists during the theory and after the theoretical action is concluded. Philosophy of science views are also discerned. Questions are asked about what the theory asserts to be true, what beliefs underlie the theory, and which positions within the philosophy of science the theory represents. These questions lead to further insights regarding congruence between statements and concepts of the theory.

The internal consistency (e.g., consistent usage of terms) of MRTs is usually less of a problem than that of more global discussions found in grand theories. Nevertheless, assessing all concepts to determine whether inconsistency in definitions occurs across the theory will assist with the evaluation of clarity. Empirical adequacy, the inherent ability to operationalize and measure aspects of a theory, is also very important in MRT. Operational definitions are needed for empirical adequacy, and these too are evaluated (i.e., are they adequate and readily applied?).

External analysis of MRT has to do with its congruence with more global and MRT theories, supporting evidence from research, and with standards of practice. Even though MRT may not directly guide practice, the relationship to professional practice is an important issue to consider.

Questions are also asked about the nursing perspective represented: Is the nursing perspective represented consistent with the *historical* view, for example, that found within nursing conceptual models? Because MRT is more readily applied than grand theory, its ethical, cultural, and social policy stances are crucial. Does the theory seem relevant to various cultural groups? Are there ethical concerns in this regard? What would be the result should social policy be based upon this theory? Finally, assessment is made of congruence with the perspective espoused by nursing, as well as with the domains of nursing that are currently accepted: Where does the theory lead nursing? What research or other empirical examination is needed to more fully develop the theory?

NURSING MODELS: ANALYSIS AND EVALUATION

The nursing models or nursings' grand theories examined in this text will continue to have a major influence on nursing. For example, products of the discipline should be examined in light of nursing models that have been developed over a long period of nursing history. The nursing conceptual models are assessed from a postmodern view; that is, with the belief that these models are in and of themselves important, are free to vary between each other, and may be utilized as sources of either practice or MRT. Unlike disciplines in which grand theories do not continue to be influential, in nursing conceptual models continue to guide various programs of research, as discussed in each of the chapters of this text. The guidelines presented for these models highlight the differences of each of the models as well as similarities across models.

Historically, Dubin (1978) described grand theory/conceptual models as composed of summative units, or very abstract concepts; partial relationship statements or propositions usually join these concepts. Oftentimes the assumptions of the models are in essence the general beliefs or understanding of nursing theorists. The guidelines presented in Table 2–3, there-

TABLE 2–3 Criteria for the Analysis and Evaluation of Nursing Conceptual Models

Introduction to the model

Basic paradigm concepts included in the model

1. What are the definitions of person, nursing, health, and environment?
2. What are the additional understandings of person?
3. What are the additional understandings of nursing?
4. What are the additional understandings of health?
5. What are the additional understandings of environment?
6. What are the interrelationships among concepts of person, nursing, health, and environment?
7. What are the descriptions of other concepts found in the model?

Internal analysis and evaluation

1. What are the underlying assumptions of the model?
2. What are the definitions of any other components of the model?
3. What is the relative importance of basic concepts or other components of the model?
4. What are the analyses of internal and external consistency?
5. What are the analyses of adequacy?

External analysis

1. Is nursing research based upon the model or related to the model?
2. Is nursing education based upon the model or related to the model?
3. Is nursing practice based upon the model or related to the model?
4. What is the relationship, if any, to existing nursing diagnoses and interventions systems?

fore, are not only analysis guidelines but also evaluation guidelines that can continue to be used by students as a model continues to be developed.

Given that nursing conceptual models are composed of the major paradigm concepts found within nursing (i.e., person, environment, health, and nursing), as well as additional concepts specific to the model, the first question addressed is the definition of these concepts. In addition to asking about the definition of person, as defined throughout the model, the interrelationships of person with the other concepts within the model, for example, are addressed. Oftentimes the way in which person is discussed in other concepts within the model fills out the description that the theorist wishes to give.

It is important to realize that although the term *person* is used within most of the models, the term *recipient of care* could be equally well used. This means that the recipient of care can be more than a single individual. The recipient may be a family, it may be a community, or it may be a group with which the nurse is working.

It is important to understand whether *nursing* is used as a verb or as a noun, and within what context it is used in either of these two ways. The description of nursing in terms of the actions taken, of the goals of nursing, and of the view of society is next addressed. How this view is alike or different from other commonly accepted views of nursing, such as that found within current organizations, is addressed. Finally, the way in which nursing addresses the care of individuals, families, groups, and communities is compared.

Health is addressed within each nursing conceptual model in overt or covert ways. If the definition of health is given, is health seen as the goal of nursing, is a definition of health from another source used, and are these definitions and discussion of the concept of nursing congruent with one another? If health is seen as some sort of steady state, then are the propositional statements regarding health consistent with the steady-state perspective, or is health seen as an open, ever-evolving state that is related to all aspects of humans and their environment? The way in which the nurse acts to bring about health is of major interest to these analyses.

The way in which environment is defined is extremely important to nursing. Florence Nightingale, in essence, saw nursing as a science of environmental management. Nightingale's early emphasis upon environment brought nursing to the realization that there are physical and emotional environments as well as other kinds of environments. It is of interest in the analysis to determine the way in which the theorist defines environment; to determine if it is directional, linear, open, or closed; and if it is interrelated with the other metaparadigm concepts.

The interrelationships among the four metaparadigm concepts are of interest because they identify the relative importance of each of these concepts. If, for example, a greater amount of time is spent within the model discussing person versus nursing, then there may be some difficulty for practice applications of the model. If the interrelationships are of equal importance, is there some implied hierarchy as these concepts are addressed? The importance of these four major concepts can be fairly well determined by reading through all portions of the model to determine how each of these concepts is described.

Within each model are found additional concepts that describe the other elements of importance. Oftentimes, the other major concepts that the theorist uses really define the model. Next, the interrelationships amongst the major concepts of the model, other than the four metaparadigm concepts, are addressed. Are these well defined? Are these relationships and various outcomes of the relationships described in detail? Is more detail needed?

In the internal analysis and evaluation, the underlying assumptions on which the model is based are important. Underlying assumptions provide data about the nature of science ascribed to, for example, pragmatism or realism. The philosophical underpinnings of the model should guide the relationship statements provided. In addition, it should be determined whether there is conflict between the philosophical position suggested and the overall perspective of nursing. A portion of the model analysis should address this.

Many times theories or subtheories are presented within a given nursing model. In what way are these elements or related elements congruent with the overall nursing model? For example, is a certain subtheory identified but not further explored? If this is the case, then both the internal and external consistency of the model is affected. If a feature of the model that is presented is not discussed, one would assume that this is of lesser importance.

Internal consistency has to do with the uniformity of discussion throughout the model. Are the concepts used in the same way at the beginning as they are at the end of the model? Are the propositional statements consistent with the assumptions of the model? Are the propositional statements and concepts consistent with one another and with the assumptions of the model? Each of these points leads to a decision regarding the level of internal consistency.

External consistency is addressed; for example, do the authors or theoreticians view the world in a manner consistent with views external to the model? Even though nursing models are not at a level that for the most part directly suggests practice procedures, these questions are important considerations. Likewise is the model view consistent with other nursing conceptual models, with other statements found within nursing, with elements such as the role of the nurse, and with nursing intervention classification systems? Each of these questions addresses the external consistency of the model.

Pragmatic adequacy is addressed; for example, does the model suggest feasible activities for nursing? Empirical adequacy asks, in essence, "Can model elements be measured?" The level of abstraction of the model certainly affects usefulness and measurement: the more abstract the model, the more difficulty exists with use and measurement. If the concepts are highly abstract, it is often difficult to "bring them down" to a practice or more concrete level without using a good deal of interpretation. Nursing models having concepts that are very much "rooted in the senses" or observable, however, may be difficult to relate back to the philosophical assumptions of the model. Finally, the external analysis of the nursing model has to do with the way that it has been used in research, education, and practice.

Although nursing diagnoses are not often stated within the nursing models, there are portions within every nursing model that have to do with practice. Often these sections of the model lend themselves to nursing diagnoses that may be derived from the model. These nursing diagnoses, however, may not be congruent with external nursing diagnosis systems. For example, using Martha Rogers' model, one might identify a problem with an individual's environment. Although Rogers herself never used the term *nursing diagnosis* with her model, a diagnosis relating to the environment might be derived. Therefore, where possible, the authors of the chapters in this text identify nursing diagnoses that might be derived from the model.

Not included in this text, but a step related to derived nursing diagnoses, is identification of nursing interventions that are compatible with the nursing model (such as those found in Nursing Interventions Classification (NIC) systems). Because the models presented here vary with respect to derivation of nursing diagnoses and interventions, it is left up to the reader in many instances to determine possible diagnoses and interventions related to the model.

One final note is that in this neomodernist era, it is realized that some of these analytical and evaluative questions may be less suitable for any one given model. When this is the case, the rationale relating to why each question is unsuitable is important, for this analysis sheds light not only upon the model, but also upon the evaluation criteria. It is hoped that the reader will enjoy this updated and more relevant journey through nursing theory presented in this chapter and the chapters that follow.

REFERENCES

Abbey, R. (2000). Charles Taylor: Philosophy now. In J. Shand (Series Ed.), *Philosophy Now,* Princeton, NJ: Princeton and Oxford Press.

Algase, D., & Whall, A. (1993). Rosemary Ellis' views on the substantive structure of nursing. *Image: Journal of Nursing Scholarship, 25*(1), 69–72.

Algase, D., & Whall, A. (1995, June). Analytic questions for emerging doctoral programs in nursing: An approach to develop culturally sensitive nursing content. *Proceedings, Nursing Forum on Doctoral Education.* Dearborn, MI: University of Michigan, School of Nursing.

Benner, P., Hooper-Kytiakidis, P., & Stannard, D. (1999). *Clinical wisdom and interventions in critical care: A thinking-in-action approach.* Philadelphia: W.B. Saunders.

Carper, B. (1978). Fundamental patterns of knowing in nursing. *Advances in Nursing Science, 1*(1), 13–23.

Dubin, R. (1978). *Theory building.* New York: Collier Macmillan.

Dulock, H., & Holzemer, W. (1991). Substruction: Improving the linkage from theory to method. *Nursing Science Quarterly, 4*(2), 83–87.

Hardy, M. (1974). Theories: Components, development, evaluation. *Nursing Research, 23,* 100–107.

Johnson, J., & Ratner, P. (1997). The nature of knowledge used in nursing practice. In S. Thorne & V. Hayes (Eds.), *Nursing praxis: Knowledge and action* (pp. 3–20). Thousand Oaks, CA: Sage.

Lakatos, I. (1977). The methodology of scientific research programmes. In J. W. G. Currie (Ed.), *Philosophical papers* (Vol. 1). Cambridge: Cambridge University Press.

Laudan, L. (1977). *Progress and its problems.* Los Angeles: University of California Press.

Merton, R. (1977). *On sociological theory.* New York: Free Press.

Phillips, D. C. (1987). *Philosophy, science, and social inquiry: Contemporary methodological controversies in social science and related applied fields of research.* New York: Pergamon Press.

Phoenix, P. (1964). *Realms of meaning.* New York: McGraw-Hill.

Reed, P. G. (1995). A treatise on nursing knowledge development for the 21st century: Beyond postmodernism. *Advances in Nursing Science, 17*(3), 70–84.

Reed, P. G. (1997). Nursing: The ontology of the discipline. *Nursing Science Quarterly, 10*(2), 76–79.

Schrag, C. O. (1997). *The self after postmodernity.* New Haven: Yale University Press.

Walker, L., & Avant, K. (1995). *Strategies for theory construction in nursing.* Norwalk, CT: Appleton & Lange.

Whall, A. (1986). *Family therapy theory for nursing: Four approaches.* Norwalk, CT: Appleton & Lange.

Whall, A. (1989). The influence of logical positivism on nursing practice. *IMAGE: Journal of Nursing Scholarship, 21*(4), 243–245.

Whall, A., & Hicks, F. (2002). The unrecognized paradigm shift within nursing: Implications, problems, and possibilities. *Nursing Outlook, 50*(2), 72–76.

Whall, A., Sinclair, M., & Paraboo, K. (2004). A philosophic analysis of evidence based nursing. Manuscript in preparation.

3

Florence Nightingale: Pioneer in Nursing Knowledge Development

Tamara L. Zurakowski

As the 21st century becomes reality, a 19th-century woman still looms over nursing and health care—Florence Nightingale. A full century after her death, authors continue to analyze, describe, and discuss her work; identify current educational uses of her writing (Gerber & McGuire, 1999); acknowledge her contributions to holistic nursing (Light, 1997; Macrae, 1995); and laud her pioneering role in outcomes-based practice (Griffiths, 1995). Nightingale first explicated what has come to be known as nursing's meta-paradigm (Fawcett, 1978) as well as the syntax for building nursing knowledge (Hayne, 1992; Ray, 1999). Her systematic organization of knowledge about person, health, and environmental phenomena as reflected in her laws of nursing provided a distinct perspective for the discipline. Furthermore, as nurses seek to validate their practices through evidence, Nightingale's groundbreaking use of data and statistics points the way for new generations of nurses who must offer state-of-the-art care to their clients.

It has been suggested that nursing became a science when Nightingale identified her laws of nursing (Barritt, 1973). It must be noted, however, that Nightingale's view of nursing encompassed a somewhat different and broader perspective than that typically regarded as professional nursing today. According to Nightingale (1859/1969), a nurse was any woman who had the "charge of the personal health of somebody," whether sick or well

(p. 3). Nightingale held a religious view of nursing as a "calling" or God's work. The nurse was to acquire and apply knowledge about God's laws of health and thus, move humankind closer to perfection. Nursing activities served as an art form through which one might develop spiritually (Cook, 1942; Welch, 1986; Widerquist, 1992). Her *Notes on Nursing: What It Is and What It Is Not* (1859/1969) were written to offer "hints for thought" and to encourage all women to learn about the laws of health through observation, experience, and reflection.

A review of Nightingale's life reveals several factors that influenced her model of nursing, including her classical education, religious beliefs about serving humankind, noted passion for statistics, and diligent study of hospitals during her travels throughout Europe. She was born to a wealthy English aristocratic family in Florence, Italy, on May 12, 1820, during an era when women did not ordinarily display any interests beyond domestic or social events. The young Nightingale clashed frequently and violently with her mother and older sister about her nonconformist beliefs and actions (Allen, 1975; Webb, 1992). She was well educated as a result of her father's efforts; she spoke several languages, read Plato in the original Greek, understood mathematics, and pursued religious and philosophical studies (LeVasseur, 1998). She was an active member of the Unitarian church and was very involved in the social reform aspect of this denomination (Widerquist, 1992). Moreover, Nightingale frequently interacted with leading scientists and educators of her day, although the education her father provided was that of a classical, rather than scientific, scholar (Allen, 1975).

On February 7, 1837, when she was 16 years old, Nightingale experienced a "calling" from God for her to serve humankind. In 1852, she experienced a second calling. Nursing, as the application of knowledge of nature's laws to help mankind, became Nightingale's means for serving God. At age 24, Nightingale identified her desire to be a nurse but was unable to actively pursue her interest until the age of 31, when she broke away from her family to train and work in nursing. She completed the 3-month probationer course in nursing at the Institution for the Training of Deaconesses in Kaisersworth, Germany. Soon after, during the Crimean War (1854–1856), Nightingale seized the opportunity to display to the world the significant impact nursing could have on reducing human mortality and morbidity. Although she was not the first British woman to be so directly involved in a war effort, Nightingale became famous for her improvements in the British military healthcare system. Through persistent attention to soldiers' basic hygiene, including wound care, sanitary food, and clean water, Nightingale reduced the mortality rate from 57% to 2% (Cohen, 1984).

Ironically, given her abhorrence of the Victorian woman's role, it has been suggested that her fame came in large part from her successful blending of that role with a military one (Wheelwright, 1987). Through her heartfelt service to God by attending to the health and welfare of humankind, Nightingale effectively reformed military health care. She emerged as a legendary leader during the Crimean War, in part because of the power of the press and the British war correspondents who helped spread her fame (Benson, 1992). The focus on her influence on military nursing, however, overshadowed her very significant progress in public health and district nursing (Baly, 1986a).

In 1856, after serving 21 months in the Crimean war and suffering with Crimean fever, Nightingale returned home without public notice, avoiding the accolades that awaited her. Woodham-Smith (1951) characterized Nightingale as a bereaved woman, haunted by men's deaths from injuries and disease. After collapsing in 1857, she confined herself to her apartment for most of her remaining 54 years of life, suffering from a variety of somatic symptoms. Ulrich (1992) suggested that Nightingale's self-imposed bedrest was the ultimate in time management techniques, in that she effectively eliminated the distractions of everyday life. Inspired by her religious beliefs about service and driven by her wartime experiences, however, she focused her energies on reforming the British military hospital system, enacting standards of public health, and establishing formal secular nursing education. She wrote more than 10,000 letters, speeches, and pamphlets. Her successes in reform were aided by her pioneering and passionate use of statistical techniques, including graphs, to demonstrate her thesis (Cohen, 1984; Kopf, 1978; Nuttall, 1983). As a result of her contributions to statistics, Nightingale became a fellow of the Royal Statistical Society and Honorary Member of the American Statistical Association (Grier & Grier, 1978).

Nursing was but one aspect of Nightingale's drive to improve social welfare. She encouraged all Englishwomen to speak up and use their influence for the "cause of social progress" (Nightingale, 1892). Nightingale was an active member of the National Association for the Promotion of Social Science and presented several papers on improving the lives and living conditions of native populations in the British colonies (Nightingale, 1863a, 1863b, 1865).

It is difficult to extract an accurate depiction of Nightingale from the published accounts of her life. Her attributes as an aristocratic woman, unmarried, and fiercely involved in such unlikely activities as healthcare administration and statistics during the Victorian era, have given rise to myths that have obscured her reality. Romantic images of Nightingale during the Crimean War, as the self-sacrificing "lady with the lamp," that dominate popular thought misrepresent her contributions to professional nursing as well as to society in general. Although compassionate and deeply religious, she was also tyrannical, calculating, and manipulative, using political networks to achieve her objectives. Her development of nursing as a respectable career for women was a slow and tedious process (Skeet, 1988), and did not happen overnight following her return from Crimea, as myths would suggest. Detailed attention to the gap between the myths and realities of Nightingale's life can be found in the publications of Baly (1986a, 1986b), Kalisch and Kalisch (1983a, 1983b), Nauright (1984), Skeet (1988), and Palmer (1981, 1983a, 1983b).

Nightingale established a school for nurses at London's St. Thomas' Hospital in 1860. The philosophy of the school with regard to the importance of formal education and nurses' accountability to nurses remains relevant today. Some point out that Nightingale's views on nursing were derived from her patrician society, in which nurses were regarded as part of the servant class (Iveson-Iveson, 1983; Palmer, 1983a). However, others describe Nightingale's vision of nursing education as a synthesis of the moral purpose of the religious orders with nonsectarian and nonclass criteria for admission, and as fostering both the educational level of upper-middle classes and the boldness of the working class (Baly, 1986a). Nightingale remained actively involved in the school until her death in 1910 (Ulrich, 1992), and the school became a model for nursing education around the world (Uhl, 1992).

BASIC CONSIDERATIONS INCLUDED IN THE MODEL

Notes on Nursing (1859/1969) represented Florence Nightingale's first effort at stating her philosophy and description of nursing in one written source. Prior to its publication, she had limited her nursing writings to personal correspondence and to pamphlets that were distributed to influential governmental officials. In addition, introductions and forewords written for other works (e.g., Nightingale, 1872a, 1892) provided her opportunities to expound on her views about nursing.

Definition of Nursing

Nursing, to Nightingale, was, above all, to "put the patient in the best condition for nature to act upon him" (Nightingale, 1859/1969, p. 133), and "service to God in the relief of man" (Nightingale, 1858b). She described two different types of nursing: sick nursing or "nursing proper," and health nursing, as well as nurse midwifery (Nightingale, 1892/1949, 1859/1969). She advised that all women practice health nursing, which required some practical teaching, its goal being the prevention of disease. It was for health nurses that *Notes on Nursing* was originally written, although the text was later used in the Nightingale school.

Nursing proper was both an art and a science, requiring organized, formal education (Nightingale, 1872a, 1892/1949). The scientific dimension grew from Nightingale's own grasp of statistics, sanitation, logistics, administration, and public health, as well as the laws of health and observation of the sick. Nursing activities were to be based not only on compassion, but on observation and experience, statistical data, knowledge of sanitation and nutrition, and administrative skills (Agnew, 1958; Andrews, 1929; Barritt, 1973; Nightingale, 1885a, 1859/1946, 1969). Nursing practice required formal education; nursing education ensured diffusion of health knowledge (Montiero, 1984).

Nightingale (1872b, 1914, 1892/1949) was explicit in defining nursing as distinct from medicine, citing as the basic difference nursing's concern as for the patient who was ill, rather than for the illness. Furthermore, nursing was to offer preventive and health-oriented care, whereas medicine offered cures for illnesses. Although nurses were to carry out physicians' orders, they were to do so only with an independent sense of responsibility for their actions. Nursing was differentiated from medicine in both theory and practice, and in the educational process and administration of the school (Nightingale, 1872b). Nightingale believed this so strongly that women who stated their aspiration to become physicians were denied entrance to the St. Thomas' school (Montiero, 1984).

Description of Nursing Activity

The focus of nursing activity for both health nurses and trained nurses was the use of "fresh air, light, warmth, cleanliness, [and] quiet, and the proper selection and administration of diet" while monitoring the patient's expenditure of energy (Nightingale, 1859/1969, p. 8). Activity was to be directed toward the patient's environment as well as the patient. In *Notes on Nursing*, Nightingale outlined 13 canons for nursing care, the first being "to keep the air he [the patient] breathes as pure as the external air, without chilling him" (1859/1969, p. 12). The other canons are listed in Table 3–1.

TABLE 3–1 Nightingale's Canons of Nursing

Ventilation and warming
Health of houses
Petty management (avoidance of)
Noise (avoidance of)
Variety (in sights, activities, foods)
Taking food
Selection of food
Bed and bedding (clean and dry)
Light
Cleanliness of rooms and walls
Personal cleanliness
Chattering hopes and advices (avoidance of)
Observation of the sick

The wider scope of practice and "careful inquiry" of trained nurses required specialized knowledge in addition to knowledge of the laws of health (Nightingale, 1859/1946, 1892/1949). Prescribed content in the Nightingale school included, among other things, observation of the sick, bandaging, making of occupied beds, application of leeches, use of surgical appliances, management of the convalescent, and preparation of gruel, arrowroot, egg flip, puddings, and drinks for the sick (Nightingale, 1885b, 1892/1949).

Nursing activities were broad and addressed maintenance of health, prevention of infection and injury, recovery from illness, health teaching, and environmental control (Nightingale, 1892/1949, 1859/1969). Moreover, one did not need to be ill to benefit from nursing knowledge, nor did one have to be wealthy. The laws of nursing had the potential to better everyone's lot in life.

Definition and Description of Person

Nightingale described the person as having physical, intellectual, emotional, social, and spiritual components. She viewed all persons as equal, transcending biologic differences, socioeconomic class, creed, and disease. People who were endowed with fewer capabilities could be shown how to improve themselves and come closer to God (Nightingale, 1863a, 1863d, 1865, 1869). Although Nightingale's laws of health focused primarily on the physical dimensions of the patient, she also presented ideas that addressed the emotional dimensions of the person (Nightingale, 1859/1969, pp. 95–104).

The centeredness of the patient in Nightingale's (1859/1969) model is evidenced in her emphasis on the natural course of events, facilitated by environmental factors, the nurse's activities, and the physician's interventions, that work in the patient to effect a cure (p. 133). Nightingale viewed the person as having both the ability and the responsibility to alter rather than conform to the existing situation. This view was evident in her nursing efforts, which focused on actively changing the environment to improve conditions for both the individual and the community.

Contrary to other scholars of her day, Nightingale did not believe in Cartesian duality, but rather that humans are an inseparable blend of mind and body (Welch, 1986). This holistic approach derived from her spiritual perspective, which linked salvation to moral, emotional, and physical well-being (Welch, 1991). Similarly, poverty was not a moral deficit, as was commonly believed, but a condition that could be addressed in part by improving cleanliness of home and body (Montiero, 1985). Deriving from her strong religious beliefs, Nightingale also posited that humans are innately good, or at least capable of progressing toward perfection through hard work and knowledge of God's laws (Welch, 1986; Widerquist, 1992). Helping persons to become physically healthy, then, was tantamount to bringing them closer to God (Nightingale, 1859/1969).

Definition and Description of Environment

In Nightingale's model, the environment referred to those physical elements external to the patient that affect the healing process and health, such as noise, air, temperature, and other meaningful stimuli. She stated most emphatically that sickness and death are the results of sanitary defects in the patient's surroundings (Nightingale, 1863c). Nightingale defined ways that the environment affected the patient's health and ways that the nurse could harness some control over the environment. She isolated five essential environmental components in the maintenance of the individual's health: pure air, pure water, efficient drainage, cleanliness, and light (Nightingale, 1859/1969). She elaborated on these components and their use in nursing interventions in great detail in many of her writings.

Nightingale's concept of the patient's environment as a major component in her model emerged, in part, from her experiences early in the Crimean War, where wounded and sick soldiers at Scutari were exposed to overcrowding, poor ventilation, and inadequate lighting. Nightingale attributed their sicknesses and deaths to the unsanitary environment, not to germs or microorganisms. She was vehement in her disbelief of the germ theory, and regarded "contagion" as a word borrowed from poets that was connected with "no end of absurdities" (Nightingale, 1859). In fact, she was deeply concerned that attention to "mystic rites" such as antisepsis and disinfection would sway people from the real problem of poor sanitation (Nightingale, 1892/1949). The significance of environment is reflected in Torres' (1980), Lobo's (1995), and Gropper's (1990) references to Nightingale's "environmental theory of nursing."

Nightingale consulted and wrote extensively on the organization, construction, and management of hospitals (Bishop, 1960; Nightingale, 1859, 1863b, 1863c, 1867, 1871, 1874). Her recommendations for hospitals were based largely on meticulously tabulated statistics on the outcomes of hospitalized patients. It may be stated that her greatest insight into the importance of the environment in the preservation of health is evidenced in her concern for the "health of houses" and her claim that one could better predict health problems if one inspected "houses, conditions, and ways of life" rather than the physical body (Nightingale, 1859/1969, p. 23).

Definition and Description of Health

Nightingale believed health to be an innate process, and the combined result of environmental, physical, and psychological factors. Health, along with illness, is experienced as part of the person's path toward spiritual fulfillment. She considered health not only the opposite of sickness, but as being "able to use well every power we have to use" (Nightingale, 1885b, p. 1043). Health could be augmented through education and the improvement of unsanitary conditions (Nightingale, 1863d), in particular as relating to the environmental factors of "dirt, drink, diet, damp, draughts, and drains" (Nightingale, 1892/1949, p. 362). Nightingale (1858b, 1863a) also recognized the health risks posed by inactivity, noting impairments resulting from an absence of occupation and exercise in the British army. In addition, she recognized that lifestyle choices also could have deleterious effects on health, citing the British army in India as an excellent example of how one's health could be ruined by one's fashion of living (Nightingale, 1863a). Disease, according to Nightingale (1859) is a reparative process—the body's attempt to correct some problem. The purpose of this process extends, as did the goal of nursing, beyond healing from sickness; illness and suffering are part of the path to salvation, happiness, and character development (Widerquist, 1992). Illness is also an opportunity to gain spiritual perspective (Nightingale's letter of April 1873, cited in Cook, 1942). Nightingale's concern for health extended beyond the hospital to setting goals for "high-level wellness" in the community (Palmer, 1983b; Montiero, 1985) and for spiritual achievement in the nurse.

INTERNAL ANALYSIS AND EVALUATION

Philosophical Bases and Assumptions

Nightingale believed that nursing knowledge could be acquired through both experience and observation. Both were considered essential to Nightingale, but, she placed greater value on experience in her search for truth. That is, abstract ideas about nursing, health, or environment should be grounded in experience and should be reformulated if they are inconsistent with the empirical world. Nightingale regarded observations that were based on one's senses as the only reliable means for obtaining and verifying knowledge of the laws of health (Palmer, 1977; Schlotfeldt, 1977). She practiced and taught nursing based on the realities as she saw them, and admonished nurses to "let experience, not theory" be their guide (Nightingale, 1859/1969, pp. 76, 122). Nightingale regarded medicine's approach to knowledge as inappropriate for acquiring understanding of the laws of nursing. Believing that which was not verified by the senses was superstition, or at least not useful for nursing, she rejected the principles of bacteriology, antisepsis, and germ theory (Huxley, 1975).

Nightingale held an eclectic philosophy about life and health. She was influenced by the empiricist tradition of Bacon, Locke, and Comte (the Fathers of Positivism), as well as by idealist and religious philosophers of her day. She believed that society could be perfected by uncovering its social and moral laws (Welch, 1991). Nightingale's classical education and religious views helped temper the dominant positivist philosophy, however, rendering her more sensitive to and knowledgeable of the whole person and factors related to health. Her views on leadership were derived from Plato, whose works she read in great detail (LeVasseur, 1998).

Nightingale regarded knowledge as a means to improve the conditions of people, and of women in particular. She promoted knowledge of the laws of nursing as emancipatory; they gave people, especially women, power over their environment, freedom to make choices, and relief from moral and physical suffering. Nightingale wrote her nursing texts for women, fulfilling a need for women to have accurate information with which to care for their families (Nightingale, 1859/1969).

Nightingale's approach to science is congruent with feminism, in that it values women's experience in inquiry and recognizes the connectedness between the physical and metaphysical; the personal, professional, and political; and health and wholeness (Campbell & Bunting, 1991). This is evident in Nightingale's explanation of disease as being a result of unsanitary conditions and eased by a connection between caring and healing, which had been validated by her personal experiences (Nightingale, 1892/1949). Nightingale's consternation about women wanting to do the same things as men (e.g., become physicians) may be viewed as antifeminist. However, feminist consciousness was clearly evident in her active commitment to encouraging women to develop their own unique gifts and not let their talents waste away under Victorian notions of propriety or under the guise of doing something "merely because men do it."

Nightingale's ontology was grounded in her religious beliefs about human beings, particularly her Unitarian beliefs in charity, expressing spiritual renewal through works for others, and concern for the ultimate salvation of all (Widerquist, 1992). Human beings were dynamic and creative, capable of learning and developing, and able to achieve release from suffering through rational thought, respect for God's laws, and hard work. The person's potential for perfection was put into operation in the reparative process, which was inherent and not to be disrupted. It was, however, within the nurse's purview to "disrupt" the environment to facilitate the reparative process in the person.

CENTRAL COMPONENTS

There are three central components in Nightingale's model: (a) *nursing*, a calling, the goal of which is to discover and use nature's laws governing health in the service of humanity; (b) the *patient*, one who is suffering but who possesses the physical, intellectual, and metaphysical attributes and potential to become healthy and be able to use every power one has; and (c) the *environment*, those elements external to and affecting the health of sick and healthy persons. These three concepts are termed *summative units* (Dubin, 1978) because they are global and abstract in their representation of reality. For example, the concept of environment represents everything from the patient's food and flowers to the nurse's verbal and nonverbal interactions with the patient. Nursing encompasses a wide range of activities related to putting the patient in the best possible condition so that nature can effect a cure. Thus, the meanings of these major components are open to a great deal of interpretation, although Nightingale's (1859/1969) 13 canons provide very concrete meanings for these abstract components and their interrelationships.

As the one who possesses the healing potential, the patient is the central focus in the model. The environment, however, is the nurse's main mode of intervention; the nurse intervenes with the environment to a greater degree than with the person in facilitating health. The direction of interaction among the three components is primarily a unidirectional movement, with the nurse affecting the environment, which in turn affects the patient's health either positively or negatively. The patient's health is a function of both the environment and the inherent reparative process (Figure 3–1).

ANALYSIS OF CONSISTENCY

Nightingale's conceptual model is judged in general to be internally consistent, the major concepts clearly and consistently defined. The relationships among these concepts flow logically from the meaning attributed to each concept and from the worldview of the concepts' creator. Nightingale's approach to knowledge development resembles Reynolds' (1971) "set-of-laws" approach in that her laws of nursing were empirical generalizations that outlined relationships between concepts but did not propose substantive explanations of the relationships. Nightingale's laws of nursing addressed relationships between the person's health experience and environmental factors such as sunlight, fresh air, and quiet.

Nightingale's laws of nursing were empirical generalizations developed according to the canons of inductive logic, induced in a consistent

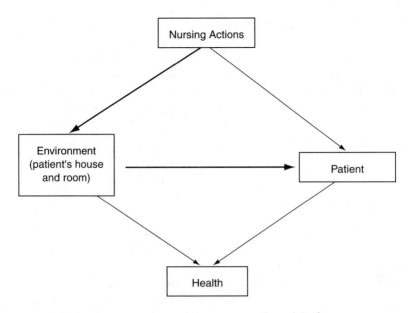

FIGURE 3-1   Nightingale's conceptual model of nursing.

and logical manner from practice situations. Thus, in general, Nightingale's approach to model building was consonant with her assumptions about the experiential basis of knowledge.

ANALYSIS OF ADEQUACY

The adequacy of Nightingale's model may be analyzed best by addressing its problem-solving ability vis-a-vis the historical context in which the model was developed. The historical approach (Silva & Rothbart, 1984) offers a broadened framework for analyzing Nightingale's model, which was developed nearly 70 years before criteria influenced by logical empiricism for evaluating theory were introduced.

Nightingale's model emerged from many sociocultural and personal influences, including her fierce rejection of superstitious beliefs, her deep convictions about God and the functioning of the universe and humanity, her personal experiences during the Crimean War and in hospitals across Europe, and her passion for systematic observation and statistical analyses. Attention to the needs of practicing nurses, by providing information to use in the care of patients, is an important aspect of nursing theory and research (Algase & Whall, 1993), and one that Nightingale used in developing her ideas. Factors such as these gave rise to Nightingale's research tradition and her perspective for solving conceptual and practice problems

(Laudan, 1977, 1981). The research tradition provides guidelines for developing theories, defines the entities that are fundamental to the domain, specifies the relationships among those entities, and delineates methods of inquiry. In many respects, research traditions are analogous to the grand level of theory described by Chinn and Kramer (1999) in that they describe broad areas of concern for a discipline. The adequacy of a research tradition is evaluated through its problem-solving ability. Within such a framework, the adequacy, as well as the limitations, of Nightingale's model become apparent.

Pragmatic Adequacy

The pragmatic adequacy of Nightingale's model is attested to by the fact that the conceptual relationships proposed by Nightingale were supported in her actual practice with sick persons (Ellis, 1969). Nightingale's methodical approach to studying nursing phenomena and her theories about environment and health generated significant solutions to the health problems of her day, most notably the drastic reduction in mortality at Scutari. Even though she rejected the theories of antisepsis that were being propagated, she achieved admirable results in the reduction of infectious diseases (Larson, 1989). She also applied her knowledge of statistics and her laws of nursing concerning the use of space, activity, diet, and water to effectively reduce the mortality rate among soldiers in India from nearly 7% to 1.9%, without ever stepping foot in India (Hays, 1989). In addition, her ideas led to the establishment of therapeutic hospital environments and undoubtedly benefited the emotional as well as physical well-being of many patients.

Although Nightingale's laws emphasized relationships that are not regarded as particularly revolutionary or complex today, her model provides a broad framework for organizing observations about a number of nursing phenomena; that is, the model has a broad scope (Ellis, 1968). It not only provides a metaparadigmatic perspective for nursing but is also meaningful at the practice level. The model's scope and usefulness support its significance and pragmatic adequacy.

The pragmatic adequacy of Nightingale's ideas is limited by its roots in Victorian attitudes and religious philosophy. Salvation could not, according to Nightingale, be achieved through grace alone; it had to be earned (Widerquist, 1992). Nursing, as a path toward salvation through service to humankind, was formulated as a profession that offered numerous opportunities to reach this goal. Nightingale specified many tasks in nursing, such as the meticulous cleaning of sheets as well as patients, scrubbing floors, dusting furniture, airing rooms, and practicing other habitual behaviors and observations (Nightingale, 1859/1969) that kept the nurse from idleness.

Rather than emphasizing women's talents for thinking or knowing, Nightingale emphasized women's talents for doing tasks and judged them by what they did. Although this emphasis was expedient for its day, placing so much value on "doing" has been deplored by contemporary writers such as Peplau (1992), Decker and Parley (1991), and Welch (1990, 1991). In the spirit of Nightingale, many contemporary nurses define nursing in terms of "doing," rather than of "thinking" or "being." This may pose significant barriers to further development of the discipline, and its potential to make valuable contributions to health care (Meleis, 1997). Unwittingly, Nightingale may have established major roadblocks to the continued growth of nursing by emphasizing tasks over thoughts.

Empirical Adequacy

Empirical adequacy is evidenced in the rate of progress in research and theory development that is engendered by the research tradition (Laudan, 1981). Nightingale's 13 canons in her *Notes on Nursing* (1859/1969) outline areas of testable propositions. The hiatus in theory development following Nightingale was due more likely to the absence of a community of nurse-scholars than to the empirical adequacy of her model, although the inadequacy of Nightingale's model in providing accurate substantive explanations for observed relationships between environmental factors and patients' health outcomes may also have been a factor. This gap between empirical generalizations and theoretical explanation at a more abstract level is demonstrative of the "precision paradox" (Dubin, 1978; Kaplan, 1964). Within this paradox, one aim of science (i.e., prediction) is achieved, whereas the second aim (i.e., understanding) is not. As others have similarly noted (Levine, 1992; Styles, 1992), Nightingale's precision in predicting relationships between environmental factors and subsequent health events was not often based upon a valid theoretical system for explaining the predicted events; "miasma" and "effluvia" did not offer explanatory power for the importance of sanitary practices in nursing.

CONCLUSIONS

The substantive structure of the discipline of nursing is still not fully explicated (Algase & Whall, 1993). However, Nightingale provided a significant starting point by enumerating person, nursing, health, and environment as critical aspects of nursing (Hayne, 1992). These concepts subsume the phenomena that are still of interest to nurse-scholars: lifestyle and health, health promotion, outcomes of care, and "tender loving care" (Algase & Whall, 1993).

Although Nightingale's rejection of bacteriologic principles limited the explanatory power of the relationships in her model, it may have enhanced identification and description of critical links between human health and environmental phenomena that might otherwise have been overlooked by other scientists of her day. Seemingly "illogical processes" can still contribute to the creative knowledge of a discipline (Silva & Rothbart, 1984).

Nightingale's research tradition thrives today regardless of the void of empirical nursing data that preceded and followed Nightingale. Relationships among environment, person, and health are an integral part of current research and theorizing. For example, Torres (1980) has suggested that the current theories on stress, need, and adaptation derive from Nightingale's model. Johnson (1992) regarded Nightingale's work on "variety" as a forerunner of scientific study of sensory deprivation and overload. More broadly, Nightingale's ideas are congruent with current-day research focuses on environmental variables that may predict health problems, from urbanization and global climate changes to genetic diversity.

Although certain ideas of Nightingale have been disregarded as outdated or inaccurate, her research tradition persists and continues to evolve. Her systematic yet humanistic approach to the study of human health and the environment has served as an exemplar for nurse-scholars. The global perspective of her model continues to provide scope for generating problem-solving theories about health-promoting environments.

EXTERNAL ANALYSIS

Nightingale's use of experiential data and statistical analysis in discovering the basic laws of nursing contributed to the identification of concepts that have since provided perspective for the development of nursing theories to guide nursing practice, education, and research.

Relationship to Nursing Research

Nightingale's work established a definition and focus of inquiry for nursing. She acknowledged that, whereas the laws of nursing were as yet unknown, nurses had to be truth seekers and continue discovering the great secrets of nursing (Montiero, 1974). Truth seeking and practice-related activities were combined, often without clear distinction between the development of theoretical knowledge and the deliberate use of knowledge in practice. Nightingale, however, subjected her clinical discoveries to systematic and careful analysis. She urged nurses to be astute observers and to indulge in "careful inquiry" (1859/1946). Her essential research strengths were recording, communicating, ordering and codifying, conceptualizing, inferring, analyzing, and synthesizing (Palmer, 1977). She engaged in historical, explanatory, descriptive, comparative, and field research. Nightingale identified the model presented in *Notes on Nursing* as being a result of data she had collected during the Crimean War and in the 14 years thereafter (1859/1969).

Nightingale not only collected and analyzed data using methods that were quite new in her day (Cohen, 1984), but she was a master at communicating her findings using statistically derived diagrams and graphs to support her arguments for needed changes in health care (Nightingale, 1858a). She regarded statistics as the science upon which all other sciences depended for its use in improving the accuracy of one's observations (Cope, 1958). Thus, Nightingale's statistical abilities were integral to the development and dissemination of knowledge for formulating healthcare decisions.

Although Nightingale's work could be the bases for many mid-range theories, few current researchers draw Nightingalian hypotheses to test. A few exceptions, though, are found. Research by McCarthy, Ouimet, and Daun (1991) on the relationship between noise stress and wound healing and Valentine's (1988) work with impaired nurses are two recent examples. Nightingale's concepts related to the environment have been found to predict variation in patients' nursing dependency, length of stay, and complications (Stratton, 1990). In addition, Dennis and Prescott (1985) demonstrated that nurses continued to incorporate Nightingale's concepts in their work, yet rarely recognize the historical import of her actions.

Two studies based on Nightingale's model warrant discussion. In the first, Pattison and Robertson (1995) studied the effects of two hospital architectural designs on patient outcomes: the "Nightingale ward" and the "bay ward." The ward design specified by Nightingale, a long room, open to view, with multiple beds, is still in use in the United Kingdom. Pattison and Robertson compared this ward layout with the more modern bay ward, with patients in units comprised of eight four-bed suites. Patients in the Nightingale ward identified significantly less ambient noise than their bay ward counterparts, and the decreased noise was positively correlated with decreased levels of anxiety. Although patients indicated that they preferred the bay wards, positive effects on their well-being were provided by the design Nightingale worked so hard to implement.

Kolcaba's program of research on comfort care is explicitly congruent with Nightingale's view of the environment (2001). Specifically, the manipulation of the environment to enhance patient health, as described by

Nightingale, is the basis for studies using Kolcaba's comfort theory to examine patient outcomes. This line of research is expected to prosper over the next period of time.

Relationship to Nursing Education

Nightingale's significant influence on nursing education remains evident today. The basic educational goal was for students to acquire the practical and theoretical knowledge bases of implementing physicians' orders and observing the consequences (Nightingale, 1872b, 1885a). Nursing judgment was a significant part of education because "nearly all physicians' orders were conditional" (Nightingale, 1885a, p. 1038). She believed that students were there primarily to learn, not to provide service to hospitals (Prince, 1984). The hospital was to function as a place for students to practice their newly learned nursing skills. These ideas were incorporated into the Nightingale school at St. Thomas' Hospital.

Techniques for educating nurses that were advocated by Nightingale remain in use today. They include keeping ward diaries, instruction by practicing nurses, and role modeling and mentorship (Skeet, 1988). Her writings on environmental health are still suggested readings for students of public health nursing (Gerber & McGuire, 1999). Regardless of her own education, however, Nightingale did not establish nursing education in the university. Palmer (1983b) suggests that Nightingale's nurses based their education in the hospitals because of the value she placed on clinical training and her failure to acknowledge the significance of higher education in her own nursing pursuits. It is of interest, in reference to hospital-based training, that Nightingale (1871) advocated separate wards for nursing and medical students, because higher mortality rates seemed to accompany the presence of medical students.

Nightingale was very clear about her position on both entry into practice and continuing education for nurses. Formal education was regarded simply as that which taught nurses how to go on learning for themselves, and provided only basic information (Nightingale, 1885a). The formal educational experience was to reflect the different careers in nursing: hospital nurses and those who would care for the ill in institutions received 1 year of schooling. District nurses who provided primary health care, midwives, and those who sought leadership or administrative roles in hospitals required 3 years of education. Consistent with her times, Nightingale viewed social class as an appropriate criterion for admission to the school at St. Thomas', and only "ladies" were matriculated in the 3-year program. Neither men nor persons of color were considered for admission.

Nightingale was strongly opposed to licensure for nursing; this resulted in part from her concern that qualities important in nurses could not be assessed on a single examination and that it was dangerous to give women unlimited license to practice. She opposed attempts to make nursing "a book and examination business" (1914); a test could not ensure the moral character, clinical expertise, or systematization Nightingale required of nursing students. Currently, many states require nurses to update their knowledge for practice, often through "mandatory continuing education." This seems wholly consistent with Nightingale's beliefs.

Relationship to Professional Nursing Practice

Concepts and ideas advocated by Nightingale continue to work in nursing practice today. The values she espoused continue to be major factors in public health nursing (Erickson, 1996). Nightingale's approach to working with the poor was to offer them nursing care that led them to new levels of physical, social, and environmental health (Erickson, 1996), a notion that resonates with current concerns of nurse-client partnerships and client empowerment. Whall, Shin, and Colling (1999) have proposed that care for persons with dementia be based on Nightingale's model. Indeed, closer examination of many models of care for persons with Alzheimer's disease reveals that they are completely consistent with Nightingale's "nursing the room" and other environmental manipulations (Selander, 1998). Whall et al., (1999) identified Nightingale's work as consistent not only with Western modalities for assisting persons with Alzheimer's disease, but is also compatible with traditional Eastern, particularly Korean, nursing thought. The emphasis on harmony with one's natural environment, a cornerstone of Korean theories of health, is also found in Nightingale's concerns that the environment be arranged to support the ill or recuperating person. Nightingale's ideas, therefore, have applications in a variety of cultural contexts (Whall et al., 1999).

Other environmental concerns, such as preservation and protection of the patient's environment, have taken on new meaning in an era of concern about water and air quality, toxic wastes, overused landfills, and biohazardous waste (Gropper, 1990). The guidelines Nightingale established for feeding the British army in the Crimea, the first such guidelines ever developed, remain adequate by today's standards (Calkins, 1989). The classifications of diseases and operations by Nightingale became the basis for the International Classification of Diseases, 9th Revision (ICD9) codes (Keith, 1988), and as stated previously, Nightingale was the pioneer in evidence-based nursing practice (Duff, 1998; Spath, 1998; Griffiths, 1995). Furthermore, current scholars point to Nightingale as the progenitor of contemporary nursing interest and practices in health promotion (Rafael, 1999), caring (Watson, 1998), addictions nursing (Naegle, 1991), naturopathy (McCabe, 2000), animal-assisted therapy (Brodie & Biley, 1999), infection control (Gallagher, 1999), and holistic care (Light, 1997). She is exulted as a role model for clinical nurse specialists (Sparacino, 1994) and nurse activists (Shames, 1993).

Nightingale's most important message to present-day practitioners was derived from her understanding of how nursing is related to the whole of society, including social and political contexts. She pushed nursing beyond its traditional boundaries to meet the variety of needs exhibited by her patients (Wintz, 1987). Nightingale (1892/1949) was clear in conveying that progress in nursing was the outgoing responsibility of nurses. She provided an excellent example of how to go about this through clear discourse to the public, use of statistical data, political activism, and collaboration with government agencies and officials.

Relationship to the Omaha System

Ray (1999) stated that evidence is used to demonstrate the validity of healthcare institutions (including nursing practices), as well as to demonstrate the value, cost effectiveness, and unique contributions of a profession. Nightingale kept voluminous records on her interventions and their results, using this information to convince others of the efficacy of nursing. The Omaha system was developed, in part, because nurses were unable to demonstrate either the efficacy of, or future needs for, nursing care (Martin & Scheet, 1992). Nightingale used evidence to establish nursing practice; Martin and Scheet sought to classify evidence so that nursing practice could be practiced, communicated, and advanced. Nightingale used an inductive approach to knowledge development; Martin and Scheet wrote "theory is born in practice" (p. 32). Nightingale's canons of nursing focused on the environment, management of patient care, and observation of the sick, whereas Martin and Scheet classified patient problems environmental, psychosocial, physiological, or health-related behaviors, and nursing interventions as health teaching, nursing treatments, case management, and surveillance. Martin and Scheet were separated from Nightingale by 140 years, but were united with her in purpose, and were consistent in their views on patients and nursing.

The Omaha system was developed in nursing practice and continually validated through research in nursing practice settings (Martin & Scheet, 1992). The system includes three major parts: Problem Classification Scheme, Intervention Scheme, and Problem Rating Scale for Outcomes. Forty nursing diagnoses are listed in the Problem Classification

Scheme, and are further classified as environmental, psychosocial, physiologic, or health behavior related. Problems can be modified as being actual, potential, or needing health promotion, and being a function of the individual client or family client. Nurses may intervene in identified problems using the four categories of health teaching, treatments and procedures, case management, and surveillance, and 63 targets of intervention. Finally, patient progress is documented using the Problem Rating Scale, and identifying progress as either in knowledge, behavior, or status.

Nightingale's model and the Omaha system are compatible with each other. The Omaha Problems are congruent with those identified in Nightingale's 13 canons, and all of the canons were represented in the Problem Classification Scheme. As an example, Nightingale's concern about the "health of houses" is represented in Problem 03, Residence. Her interventions of ensuring "pure air, pure water, efficient drainage, cleanliness, and light" (Nightingale, 1859/1969, p. 24) could be classified as health teaching (if the patient was taught how to clean), and treatments (if the nurse did the cleaning herself), with a target of 18, Environment. The outcomes could be followed using Knowledge (what the patient knows about the health of the house), Behavior (the patient's cleaning activities), and Status (the health of the house). Similarly, "personal cleanliness" is congruent with Problem 38, Personal Hygiene, in the Health-Related Behaviors Domain, "variety" with Problem 07, Social Contact in the Psychosocial Domain, and "taking food" with Problem 30, Digestion-Hydration in the Physiologic Domain. Given Nightingale's concern about removing unnecessary tasks from the nurse's workload (Nightingale, 1863b), it is likely she would approve of the economies of an integrated chart and use of checklists. Moreover, she encouraged nurses to be clear thinkers (1885a), and the notion of "classification" would most likely appeal to her.

Relationship to Theory-Driven, Evidence-Based Practice

Nightingale believed that "experience, not theory" should guide all things (1859/1969, p. 76). However, she was also classically educated, and very familiar with rationalism and able to engage in philosophical debate (LeVasseur, 1998). "Experience," then, should not be construed as only empirical evidence, but also aesthetic, ethical, and personal evidence. All of these patterns of knowing are evident in her writings, and all are included in the body of knowledge Nightingale prescribed for nurses.

Fawcett, Watson, Neuman, Walker, and Fitzpatrick (2001) have raised important questions about what constitutes evidence for nursing practice. Empirics have constituted the bulk of theorizing in nursing over the last 50 years, paralleling a societal fascination with science (Feyerabend, 1981). Nightingale, however, lived in the waning days of rationalism and waxing days of empiricism. A master of statistics, an empirical modality, she was well educated in the Unitarian tradition (personal and ethical knowing), the arts and humanities (aesthetic knowing), and Greek philosophies (aesthetic and ethical knowing). She developed and propagated empirical theories, such as those related to adequate ventilation and its effects on mortality at Scutari. These are the theories for which she was best known in her own time, although her ethical and aesthetic theories were her greatest legacy in the mid-20th century, as generations of nurses were instructed in Nightingalian standards of "ladylike" deportment (Baly, 1988). Rules about nurses' dormitories, dating and courtship, and proper attire were based on aesthetic theories developed by Nightingale. Nightingale's personal theories are the least well developed, and least well known.

Nightingale's writings contain evidence from all four patterns of knowing (Carper, 1978). *Notes on Nursing* (1859/1969) was based, in part, on Nightingale's empirical knowledge, gained in Scutari, and carefully recorded and analyzed into a body of "facts." Personal anecdotes, soul searching, and explication of her religious beliefs are found in the many letters and pamphlets that comprise the majority of Nightingale's writings. These are the autobiographical stories that provide evidence for her personal theories. Standards of practice are also plentiful in *Notes on Nursing;* this is evidence of her ethical theories, including the primacy of the patient. Finally, aesthetic theories of nursing are also described in *Notes on Nursing*, particularly in the section on "Observation of the Sick." Examples and stories are presented, each highlighting a particular aspect of observation, and nurses are advised to learn from them, to practice, and become expert with time.

Perhaps Nightingale continues to be such a driving force in nursing because her evidence-based model is so complete, containing all patterns of knowing, and interweaving them so skillfully.

SUMMARY

Nightingale proposed a model of nursing that continues to influence professional nursing nearly 100 years after her death. She identified the essential elements of nursing (person, nursing activity, environment, and health), but more than that, she identified how these elements fit together. In establishing an evidence-based theory, Nightingale wove together all four patterns of knowing in nursing. She is often credited with establishing science in nursing (Barritt, 1973), but she also established art, ethics, and personal knowing in nursing.

It is noteworthy that practitioners, scholars, and scientists in nursing continue to contemplate Nightingale's work. Some look to her pioneering role, whereas others seek her insights into current concerns. There can be no doubt that much of what we consider professional nursing practice had its start in a visionary, sometimes frustrated and angry woman named Florence Nightingale.

REFERENCES

Agnew, L. R. C. (1958). Florence Nightingale—Statistician. *American Journal of Nursing, 58*, 664–665.

Algase, D. L., & Whall, A. F. (1993). Rosemary Ellis' views on the substantive structure of nursing. *Image: Journal of Nursing Scholarship, 25*, 69–72.

Allen, D. R. (1975). Florence Nightingale: Toward a psychohistorical interpretation. *Journal of Interdisciplinary History, 6*(1), 23–45.

Andrews, M. R. S. (1929). *A lost commander: Florence Nightingale*. New York: Doubleday, Doran.

Baly, M. E. (1986a). *Florence Nightingale and the nursing legacy*. Dover, NH: Croom Helm.

Baly, M. E. (1986b). Shattering the myth. *Nursing Times, 82*(24), 16–18.

Baly, M. E. (1988). Florence Nightingale and "her" schools of nursing. *Humane Medicine, 4*(1), 45–51.

Barritt, E. R. (1973). Florence Nightingale's values and modern nursing education. *Nursing Forum, 12*(1), 7–47.

Benson, E. R. (1992). On the other side of the battle: Russian nurses in the Crimean War. *Image: Journal of Nursing Scholarship, 24*(1), 65–68.

Bishop, W. J. (1960). Florence Nightingale's message for today. *Nursing Outlook, 8*(5), 246–249.

Brodie, S. J., & Biley, F. C. (1999). An exploration of the potential benefits of pet-facilitated therapy. *Journal of Clinical Nursing, 8*, 329–337.

Calkins, B. M. (1989). Florence Nightingale: On feeding an army. *American Journal of Clinical Nutrition, 50*, 1260–1265.

Campbell, J. C., & Bunting, S. (1991). Voices and paradigms: Perspectives on critical and feminist theory in nursing. *Advances in Nursing Science, 13*(3), 1–15.

Carper, B. A. (1978). Fundamental patterns of knowing in nursing. *Advances in Nursing Science, 1*(1), 13–23.

Chinn, P. L., & Kramer, M. K. (1999). *Theory and nursing: Integrated knowledge development* (5th ed.). St. Louis: Mosby.

Cohen, I. B. (1984). Florence Nightingale. *Scientific American, 250*, 128–133, 136–137.

Cook, E. (1942). *The life of Florence Nightingale* (Vols. I and II). New York: Collier MacMillan.

Cope, Z. (1958). *Florence Nightingale and the doctors*. Philadelphia: Lippincott.

Decker, B., & Parley, J. K. (1991). What would Nightingale say? *Nurse Educator, 16*(3), 12–13.

Dennis, K. E., & Prescott, P. A. (1985). Florence Nightingale: Yesterday, today, and tomorrow. *Advances in Nursing Science, 7*, 66–81.

Dubin, R. (1978). *Theory building* (Rev. ed.). New York: Collier MacMillan.

Duff, E. (1998). Florence Nightingale: Basing care on evidence. *RCM Midwives Journal, 1*(6), 192–193.

Ellis, R. (1968). Characteristics of significant theories. *Nursing Research, 17*(3), 217–222.

Ellis, R. (1969). The practitioner as theorist. *American Journal of Nursing, 69*(7), 1434–1438.

Erickson, G. P. (1996). To pauperize or empower: Public health nursing at the turn of the 20th and 21st centuries. *Public Health Nursing, 13*(3), 163–169.

Fawcett, J. (1978). The what of theory development. In *Theory development: What, why, how?* (pp. 17–34). New York: National League for Nursing.

Fawcett, J., Watson, J., Neuman, B., Walker, P. H., & Fitzpatrick, J. J. (2001). On nursing theories and evidence. *Journal of Nursing Scholarship, 33*(2), 115–119.

Feyerabend, P. (1981). How to defend society against science. In I. Hacking (Ed.), *Scientific revolutions* (pp. 156–167). New York: Oxford University Press.

Gallagher, R. (1999). Infection control: Public health, clinical effectiveness and education. *British Journal of Nursing, 8,* 1212–1214.

Gerber, D. E., & McGuire, S. L. (1999). Teaching students about nursing and the environment: Part I—Nursing role and basic curricula. *Journal of Community Health Nursing, 16*(2), 69–79.

Grier, B., & Grier, M. (1978). Contributions of the passionate statistician. *Research in Nursing and Health, 1,* 103–109.

Griffiths, P. (1995). Progress in measuring nursing outcomes. *Journal of Advanced Nursing, 21,* 1092–1100.

Gropper, E. I. (1990). Florence Nightingale: Nursing's first environmental theorist. *Nursing Forum, 25*(3), 30–33.

Hayne, Y. (1992). The current status and future significance of nursing as a discipline. *Journal of Advanced Nursing, 17,* 104–107.

Hays, J. C. (1989). Florence Nightingale and the India sanitary reforms. *Public Health Nursing, 6*(3), 152–154.

Huxley, E. (1975). *Florence Nightingale.* New York: Putnam.

Iveson-Iveson, J. (1983). A legend in the breaking. *Nursing Mirror, 156*(19), 26–27.

Johnson, D. E. (1992). The origins of the behavioral system model: Commentary on Nightingale. In *Florence Nightingale's Notes on Nursing: What it is and what it is not* (Commemorative ed., pp. 23–27). Philadelphia: Lippincott.

Kalisch, B. J., & Kalisch, P. A. (1983a). Heroine out of focus: Media images of Florence Nightingale (Part I). *Nursing and Health Care, 4*(4), 270–278.

Kalisch, B. J., & Kalisch, P. A. (1983b). Heroine out of focus: Media images of Florence Nightingale (Part II). *Nursing and Health Care, 4*(5),181–187.

Kaplan, A. (1964). *The conduct of inquiry.* New York: Crowell.

Keith, J. M. (1988). Florence Nightingale: Statistician and consultant epidemiologist. *International Nursing Review, 35*(5), 147–150.

Kolcaba, K. (2001). Evolution of the mid-range theory of comfort for outcomes research. *Nursing Outlook, 49,* 86–92.

Kopf, E. W. (1978). Florence Nightingale as statistician. *Research in Nursing and Health, 1,* 93–102.

Larson, E. (1989). Innovations in health care: Antisepsis as a case study. *American Journal of Public Health, 79,* 92–99.

Laudan, L. (1977). *Progress and its problems: Towards a theory of scientific growth.* Berkeley: University California Press.

Laudan, L. (1981). A problem-solving approach to scientific progress. In I. Hacking (Ed.), *Scientific revolutions* (pp. 144–155). New York: Oxford University Press.

LeVasseur, J. (1998). Plato, Nightingale, and contemporary nursing. *Image: Journal of Nursing Scholarship, 30,* 281–285.

Levine, M. E. (1992). Nightingale redux. In *Florence Nightingale's Notes on Nursing: What it is and what it is not* (Commemorative ed., pp. 39–43). Philadelphia: Lippincott.

Light, K. M. (1997). Florence Nightingale and holistic philosophy. *Journal of Holistic Nursing, 15*(1), 25–40.

Lobo, M. L. (1995). Florence Nightingale. In J. B. George (Ed.), *Nursing theories: The base for professional nursing practice* (4th ed., pp. 33–48). Norwalk, CT: Appleton & Lange.

Macrae, J. (1995). Nightingale's spiritual philosophy and its significance for modern nursing. *Image: Journal of Nursing Scholarship, 27,* 8–10.

Martin, K. S., & Scheet, N. J. (1992). *The Omaha system: Applications for community health nursing.* Philadelphia: W. B. Saunders.

McCabe, P. (2000). Naturopathy, Nightingale, and nature cure: A convergence of interests. *Complementary Therapies in Nursing and Midwifery, 6*(1), 4–8.

McCarthy, D. O., Ouimet, M. E., & Daun, J. M. (1991). Shades of Florence Nightingale: Potential impact of noise stress on wound healing. *Holistic Nursing Practice, 5*(4), 39–48.

Meleis, A. I. (1997). Theoretical nursing: Development and progress (3rd ed.). Philadelphia: Lippincott-Raven.

Montiero, L. A. (Ed.). (1974). *Letters of Florence Nightingale.* Boston: Nursing Archives.

Montiero, L. A. (1984). On separate roads: Florence Nightingale and Elizabeth Blackwell. *Signs: Journal of Women in Culture and Society, 9,* 520–533.

Montiero, L. A. (1985). Florence Nightingale on public health nursing. *American Journal of Public Health, 75,* 181–186.

Naegle, M. (1991). Florence Nightingale: Addiction's nursing pioneer. *Addiction's Nursing Network, 3*(4), 124–125.

Nauright, L. (1984). Politics and power: A new look at Florence Nightingale. *Nursing Forum, 21*(1), 5–8.

Nightingale, F. (1858a). *Mortality of the British army.* London: Harrison.

Nightingale, F. (1858b). *Subsidiary notes as to the introduction of female nursing in military hospitals in peace and war.* London: Harrison.

Nightingale, F. (1859). Notes on the sanitary condition of hospitals, and on the defects in the construction of hospital wards. In G. W. Hastings (Ed.), *Transactions of the National Association for the Promotion of Social Science* (pp. 462–482). London: Parker.

Nightingale, F. (1863a). *How people may live and not die in India.* London: Emil Faithfull.

Nightingale, F. (1863b). *Notes on hospitals.* London: Longman, Greer, Longman, Roberts, and Green.

Nightingale, F. (1863c). *Observations on the evidence contained in the stational reports. Submitted by her to the Royal Commission on the Sanitary State of the Army in India.* London: Edward Stanford.

Nightingale, F. (1863d). *Sanitary statistics of native colonial schools and hospitals.* London: George E. Eyre & William Spottiswoode.

Nightingale, F. (1865). *A note on the aboriginal races of Australia.* London: Emil Faithfull.

Nightingale, F. (1867). Suggestions on the subject of providing, training, and organizing nurses for the sick poor in workhouse infirmaries. In *Government Report of the Committee to Consider the Cubic Space of Metropolitan Workhouses* (Paper No. XVI, Parliamentary Blue Book, pp. 64–79). London: Parliament of the United Kingdom.

Nightingale, F. (1869). A note on pauperism. *Fraser Magazine, March,* 281–290.

Nightingale, F. (1871). *Introductory notes on lying-in institutions.* London: Longmans, Green.

Nightingale, F. (1872a). Introduction. In *Una and her paupers: Memorials of Agnes Elizabeth Jones by her sister* (pp. i–xvii). New York: Routledge.

Nightingale, F. (1872b). Letter to Dr. W. Gill Wylie.

Nightingale, F. (1874). *Life or death in India.* London: Harrison.

Nightingale, F. (1885a). Nurses, training of. In R. Quain (Ed.), *A dictionary of medicine* (9th ed., pp. 1038–1043). New York: Appleton.

Nightingale, F. (1885b). Nursing the sick. In R. Quain (Ed.), *A dictionary of medicine* (9th ed., pp. 1043–1046). New York: Appleton.

Nightingale, F. (1892). Introduction. In D. Gidumal (Ed.), *Behramji M. Malabari: A biographical sketch*. London: T. Fisher Unwin.

Nightingale, F. (1914). Letter. In *Florence Nightingale to her nurses*. London: Collier MacMillan. (Original work dated May 1888.)

Nightingale, F. (1946). *The art of nursing*. London: Claud Morris. (Original work published 1859.)

Nightingale, F. (1949). Sick nursing and health nursing. In I. A. Hampton (Ed.), *Nursing of the sick, 1893*. New York: McGraw-Hill. (Original work published 1893.)

Nightingale, F. (1969). *Notes on nursing: What it is and what it is not*. New York: Dover. (Original work published 1859.)

Nuttall, P. (1983). The passionate statistician. *Nursing Times, 79*(39), 25–27.

Palmer, I. S. (1977). Florence Nightingale: Reformer, reactionary, researcher. *Nursing Research, 26*(2), 84–89.

Palmer, I. S. (1981). Florence Nightingale and the international origins of modern nursing. *Image, 13*, 28–31.

Palmer, I. S. (1983a). Florence Nightingale: The myth and the reality. *Nursing Times, 79*(31), 40–42.

Palmer, I. S. (1983b). Nightingale revisited. *Nursing Outlook, 31*, 229–233.

Pattison, H. M., & Robertson, C. E. (1995). The effect of ward design on the well-being of postoperative patients. *Journal of Advanced Nursing, 23*, 820–826.

Peplau, H. E. (1992). Notes on Nightingale. In *Florence Nightingale's Notes on nursing: What it is and what it is not* (Commemorative ed., pp. 48–57). Philadelphia: Lippincott.

Prince, J. (1984). Education for profession: Some lessons from history. *International Journal of Nursing Studies, 21*, 153–163.

Rafael, A. R. F. (1999). The politics of health promotion: Influences on public health promoting nursing practice in Ontario, Canada from Nightingale to the nineties. *Advances in Nursing Science, 22*(1), 23–39.

Ray, L. (1999). Evidence and outcomes: Agendas, presuppositions, and power. *Journal of Advanced Nursing, 30*, 1017–1026.

Reynolds, P. D. (1971). *A primer in theory construction*. Indianapolis: Bobbs-Merrill.

Schlotfeldt, R. M. (1977). Nursing research: Reflection of values. *Nursing Research, 26*(1), 4–9.

Selander, L. C. (1998). The power of environmental adaptation: Florence Nightingale's original theory for nursing practice. *Journal of Holistic Nursing, 16*, 247–263.

Shames, K. H. (1993). *The Nightingale conspiracy: Nursing comes to power in the 21st century*. Montclair, NJ: Enlightenment Press.

Silva, M. C., & Rothbart, D. (1984). An analysis of changing trends in philosophies of science on nursing theory development and testing. *Advances in Nursing Science, 6*(2), 1–13.

Skeet, M. (1988). Florence Nightingale: A woman of vision and drive. *World Health Forum, 9*, 175–177.

Sparacino, P. S. A. (1994). Florence Nightingale: A CNS role model. *Clinical Nurse Specialist, 8*(2), 64.

Spath, P. L. (1998). Nursing performance measures go public. *Outcomes Management for Nursing Practice, 2*, 124–129.

Stratton, L. A. (1990). *The relationship between dimensions of a hospital organizational climate and peer culture, the empowerment of nurses, and client outcome*. Unpublished doctoral dissertation, Case Western Reserve University, Cleveland.

Styles, M. M. (1992). Nightingale: The enduring symbol. In *Florence Nightingale's Notes on Nursing: What it is and what it is not* (Commemorative ed., pp. 72–75). Philadelphia: Lippincott.

Torres, G. (1980). Florence Nightingale. In *Nursing theories: The base for professional nursing practice* (pp. 27–38). Englewood Cliffs, NJ: Prentice Hall.

Uhl, J. E. (1992). Nightingale—The international nurse. *Journal of Professional Nursing, 8*(1), 5.

Ulrich, B. T. (1992). *Leadership and management according to Florence Nightingale.* Norwalk, CT: Appleton & Lange.

Valentine, N. M. (1988). The genesis of Nightingale: Alternative treatment for female health care providers. *Holistic Nursing Practice, 2*(4), 45–55.

Watson, J. (1998). Reflections: Florence Nightingale and the enduring legacy of transpersonal caring. *Journal of Holistic Nursing, 16*, 292–294.

Webb, C. (1992). Mothers and daughters: A powerful spell. *Journal of Advanced Nursing, 17*, 1334–1342.

Welch, M. (1986). Nineteenth century philosophic influences on Nightingale's concept of the person. *Journal of Nursing History, 1*(2), 3–11.

Welch, M. (1990). Florence Nightingale—The social construction of a Victorian feminist. *Western Journal of Nursing Research, 12*, 404–407.

Welch, M. (1991). The context of feminism and nursing in 19th century Victorian England. In R. M. Neil & R. Watts (Eds.), *Caring and nursing: Explorations in feminist perspectives* (pp. 67–75). New York: National League for Nursing monograph (Pub. no. 14-2369).

Whall, A. L., Shin, Y., & Colling, K. B. (1999). A Nightingale-based model for dementia care and its relevance for Korean nursing. *Nursing Science Quarterly, 12*, 319–323.

Wheelwright, J. (1987). "Amazons and military maids": An examination of female military heroines in British literature and the changing construction of gender. *Women's Studies International Forum, 10*, 489–502.

Widerquist, J. G. (1992). The spirituality of Florence Nightingale. *Nursing Research, 41*(1), 49–55.

Wintz, L. (1987). Career paths of nurses: When is a nurse no longer a nurse? *Journal of Nursing Administration, 17*(4), 33–37.

Woodham-Smith, C. (1951). *Florence Nightingale.* New York: McGraw-Hill.

4

Peplau's Theory of Interpersonal Relations

Pamela G. Reed

Hildegard Elizabeth Peplau's leadership as a nursing scholar was clearly established with the 1952 publication of her formal treatise on nursing in her book, *Interpersonal Relations in Nursing.* Springer Publishing Company reissued the book in 1991. Although Nightingale had provided the emerging discipline with a relatively well-defined conceptualization of nursing, the momentum of her accomplishments slowed to a near standstill as many practicing nurses, lacking a sound nursing knowledge base and political power, assumed the medical model of health care. Peplau (1986) was an active participant in shifting the worldview about nursing toward a focus on its scientific as well as humanistic contributions to society. Since then, nursing has been struggling to embrace fully the theoretical and educational standards put forth by Peplau for the discipline to become an autonomous profession and a visible science of the 21st century.

BIOGRAPHICAL INFORMATION

Peplau was born September 1, 1909, in Reading, Pennsylvania, as one of six children of German immigrants, Gustav and Ottylie Peplau. She received her nursing diploma from Pottstown Hospital School of Nursing in Reading at the age of 22. She worked in general duty, private practice, supervision, and camp nursing prior to accepting a position as Executive Officer, College of Health Science, Bennington College, Vermont. She held this position during her college years at Bennington, where she studied psychiatric nursing. While there, she studied with Erich Fromm and attended lectures by Harry Stack Sullivan, both of whom were among the outstanding scientists who influenced her theory and practice. In 1943, upon receiving her Bachelor of Arts degree in Interpersonal Psychology from Bennington, Peplau was commissioned 1st Lieutenant in the United States Army Nurse Corps. She was assigned to the 312th Field Station Hospital in England, serving in neuropsychiatry in London from 1943 to 1945.

Peplau received a Master of Arts degree in Psychiatric Nursing from Teachers College, Columbia University, at the age of 38. From 1948 to 1953, Peplau instituted and directed a graduate program in Psychiatric Nursing at Teachers College. During this time, she completed her book on interpersonal relations theory, which was delayed 3 years in publication because it was considered too revolutionary for a nurse to publish (O'Toole & Welt, 1989). In 1953, Peplau received a Doctorate in Education from Teachers College, Columbia University. Peplau worked as a private duty nurse from 1953 to 1955 in New York City. In 1955, she assumed a full-time position at Rutgers, the State University of New Jersey, where she established and chaired one of the first clinical specialist Masters Degree programs in psychiatric nursing. She was promoted to professor in 1960, and remained at Rutgers until retirement in 1974. She not only contributed to the development of graduate-level education nationally and internationally, but she facilitated the movement of the profession into graduate-level education in specialized fields of practice (Gregg, 1999).

Peplau served on many committees and commissions at federal and international levels; she served as consultant to the National Institute of Mental Health and the World Health Organization, Vice President of the International Council of Nurses (ICN), and as both Executive Director and President of the American Nurses Association (ANA). She was a member of the ANA Congress of Nursing Practice Task Force, which developed nursing's social policy statement. She was an elected fellow of the American Academy of Nursing (AAN) and a member Sigma Theta Tau. Peplau was honored by the AAN as a Living Legend, by the ICN with the Christiana Reimann Award, and by the ANA, which inducted her into its Hall of Fame in 1998. Peplau was awarded 12 honorary doctoral degrees from various universities, including Duke, Indiana, Ohio State, Rutgers, and the University of Ulster in Ireland. Peplau died at her home (in Sherman Oaks, CA) on March 17, 1999, at the age of 89. The archives of her life and work are housed at the Radcliffe College Schlesinger Library at Harvard University.

Peplau is well known for her 1952 book and numerous other articles as well as many unpublished writings and presentations (e.g., O'Toole & Welt, 1989). Her writings were directed toward the clarification of clinical nursing phenomena, theory development, and interventions. She was regarded as an ambassador for advanced nursing education and as an advo-cate for the mentally ill. Peplau's theoretical and metatheoretical contribu-tions to nursing are now widely acknowledged (e.g., Forchuk, 1991; Nursing Development Conference Group, 1979; Reed, 1996; Welt & O'Toole, 1989).

Sills (1978) described the impact of Peplau's contribution as responsi-ble for a "second order change in the nursing culture" (p. 124). Placing the contribution in chronological history, Peplau's interpersonal model initiated a move from an intrapsychic emphasis within psychiatric mental health nursing and a dominant focus on technical and physical care within general nursing, to an interpersonal focus in both. Following after Peplau were Hen-derson, Orlando, King, and other noted theorists who emphasized the inter-personal process in nursing. Until recently, Peplau's influence on education and practice in nursing was not given its due recognition. Once a contribu-tion becomes a part of the public domain, it is difficult to recognize its im-pact on the larger society. Peplau's contribution is now increasingly acknowledged as nurses gain insight into the historical, philosophical, clin-ical, and theoretical underpinnings of their discipline.

BASIC ELEMENTS

Peplau's views regarding the metaparadigm concepts provide a conceptual foundation for her nursing practice theory. The definitions and descriptions of these concepts also provide insight into the philosophical foundation of her theory.

Definition and Description of Nursing

Peplau (1987b) defined nursing as "a service for people that enhances heal-ing and health by methods that are humanistic and primarily non-invasive" (p. 32). More specifically, nursing was a "significant therapeutic interper-sonal process which functions cooperatively with other human processes that make health possible for individuals" (Peplau, 1952, p. 16). Peplau conceptualized nursing as an integration of art and science, evident in her description of practicing nurses as *working scientists* and the nursing process as an *investigative approach* (Peplau, 1988a). Peplau wrote about the combined application of scientific data and subjective, interpersonal data as *indirect nursing* and *direct nursing*, respectively. Thus, science is used to delineate *regularities* or universal characteristics about a phenom-enon from an objective, theoretical, *tough-minded* stance. Art and aesthetic knowledge are used to understand the observed phenomenon from an in-dividualized, ethical, and contextually sensitive, *tender-hearted* stance (Peplau, 1988a). Through the interpersonal process, clinical judgment then is used to integrate scientific and artistic aspects to define and intervene in the patient's problem.

The interpersonal process between patient and nurse represents the critical nursing phenomenon of focus, bringing together the six roles of the nurse, the various patterns of the patient, and the pattern integrations between the two. Biophysical and biochemical human patterns are excluded from Peplau's description of the focus of nursing; she regarded these as potentially important but more within the purview of medicine and pharmacology (Peplau, 1992b).

Basic to her description of nursing is her developmental perspective of human phenomena; nursing was defined as "a maturing force and educative instrument" (Peplau, 1952, p. 8). The goal of nursing is to move patients toward enhanced health via increased awareness of problematic psychosocial patterns and development of more useful "growth-continuing patterns" (Peplau, 1992b, p. 15).

Communication as a Basic Concept

Clear and supportive communication is a key tool in nursing. The significance attributed to communication in Peplau's theory (1952) is reflected in her reference to Benjamin Whorf's (1956) theory about language as a mediator of thought (Peplau, 1968). Language is attributed major importance in Peplau's theory because it influences the person's thinking, which influences actions. Therapeutic talking with patients helps them to learn from their dysfunctional thinking patterns and develop cognitive perspectives that influence productive behaviors (Peplau, 1966, cited in Welt & O'Toole, 1989).

Communication with others helps one attend to and clarify one's perception of reality, and to achieve a sense of understanding with another person (Peplau, 1952). This involves an awareness of nonverbal and verbal communication and the symbolic meanings behind these communications. It is one of the nurse's responsibilities to assess these factors and to influence the patient's communications in a way that contributes to healthy modes of thought.

Definition and Description of a Person

The person, according to Peplau, is a developing self-system composed of biochemical, physiological, and interpersonal characteristics and needs. Development occurs as a result of interactions with significant others that educe the person's innate capabilities. The power to change originates in the person and can be facilitated by the nurse (Peplau, 1992a). Developmental competencies (tools) are acquired as three sets of self-views emerge in development (Peplau, 1979, pp. 35–37). These self-views influence the person's actions and range from those of which the person is consciously aware to those that are highly anxiety producing and, therefore, repressed from conscious awareness. To a large degree, the self-views consist of a synthesis of appraisals by others that have been introjected by the person.

The prototaxic, parataxic, and syntaxic modes of experiencing, initially described by Sullivan (1952), are theoretical constructs used by Peplau to describe the person. The prototaxic mode refers to the sense of experiencing, characteristically found in infants that are limited to the present moment without relationship to the past or future. Parataxic thinking emerges as linkages between past, present, and future experiences develop and a familiar element can be identified to relate the three time dimensions. Persons experiencing severe anxiety may have difficulty perceiving these linkages and the continuity between present and past events. The individual in the syntaxic mode is able to recognize the uniqueness of a given situation as well as its relationship to the past and future. As each of these modes becomes available, the person's abilities to perceive and communicate with environmental resources, and to solve problems, are enhanced.

The mature person is viewed as capable of meeting his or her own needs and integrating a variety of experiences. Human needs are organized hierarchically and give rise to transformations of energy into observable patterns of behavior designed to meet these needs. An individual's behavior patterns in part are determined by past developmental experiences, present contextual variables, and future expectations and goals. It is, however, the person's perception of these factors that is particularly important in determining behavior.

Peplau stated (1952) that persons live in an unstable equilibrium and have two basic goals, identified previously by Symonds: "those of self-maintenance and perpetuation of the species" (1946, p. 79). All behavioral activities are purposeful and directed toward the transformation of anxiety generated from unmet needs and toward facilitating emergence of higher needs. These activities are based upon the interpersonal nature of the person. Human beings thrive on interpersonal relations. Such interpersonal experiences are significant in both identifying solutions to anxiety situations for self-maintenance, and in contributing to the development of additional anxiety.

Anxiety as a Basic Concept

Anxiety is integral to Peplau's conceptualization of the person. It is an energy source inextricably related to human development from infancy to death and is required for biological and emotional growth (Peplau, 1963b,

1992b). The theoretical frameworks of May (1950) and Sullivan (1952) are used to explicate this concept. "The self-system is an anti-anxiety system" (Peplau, 1979, p. 36); directions for development are selected in reference to behaviors that prevent excessive anxiety by addressing intrapersonal issues, social expectations, and biological needs.

Anxiety is produced when communications with others threaten the biological or psychological security of the individual (Peplau, 1963b). The presence and degree of anxiety heighten the person's sensitivity to the environment such that more information can be assimilated. The perceptual field becomes constricted as the degree of anxiety increases to the point when, in a state of panic, the ability to test reality is seriously impaired. Identifiable behavior patterns emerge as the energy from varying degrees of anxiety is transformed. Some patterns such as somaticizing or withdrawing are less effective in relieving anxiety than others that reflect more active attempts to engage in problem solving.

Debilitating behaviors are manifested during illness. In illness, and particularly during hospitalization, growing needs and behavioral characteristics of less mature developmental stages are predominant. Illness is a time of regression and retreat to mobilize energy for use in reducing tension generated by unmet needs and conflicting goals.

Definition and Description of Environment

The concept of environment is addressed primarily in reference to those external factors considered to be essential to human development. These include the presence of caring adults, secure economic status of the family, and a healthy prenatal environment (Peplau, 1952, p. 163). More importantly, Peplau presented interpersonal situations as an environmental microcosm within which health is promoted. Interactions between person and family, child and parent, or patient and nurse are examples of this interpersonal environment. Extension of the self into the community "and on into the ongoing stream of civilization" is required for the affirmation and fulfillment of human goals (Peplau, 1952, p. 79). Cultural forces are other environmental factors by which societal values and mores significant to personality development are transmitted throughout life.

Peplau also defined the treatment setting as a physical and social environment and viewed it, along with the nurse-patient interpersonal environment, as a primary responsibility of the nurse. Peplau (1982a, 1983a) explained that the treatment milieu can serve to either perpetuate illness-maintenance patterns or promote healthy interactional patterns in clients. She categorized aspects of the milieu into structured and unstructured.

Structured aspects refer to the physical and social arrangements that are preplanned or formalized in some way; for example, furniture arrangement, mealtimes, therapies, and ward rules. She expressed particular interest in the unstructured component of the milieu—the "people interactions"— as more important, but noted that it receives less attention than the structured aspects. Interactional patterns or "pattern integrations" among staff and clients that promote self-knowledge and self-care are considered by her to be critical environmental influences in clients' mental health (Peplau 1983a, 1992b). In summary, Peplau (1982a) envisioned the nurse as investigator and facilitator of a milieu environment that "evokes pattern awareness and change in patients" (p. 23).

Definition and Description of Health

Health is linked to the phenomenon of human development. The word *health* is a symbol that implies "forward movement of personality and other ongoing human processes in the direction of creative, constructive, productive, personal, and community living" (Peplau, 1952, p. 12). Derived from the basic human experiences of anxiety, human energy can be transformed into either health-promoting or debilitating behaviors.

Illness is regarded as a manifestation of "undeveloped potential," a pathological facade pointing toward an opportunity for growth of particular competencies (Peplau, 1965, in Welt & O'Toole, 1989). Acquisition of interpersonal competencies, an indicator of health, is a by-product of the developmental process, which Peplau (1992c) likened to Parse's (1992) process of "becoming" (p. 87).

Peplau's theory places health and illness on a continuum. This health-illness continuum parallels Sullivan's (1947) conceptualization of a continuum of anxiety that Peplau (1952) depicts as ranging from pure euphoria to varying degrees of anxiety. Beeber, Anderson, and Sills (1990) identified this "anxiety gradient" as a key element in Peplau's theory. The person's degree of health is related to the degree of anxiety experienced and the ability to transform this anxiety into productive, asymptomatic behavior.

This anxiety-transformative ability resides within the person. In illness, nursing interventions are required that are sustained as long as needed to educe this capability once again, and help the person progress to a higher level of development (Peplau, 1987b; Peplau, 1985b cited in Welt & O'Toole, 1989). Mental health is dependent upon communications that facilitate an accurate perception of the problematic situation, identification and integration of related feelings and cognitions, and attainment of developmental skills in handling intrapersonal anxiety. Through the interpersonal relationship with the nurse, the person can develop communication skills and self-awareness that function to maintain a productive amount of anxiety in the self-system.

INTERNAL ANALYSIS AND EVALUATION

Metatheoretical Assumptions

Although Peplau developed her theory of interpersonal relations in the 1940s and 1950s during an era of positivist philosophical thought, Peplau advocated the integration of science and art in nursing to promote a scholarly yet humanistic approach to nursing practice (e.g., Peplau, 1954, cited in O'Toole & Welt, 1989; Peplau, 1988a). Peplau's assumptions underlying her approach to nursing intervention and the interpersonal process parallel those reflected in her approach to development of nursing theory and knowledge in general. That is, acquiring knowledge, whether for theory building or assessing a patient, requires the elements of both science and art (Peplau, 1988a).

In reference to the science dimension, Peplau incorporated established knowledge, which she regarded as "scientific," in development of her nursing theory. She viewed this knowledge as belonging to nursing when it facilitated selection and organization of a number of concepts into a larger component: (a) that delineates a serial ordering or a process of particular behavior, as in Sullivan's (1952) outline of developmental tasks; (b) from which patient behavior can be understood and predicted; and (c) from which nursing interventions can easily be derived (Peplau, 1969a, pp. 34–36). Thus, Peplau's theory represents the organization of selected extant concepts into a larger component describing a sequence of behaviors that can be expected to occur in the context of interpersonal relations. Peplau incorporated in her theory building approach, as Ellis (1968) and Hardy (1974) later advocated, a critical evaluation of "scientific" knowledge for its relevance to nursing.

In addition to these scientific concepts, which Peplau regarded as more or less "universal" human processes, she also assumed that there is an art of nursing. Within the art perspective, one valued patterns of the inherent individual variability in the person's context and in the extent to which the universal processes had developed into "usable competencies" (Peplau, 1987a, p. 206). An understanding of these unique patterns was obtained through personal contact with the patient, self-reflection, and expert observation and assessment. Peplau believed that "nursing situations provided a field of observations from which unique nursing concepts could be derived and used for the improvement of the professional's work" (Peplau, 1969a, p. 36).

Nursing concepts, then, as distinguished from purely scientific concepts, are derived from empirical observations of patterns of phenomena. These patterns are held up against extant knowledge for identification of relevant theoretical concepts. The theoretical concepts are then examined for validity in the context of the interpersonal process. Peplau's approach to development of nursing knowledge is similar to Strasser's (1985) "hermeneutic spiral" by which scientific knowledge emerges from formulation and practical application of theoretical concepts that explain empirical observations. For Peplau, nursing knowledge involved an ongoing process of sifting theoretical ideas through the inspiration and validation of clinical experience and judgment. In addition, nursing knowledge was to be used not as the ultimate source of truth for the patient, but as an emancipatory instrument to help patients "express and amplify their powers" (Peplau, 1969a, 1992b).

Central Components

There are three central components of Peplau's model: *interpersonal process, nurse,* and *patient anxiety.* The interpersonal process is the central component of the model and describes the method by which the nurse facilitates useful transformations of the patient's energy or anxiety. The interpersonal process represents the point at which the nurse and patient interface in the interest of the patient's health. Characteristics of the nurse and patient are defined primarily in reference to those considered relevant to the communication and changes that occur in human relationships, and particularly in the nurse–patient relationship.

Interpersonal Process

The interpersonal process is based upon a participatory relationship between nurse and patient in which the nurse governs the purpose and the process, and the patient controls the content. The nurse's interventions are focused primarily upon the process of establishing and maintaining a trusting and goal-oriented relationship with the patient, that goal being to move the patient toward more productive interpersonal functioning. The interpersonal process is operationally defined in terms of four distinct phases: *orientation, identification, exploitation,* and *resolution.* Although it is described as having distinct phases, overlap is expected throughout the relationship. The first phase, orientation, has as its major focus assisting the patient to become aware of the availability of and trust in the nurse's abilities to participate effectively in his or her health care.

Identification, the second phase, occurs when the nurse facilitates the patient's expression of whatever feelings are experienced, and remains able to provide the nursing care needed. This expression without rejection permits the experiencing of illness as an opportunity to reorient feelings and strengthen the positive forces of the personality. Patients may respond to this experience as either an independent participant in the relationship with the nurse, an independent person in isolation from the nurse, or a person who is helplessly dependent upon the nurse.

The major working phase of the relationship is exploitation. This third phase provides the situation in which the patient may derive full value from the relationship in accordance with the view or perception of the situation. Forchuk (1991) suggested combining the second and third phases into one phase, conceptualized as the working phase. Nevertheless, identification and exploitation are important distinctions in describing the interpersonal process.

This leads to the final phase, resolution, during which the patient is gradually freed from the identification with the helping professional. Resolution permits the generation and strengthening of the ability to meet one's own needs and channel energy toward realization of potentialities (Peplau, 1952). Thus, these four phases characterize a coherent developmental process in which the nurse guides the patient from dependent toward increasingly interdependent interactions with the social environment.

Nurse

The nurse is a component of the Peplau model and is clearly activated as a process in terms of any or all six identified roles. The nurse, like the patient, is a moderating factor in the interpersonal process. The first role of the nurse, that of a stranger, includes the sharing of respect and positive interest in the patient. In the *stranger role*, the nurse is at first nonpersonal and offers the same ordinary courtesies that are accorded a guest when introduced into any new situation. These include acceptance of the person as she or he is and relating to the patient as an emotionally able stranger unless there is evidence to support expectations of limitations in this area of functioning.

The second role is that of *resource person*. As a resource person, the nurse provides specific answers to questions usually formulated to address a larger problem. Answering these questions may lead to the emergence of more pertinent areas that require assistance. The third identified role, that of *teacher,* is viewed as a combination of all other roles. *Leadership,* the fourth role, is directed toward the development of a democratic relationship, encouraging the patient's active participation in the direction of care. The nurse assumes the role of *surrogate* in situations requiring resolution of existing interpersonal conflicts. Psychological or emotional-age factors caused by arrests in development or feelings reactivated through the experience of illness may demand the assumption of surrogate roles. Through this, the nurse helps patients to learn that there are similarities and differences between individuals, and by being herself or himself, the nurse assists with the needed resolution of interpersonal conflicts.

The sixth role, that of *counselor,* is of major importance in all nurse-patient relationships. It is through this role that the nurse promotes experiences leading to health. Increasing a patient's awareness of conditions required for health and providing these when possible, identifying threats to health, and facilitating learning through the use of evolving interpersonal events are components of this role. Through all of these roles, nursing behaviors emphasizing unconditional acceptance of the patient, self-awareness, and emotional neutrality are requisites (Peplau, 1952). Hence, these six roles describe mechanisms the nurse uses throughout the interpersonal process. These roles imply, however, that the patient has the primary responsibility in reducing anxiety to a healthy level.

Patient Anxiety

Peplau addresses the patient primarily in terms of his or her anxiety as experienced in illness. Anxiety is manifested in various communications and affects the patient's ability to learn and function effectively. Peplau's (1968) assumption of human potentiality is evident in her theory in that it is emphasized that only the person can change the self and move toward health. Peplau was quite specific in her focus on patients who have unhealthy levels of anxiety; patients with other health problems generally fall outside the boundary of her theory.

Anxiety is a pivotal concept in Peplau's model. Anxiety is basic to human development. Anxiety, whether intrapsychic or interpersonal, is a main source of energy in both healthy and problematic behavior (Peplau, 1992b). There is a direct link between anxiety and illness. In illness, energy from anxiety needed for growth is instead bound in nonhealthy symptoms (Peplau, 1952). Major goals of nursing are to assess the degree of anxiety existing in a patient's life, the ways in which anxiety is communicated by both patient and nurse, and the effects of anxiety upon the patient's ability to learn and develop, and to facilitate strategies that effectively transform debilitating levels of anxiety.

Summary of Relationships among Components

The interpersonal process is the primary component in the theory, and includes the interaction between the nurse's patterns, defined in terms of the six professional roles, and the patient experiencing symptomatic anxiety manifested in dysfunctional behavior patterns. Levels of anxiety are manifested in various observable patterns, which indicate areas of focus and opportunities for growth. Pattern integrations may occur between patient and nurse if they share mutual, complementary, or antagonistic patterns of thinking, feeling, or acting (Peplau, 1987a, 1992a). The interpersonal process is characterized by the "investigative" approach, which combines a retrospective review of contextual factors with assessment of the self-views that are operative in the patient's life. Investigative counseling combines a systematic, objective (scientific) approach with participatory, reflexive, subjective (art) methods in the interpersonal process. The patient possesses the necessary data, in the form of subconscious meanings, personal knowledge, and undeveloped or unused competencies, whereas the nurse possesses the method to access the data through the interpersonal process (Martin, Forchuk, Santopinto, & Butcher, 1992; O'Toole & Welt, 1989).

The nurse manages the relationship, not the patient (Peplau, 1969a). Through investigative interviewing, the nurse works to uncover and educe the patient's "latent potentialities" or "dormant powers," and to help the patient realize and implement these capacities for recovery (Peplau, 1988b). "Interpersonal techniques rest on a one-way focus," whereby the concern is the development of the patient, not of the nurse (Peplau, 1992a, p. 18). However, mutual learning and self-understanding have been cited as common outcomes for both the patient and nurse (Beeber, Anderson, & Sills, 1990; Peplau, 1952).

Through interpersonal interaction with the patient, the nurse facilitates the patient's ability to transform symptom-bound anxiety into problem-solving energy. Latent capacities become realized competencies, which are used by the patient to continue development. The resultant transformation of anxiety moves the patient toward health, and outside of the boundary of the nurse–patient relationship.

Analysis of Consistency

Because Peplau was committed to theory-based nursing practice at a time when theory development was relatively unknown and when reductionistic conceptualizations were the norm, mechanistic depictions of the central components and their relationships may, particularly if taken out of context, be identified in Peplau's writings. Theories that were available for integration into her theory at that time portrayed human behavior within the perspectives of biologically based psychoanalytic theory, stimulus-response learning models, and closed-system notions of tension reduction and equilibrium maintenance. Persons seeking health care were approached in terms of their illness rather than as Nightingale had originally conceived, in terms of their inherent potentialities. However, Peplau's ideas overall indicate an open and interactive view of the person, wherein the nursing focus is more on the transformation rather than the reduction of anxiety, and on the facilitation of patients' latent abilities rather than on the fixing of a problem.

What may appear to be inconsistency in Peplau's theory may be more accurately viewed as the result of an early attempt to reformulate existing closed-system theories of human development in a way that would account for the nursing perspective she acquired in practice and through her own genius. Peplau's incorporation of the interpersonal process as a central component in her theory initiated a shift in emphasis from an intrapsychic to interpersonal perspective of human health and a broadening perspective of significant factors beyond the biological toward the contextual. Peplau (1992a) described the shift toward interpersonal theory as pivotal in development of nursing science, in that it moved nursing toward theory-based practice and a theoretical basis for understanding of patient problems. Integral to her psychodynamic theory were interpersonal and social factors, ongoing energy transformation, patients' unlimited potential for health, and the facilitative role of the nurse.

Peplau's writings clearly indicate conceptual movement away from earlier reductionistic principles in a way that extends the theoretical base of her 1952 theory. For example, Peplau's exposition (1963a) on learning implies a reconceptualization of the learning principles of Miller and Dollard (1941) she initially used as a theoretical base for explicating phases of the interpersonal process (Peplau, 1952, p. 34). In her later writings, she portrayed patients as the initiator of change rather than as "follower" of the nurse as "leader." Other writings reflect an increasing focus upon the social significance of the environment and of nursing's role in health maintenance as well as illness recovery (Peplau, 1970, 1982a, 1982b, 1983a, 1983b). Most noteworthy perhaps, is that as early as 1954, Peplau (cited in O'Toole & Welt, 1989) appealed for "dynamic" rather than "mechanistic" approaches to patients. She advocated treating patients as participants and recognizing the multiple person and contextual factors that influence behavior. Thus, in an important sense, Peplau's 1952 publication marked a beginning, not an end, to the development of her theoretical ideas.

Developmental-Contextual World View

The definitions and relationships of the components of Peplau's theory are consistent with a "developmental-contextual" worldview (Ford & Lerner, 1992). This worldview synthesizes elements from the organismic and contextual views originally proposed in Pepper's (1942) classic book on world hypothesis. Within the developmental-contextual worldview, the focus is on the dynamic, reciprocal interaction between selected variables of the person and significant context. The person is assumed to have inherent developmental and self-organizing capacities, and to exist mutually in a dynamic environment.

Peplau's (1952, 1963a, 1979, 1984) definition of nursing as an "educative instrument" is consistent with this developmental-contextual worldview. Her developmental perspective is operationalized in the four phases of the interpersonal process—the context of healing for the patient. The phases depict a logical progression of the nurse-patient relationship, and are consistent with basic individual developmental principles (e.g., learning to trust, to set realistic limits, to gain self-identity, and to validate oneself and participate within a community of others) (Peplau, 1952, 1969b). More broadly, the interpersonal process is used to evoke the developmental potential of the patient assumed in the developmental-contextual view. This involves "educing"—a root of the word *education*—from the patient thoughts and feelings needed to initiate change and problem-solving activities (Peplau, 1968, p. 278). Furthermore, the "reparative process" originally described by Nightingale (1859) was conceptualized by Peplau (1992a) as a complex learning process in the patient. Finally, Peplau's description of the patient as possessing the power to change oneself, an assumption within the worldview, is elucidated in her repeated emphasis on the nurse as facilitator as well as educator in the interpersonal relationship. More recently, Peplau (1988a) has defined nursing as "an enabling, empowering, or transforming art" (p. 9).

Analysis of Adequacy

Peplau provided nursing with a pragmatic theory for practice and research. The interpersonal relationship, the central component of Peplau's theory, is basic to nursing's metaparadigm, which stipulates that, as part of understanding and promoting human health, interaction must occur at some level between the patient, as "person," and the nurse. Peplau has operationalized the components of the interpersonal relations theory in a way that supports the adequacy of her theory. The level of abstraction of the concepts allows for ongoing theory testing, revision, refinement, or refutation.

Peplau's (1988b) "reduction" of human beings in interpersonal relations to observable components (e.g., interpersonal process phases, nurse roles, patient patterns, or anxiety levels) enhances the theory's applicability in nursing practice and research. Phases of the relationship, roles of the nurse, and behavior patterns and proposed serial ordering of developmental processes of the patient are clearly and logically described. Pattern integrations that may occur between patient and nurse can be "observed, studied, explained, and, if detrimental, changed" (Peplau, 1992b, pp. 14–15).

Because of the nature of the interpersonal process as defined by Peplau, it can be translated across a wide variety of nursing practice situations. Furthermore, her incorporation of developmental principles (e.g., developmental tools and tasks) enhances its application to patients of various ages. Application of the interpersonal relationship is not dependent upon specific health conditions; rather, it is dependent upon the use of verbal and nonverbal language symbols, a human characteristic that, creatively defined, transcends health condition or age of a person. Finally, it is conceivable that Peplau's theory has greater scope than is typically assumed in that the interpersonal process associated with the patient in relation to the nurse can be applied to interpersonal relations between person and nonnurse, and between person and things (Peplau, 1987a).

EXTERNAL ANALYSIS

Relationship to Nursing Research

Peplau's theory is not widely used as a basis for research. One notable exception, however, is research by Forchuk and her colleagues (1991, 1992, 1994a, 1994b, 1998), which established a focus on Peplau's phases of the interpersonal relationship as related to psychiatric nursing practice. She studied characteristics of the orientation phase of the nurse-patient relationship among persons with chronic mental illness. She identified specific person and context factors that influence the duration of this phase. Her findings have enhanced understanding about the significance of orientation and its relationship to psychotherapeutic outcomes of clients.

Peden (1993) conducted qualitative research into the process of recovering among depressed women. Her findings supported Peplau's ideas about the inner developmental resources of patients, the growth-promoting potential of the illness experience, and the primary role of the patient in attaining health through the interpersonal process. Her participants reported increased levels of self-understanding and self-esteem as a result of their depression. Morrison, Shealy, Kowalski, Lamont, and Range (1996) conducted research on the behavioral indicators and the prevalence of Peplau's nurse roles across nurse relationships with children, adolescents, and adults under psychiatric care. Among their findings, they discovered that, in accord with Peplau's (1964) proposal, the counselor was the primary role of the nurse. More recently, applications of Peplau's theory to research are found in passing references to her work, as for example, to support research on related concepts such as therapeutic intimacy (Williams, 2001); empathy (Reynolds & Scott, 2000); and forming partnerships in health care (McQueen, 2000).

Relationship to Nursing Education

Peplau's theory has been used extensively in educating both undergraduate and graduate nursing students about a major component of nursing activities—the interpersonal relationship. Her theory provides knowledge for understanding the conceptual basis and practical applications of the nurse–patient relationship and nursing psychotherapy. Peplau's (1952) "process recording" tool is used extensively in teaching students a self-reflective process and other critical approaches to their encounters with patients.

In particular, her works have provided theory-based knowledge for nursing specialization in psychiatric settings in which the one-to-one relationship is the primary nursing method. Peplau's theoretical ideas are also applicable to other interpersonal contexts of practice, such as milieu, family, and group therapies. Knowledge of the dynamics underlying interpersonal relations is essential in educating nurses for all settings in which nurses and patients interact.

Relationship to Nursing Practice

Peplau's model has served as a conceptual framework for psychodynamic nursing since 1952 and continues to be a relevant model for nursing psychotherapy today in clinical work with a variety of clients, ranging from family groups, to depressed and terminally ill clients (Sills, 1977, 1978; Beeber, Anderson, & Sills, 1990; Beeber, 1996, 1998; Forchuk & Dorsay, 1995; Yamashita, 1997). Martin et al. (1992) outlined an example of the application of Peplau's theory in intervention with a dying woman. Consistent with Peplau's theory, their example highlighted a focus on the "interpersonal" phenomena rather than individual factors. The authors also clearly portrayed the significance of the nurse as directing the "process" and the patient as directing the "content" of the relationship.

Peplau's theory provides direction to nursing practice through the six roles and the four phases of the interpersonal process. Nursing should use these to clarify nursing's unique focus in health care as well as to facilitate collaboration with other healthcare professionals.

Peplau's theoretical ideas promoting effective communication between nurse and patient are applicable to all nursing practice. Communication is a major tool in the implementation of the interpersonal process. An awareness and understanding of verbal and nonverbal communication of both the nurse and patient are considered basic to the nursing process. Through various communication skills, the nurse can convey interest and concern to the patient, clarify and validate assumptions about the patient, assist the patient to formulate the meaning of the identified problems, and generally guide the person in transforming anxiety-based energy into positive experiences.

Relationship to Nursing Classification Systems

Both philosophically and pragmatically, Peplau's model is compatible with the North American Nursing Diagnosis Association (NANDA, 1999) classification efforts. The practice-based inductive approach, combined with work to provide research-based concepts in developing nursing diagnoses, is similar to the knowledge-building approach within Peplau's model. Clinically relevant diagnoses can be derived from patterns of behavior identified within Peplau's model and then related to one of the nine human response patterns within the NANDA classification system. Nursing diagnosis, according to Peplau (1987a, 1992c) is useful in delineating universal patterns of behavior of concern to nurses. In nursing diagnoses, the focus is on naming the "regularities" observable across patients who manifest a particular phenomenon (Peplau, 1988a, p. 12). However, practice is not solely guided by the diagnosis. Peplau (1988a) regarded nursing diagnoses as a "launching pad" for beginning to understand problematic behaviors, as they emerge either within the patient or in patient interrelations. Nurses use practice and research to delve deeper into understanding the unique meanings of the diagnoses for the particular patient.

Peplau's model promoted action as well as theoretical knowledge. Her model is also compatible with the Nursing Interventions Classification (NIC) System (McCloskey & Bulechek, 2000), particularly with the efforts to link NANDA diagnoses with specific interventions, given that theory-based knowledge and practice are linked within Peplau's model. There are many examples of areas in which NANDA diagnoses have supporting NIC interventions that relate to Peplau's model.

For example, NIC has identified specific interventions for each of the following NANDA diagnoses of Impaired Social Interaction, Sensory/Perceptual Alterations, and Hopelessness. These diagnoses all relate to Peplau's postulations about disordered thinking patterns and their clinical manifestations. Disordered thinking Patterns refer to thinking and feeling behaviors that reflect an immaturity of development of language-thought processes, manifested in problems in communication, sensory experiences, and perception of oneself.

The NANDA diagnoses of Potential for Violence (Self-Directed or Directed at Others) and Social Isolation also have accompanying NIC interventions. These two NANDA diagnoses effectively label Peplau's descriptions about the transformation of anxiety into unhealthy attempts to vent or express oneself. The defining characteristics range from dysfunctional behaviors (directed toward self or others) that are overtly hostile, to those that are more passive or covert. Other NANDA diagnoses that could be derived from Peplau's model and that have corresponding NIC interventions are Anxiety, Self-Esteem Disturbance, and Risk for Altered Development. These diagnoses identify problems that are basic to Peplau's conceptualization of mental health problems. The NIC interventions of anxiety reduction, self-esteem enhancement, and development enhancement reflect many of Peplau's interpersonal strategies. It was Peplau's (1988b, 1989, 1992b) plan that naming the clinical phenomena of interest to nurses, through nursing diagnoses, would facilitate research into and the ultimate understanding of nursing phenomena. Because of Peplau's clinically based approach to theory development, many diagnostic categories and interventions derived from her theory likely could be readily applied in mental health nursing practice.

Relationship to Theory-Driven, Evidenced-Based Practice

Peplau was explicit in promoting theory-driven, evidence-based nursing practice (1969a, 1970, 1985a). Her early writings indicated support of theory-building research in that she identified the need for reformulation of theories from other disciplines. She also emphasized the need for more research into nursing's phenomena of health-related responses as a source of nursing theory. Her theory, as a coherent synthesis of theories about communication, learning, anxiety, and human development, provides a theoretical framework for creative research on mental health nursing.

Peplau's model provides a theory base for generating evidence to support the relational nature of nursing and interpersonal therapies that enhance mental health and well-being. Sources of evidence, according to Peplau, are found primarily in the link between empirical research and practice knowledge. Her model also informed nursing that a sound base of practice must include knowledge of self, particularly as this influences the nurse-patient relationship, and a philosophical and moral commitment to the professionalization of nursing (Sills, 1998). It is with a clear sense of urgency that Peplau (1986) stated that nursing has both a social right and public obligation to develop nursing science to support an autonomous practice. Sources of evidence for practice based upon Peplau reached beyond traditional applications of the scientific method to embrace many patterns of knowing relevant to nursing—ethical, political, personal, and empirical (Gastmans, 1998; Reed, 1996). Peplau's works initiated a shift from the prevailing paradigm of technical practice to a paradigm of theory-based advanced nursing practice. She led the development of psychiatric nursing as an important specialty area within nursing (Church, 2000).

SUMMARY

Peplau has developed a nursing theory that is useful in a variety of nursing contexts in which the nurse engages in a therapeutic relationship with a patient. The theory is parsimonious and relates a limited number of concepts in an understandable way. It can be described as a practice theory, applicable to clinical practice and demonstrating pragmatic adequacy. Her concepts of interpersonal process, anxiety, and communication define broad areas that continue to be relevant to nursing practice today.

Peplau has been exemplary in her approach to using theories originating in other disciplines in model building. Her ideas reflected a process of reformulating existing theories of renowned psychologists in a way that enriched the conceptual base of nursing practice. These reformulations contributed to the development and refinement of Peplau's interpersonal relations theory of nursing. On a theoretical level, Peplau contributed significantly to the shift in paradigms from the intrapsychic to the interpersonal approach in the therapeutic relationship. Although initially controversial, the interpersonal process has been integrated into nursing education and practice, often without appropriate acknowledgment of its originator. This analysis and evaluation of Peplau's model acknowledge the historical significance of the theory, its continuing relevance to nursing today, and its encouragement for nurses to anticipate the emergence of other definitive interpersonal theories in nursing in the near future.

REFERENCES

Beeber, L. S. (1996). Pattern integration in young depressed women: Pts. I and II. *Archives of Psychiatric Nursing, 10*(3), 151–164.

Beeber, L. S. (1998). Treating depression through the therapeutic nurse–client relationship *Nursing Clinics of North America, 33*(1), 153–157.

Beeber, L., Anderson, C. A., & Sills, G. M. (1990). Peplau's theory in practice. *Nursing Science Quarterly, 3*(1), 6–8.

Church, O. M. (2000). Hildegard E. Peplau's leadership and achievements in the advance of psychiatric nursing: The right person in the right time and place. *Journal of the American Psychiatric Nurses Association, 6*(1), 16–24.

Ellis, R. (1968). Characteristics of significant theories. *Nursing Research, 173,* 217–222.

Forchuk, C. (1991). Peplau's theory: Concepts and their relations. *Nursing Science Quarterly, 4*(2), 54–60.

Forchuk, C. (1992). The orientation phase of the nurse–client relationship: How long does it take? *Perspectives in Psychiatric Care, 28*(4), 7–10.

Forchuk, C. (1994a). Peplau's theory-based practice and research. *Nursing Science Quarterly, 7*(3), 110–112.

Forchuk, C. (1994b). The orientation phase of the nurse–client relationship: Testing Peplau's theory. *Journal of Advanced Nursing, 20,* 1–6.

Forchuk, C., & Dorsay, J. P. (1995). Hildegard Peplau meets family systems nursing: Innovation in theory-based practice. *Journal of Advanced Nursing, 21*(1), 110–115.

Forchuk, C., Westwell, J., Martin, M., Azzapardi, W. B., Kosterewa-Tolman, D., & Hux, M. (1998). Factors influencing movement of chronic psychiatric patients from the orientation to the working phase of the nurse–client relationship. *Perspectives in Psychiatric Care, 34*(1), 36–44.

Ford, D. H., & Lerner, R. M. (1992). *Developmental systems theory: An integrative approach.* Newbury Park, CA: Sage.

Gastmans, C. (1998). Interpersonal relations in nursing: A philosophical-ethical analysis of the work of Hildegard E. Peplau. *Journal of Advanced Nursing, 28*(6), 1312–1319.

Gregg, D. E. (1999). Hildegard E. Peplau: Her contributions. *Perspectives in Psychiatric Care, 35*(3), 10–12.

Hardy, M. E. (1974). Theories: components, development, evaluation. *Nursing Research, 23*(2), 188–197.

Martin, M., Forchuk, C., Santopinto, M., & Butcher, H. K. (1992). Alternative approaches to nursing practice: Application of Peplau, Rogers, and Parse. *Nursing Science Quarterly, 5*(2), 80–85.

May, R. (1950). *The meaning of anxiety.* New York: Ronald Press.

McCloskey, J. C., & Bulechek, G. M. (2000). *Nursing interventions classification (NIC)* (3rd ed.). New York: Mosby.

McQueen, A. (2000). Nurse–patient relationships and partnership in hospital care. *Journal of Clinical Nursing, 9*(5), 723–731.

Miller, N. E., & Dollard, J. (1941). *Social learning and imitation.* New Haven, CT: Yale University Press.

Morrison, E. G., Shealy, A. H., Kowalski, C., Lamont, J., & Range, B. A. (1996). Workroles of staff nurses in psychiatric settings. *Nursing Science Quarterly, 9*(1), 17–21.

Nightingale, F. (1859). *Notes on nursing: What it is, and what it is not.* London: Harrison & Sons.

North American Nursing Diagnosis Association. (1999). *NANDA Nursing Diagnoses: Definitions and classification 1999–2000.* Philadelphia: North American Nursing Diagnosis Association.

Nursing Development Conference Group. (1979). *Concept formalization in nursing: Process and product* (2nd ed.). Boston: Little, Brown.

O'Toole, A. W., & Welt, S. R. (1989). *Interpersonal theory in nursing practice: Selected works of Hildegard E. Peplau.* (Unpublished writings and presentations by Peplau, 1954, 1975, 1985). New York: Springer.

Parse, R. R. (1992). Human becoming: Parse's theory of nursing. *Nursing Science Quarterly, 5*(2), 35–42.

Peden, A. R. (1993). Recovering in depressed women: Research with Peplau's theory. *Nursing Science Quarterly, 6*(3), 140–146.

Peplau, H. E. (1952). *Interpersonal relations in nursing.* New York: Putnam.

Peplau, H. E. (1962). Interpersonal techniques: Crux of psychiatric nursing. *American Journal of Nursing, 62*(6), 50–54.

Peplau, H. E. (1963a). Process and concept of learning. In S. F. Burd & M. A. Marshall (Eds.), *Some clinical approaches to psychiatric nursing* (pp. 333–336). New York: Collier Macmillan.

Peplau, H. E. (1963b). A working definition of anxiety. In S. F. Burd & M. A. Marshall (Eds.), *Some clinical approaches to psychiatric nursing* (pp. 323–327). New York: Collier Macmillan.

Peplau, H. E. (1964). *Basic principles of patient counseling.* Philadelphia: Smith, Kline & French.

Peplau, H. E. (1968). Psychotherapeutic strategies. *Perspectives in Psychiatric Care, 6*(6), 264–278.

Peplau, H. E. (1969a). Theory: The professional dimension. In C. Norris (Ed.), *Proceedings of the First Nursing Theory Conference.* Kansas City: University of Kansas Medical Center, Department of Nursing Education.

Peplau, H. E. (1969b). Professional closeness. *Nursing Forum, 8,* 342–359.

Peplau, H. E. (1970). ANA's new Executive Director states her views. *American Journal of Nursing, 70*(1), 84–88.

Peplau, H. E. (1979). In W. E. Field (Ed.), *The psychotherapy of Hildegard E. Peplau.* New Braunfels, TX: PSF Productions.

Peplau, H. E. (1982a). *Some ideas about nursing in the psychiatric milieu.* Paper presented at the Boulder Psychiatric Institute, Boulder, CO.

Peplau, H.E. (1982b). Some reflections on earlier days in psychiatric nursing. *Journal of Psychological Nursing and Mental Health Services, 20,* 17–24.

Peplau, H.E. (May, 1983a). *Milieu.* Paper presented at the Vista Sandia Hospital Psychiatric Nursing Seminar, Albuquerque, NM.

Peplau, H. E. (April, 1983b). *Some dimensions on the concept of prevention.* Paper presented at the Annual Nurse Scholar Series, First Endowed Hildegard E. Peplau Lecture, Rutgers, NJ.

Peplau, H. E. (1984, April). *Historical reasons for a new definition of nursing.* Paper presented at the banquet meeting of nurses, Sydney, Australia.

Peplau, H. E. (1985a). Is nursing's self-regulatory power being eroded? *American Journal of Nursing, 85,* 141–143.

Peplau, H. E. (1985b). The power of the dissociative state. *Journal of Psychosocial Nursing, 23*(8), 31–33.

Peplau, H. E. (1986). Nursing science: A historical perspective. In R. R. Parse (Ed.), *Nursing science: Major paradigms, theories, and critiques* (pp. 13–29). New York: Saunders.

Peplau, H. E. (1987a). Interpersonal constructs for nursing practice. *Nursing Education Today, 7*(5), 201–208.

Peplau, H. E. (1987b). Psychiatric skills: Tomorrow's world. *Nursing Times, 83*(1), 29–32.

Peplau, H. E. (1988a). The art and science of nursing: Similarities, differences, and relations. *Nursing Science Quarterly, 1*(1), 8–15.

Peplau, H.E. (1988b). Perspectives on nursing science (interview by M. J. Smith). *Nursing Science Quarterly, 1*(2), 80–85.

Peplau, H. E. (1989). Future directions in psychiatric nursing from the perspective of history. *Journal of Psychosocial Nursing and Mental Health Services, 27*(2), 18–21, 25–28, 39–40.

Peplau, H. E. (1992a). Notes on Nightingale. In F. Nightingale, *Notes on Nursing: What it is, and what it is not* (Commemorative ed., pp. 48–57). Philadelphia: J.B. Lippincott.

Peplau, H. E. (1992b). Interpersonal relations: A theoretical framework for application in nursing practice. *Nursing Science Quarterly, 5*(1), 13–18.

Peplau, H. E. (1992c). Perspectives on nursing knowledge (interview by T. Takahashi). *Nursing Science Quarterly, 5*(2), 86–91.

Pepper, S. (1942). *World hypotheses.* Berkeley: University of California Press.

Reed, P. G. (1996). Transforming practice knowledge into nursing knowledge: A revisionist analysis of Peplau. *Image: Journal of Nursing Scholarship, 28*(1), 29–33.

Reynolds, W., & Scott, B. (2000). Do nurses and other professional helpers normally display much empathy? *Journal of Advanced Nursing, 31*(1), 226–234.

Sills, G.M. (1977). Research in the field of psychiatric nursing 1952–1977. *Nursing Research, 26*(3), 281–287.

Sills, G. M. (1978). Hildegard E. Peplau: Leader, practitioner, academician, scholar, and theorist. *Perspectives in Psychiatric Care, 16*(3), 5–9.

Sills, G. M. (1998). Peplau and professionalism: The emergence of the paradigm of professionalization. *Journal of Psychiatric and Mental Health Nursing, 5,* 167–171.

Strasser, S. (1985). *Understanding and explanation: Basic ideas concerning the humanity of the human science.* Pittsburgh: Duquesne University Press.

Sullivan, H. S. (1947). *Conceptions of modern psychiatry.* Washington, DC: W. Alanson White Psychiatric Foundation.

Sullivan, H. S. (1952). *The interpersonal theory of psychiatry.* New York: W.W. Norton.

Symonds, P. (1946). *The dynamics of human adjustment.* New York: Appleton Century Crofts.

Welt, S. R., & O'Toole, A. W. (1989). Hildegard E. Peplau: Observations in brief. *Archives of Psychiatric Nursing, 3*(5), 254–264.

Whorf, B. (1956). *Language, thought and reality.* New York: Wiley.

Williams, A. (2001). A literature review on the concept of intimacy in nursing. *Journal of Advanced Nursing, 33*(5), 660–667.

Yamashita, M. (1997). Family caregiving: Application of Newman's and Peplau's theories. *Journal of Psychiatric and Mental Health Nursing, 4,* 401–405.

5

Henderson's Conceptualization of Nursing

Mary J. Thorson and Edward J. Halloran

In the opening paragraph of *Principles and Practice of Nursing* (6th ed.), Virginia Henderson (Henderson & Nite, 1978) says that those who practice, administer, teach, study, conduct research on, and legislate for nursing must answer the following questions: What is nursing? and What is the function of the nurse? If the answers to these questions are clear and valid, she says, it can guide them to consistent and constructive action; if the answers are confused and uninformed, it can lead to inconsistent, ineffective, or even harmful action.

Her search for clarity on the nature of nursing is described in her book of the same title (Henderson, 1966, 1991). *The Nature of Nursing,* however, provides only a glimpse into the mind of the 20th century's most important nurse. Ferreting out what was on Henderson's mind is a matter of examining the record; everything she thought about nursing is documented and shared in her writings. Although her struggle with the nature of nursing began with her training, Henderson's labor reflected her unique person and the era in which she lived.

HENDERSON AND HER ERA

Virginia Avernal Henderson was born in Kansas City, MO, on November 30, 1897, and named for the state her mother longed for. She died at the age of 98 on March 16, 1996, at the Connecticut Hospice, Branford, CT. The fifth of eight children of Daniel B. and Lucy Minor (Abbot) Henderson, Virginia spent her school years at Bellevue, a boarding school near Bedford, Virginia, where her grandfather, William Richardson Abbot, Principal, prepared boys for the University of Virginia (Southall, 1955). Her father, Daniel B. Henderson, a former teacher at Bellevue and an attorney for Native American Indians, established the family home at Trivium, near the Bellevue estate, after returning from the West. Extended absences by her father (who later was a lawyer in Washington, DC, who won a major case for the Klamath Indians against the U.S. Government in 1937), placed her under the influence of her teachers, especially an aunt, Anne Minor, and Mr. Abbot. The boarding school was closed in 1909 and her schooling continued at home, at one point by her sister Jane, a graduate of Sweet Briar College. All four Henderson women had professional careers—Lucy and Jane in education, Frances as a staff member for the American Federation of Arts, and Virginia as nurse and educator.

Education was the business of the extended Abbot, Minor, and Henderson clans. If the members were not providing it, they were its recipients. At a crucial juncture in Henderson's life, the Great War raged in Europe and patriotism abounded. Henderson combined her own patriotic fervor with the desire for more education by enrolling in the Army Nursing School and thus she happened on a career in nursing. She said she was treated like a West Point Cadet in the Army School and recounts that Vice President Coolidge attended the graduation of the last Army School class in 1921 (Smith, 1989). Annie W. Goodrich, the School Director, gave the students a sense of the social and ethical significance of nursing (Henderson, 1955). Henderson, like her forebears, went on to a distinguished career in education at Teacher's College in New York. While there, she was asked to continue the textbook Bertha Harmer had authored for three editions (1922, 1928, 1934). The 4th edition, Henderson's first, required relatively little work on Henderson's part because Harmer had done such a thorough job in the previous edition (Harmer & Henderson, 1939). However, the 5th edition of the *Textbook of the Principles and Practice of Nursing* (Harmer & Henderson, 1955) was completely revised between 1949 and 1954 and was the first edition to be written around Henderson's definition of the unique function of the nurse. Her career at Yale in nursing research commenced in 1953, where she worked full time as research associate for another 30 years.

The era in which Henderson wrote was at the end of one of the most tumultuous centuries (1850–1950) the world had ever witnessed. It opened with the Crimean War and included America's Civil War and two World Wars. The need for the trained nurse was demonstrated in the Crimean and confirmed in the Civil War, both of which prompted reforms leading to the modern hospital. Nightingale's research supported the widespread use of cleanliness, hygiene, air circulation, nutrition, and comfort to prevent illness and to minister to the ill. A mere 40 years later (1860–1900), no hospital in the Western world could do without trained nurses (Thompson & Goldin, 1975). During the next 50 years (1900–1950), nurses' contributions to disease prevention were slowly eclipsed, however. Asepsis, the prevention of disease through cleanliness (and equally at home in miasmic and germ theories of disease causation) was replaced with antisepsis, in the form of vaccines and antibiotics. Nightingale's science, which had served the nursing profession well for nearly 100 years, yielded to a view that nursing was an arm of the medical profession (Abel-Smith, 1964).

A DEFINITION, A TEXTBOOK, AND NURSE EDUCATION

Henderson thought differently and articulated a vision that called upon nurses to help people, sick or well, in the performance of those activities contributing to health and its recovery (or to a peaceful death) that they would perform unaided if they had the necessary strength, will, or knowledge. It is likewise the function of nurses to help people become independent as rapidly as possible (Harmer & Henderson, 1955, p. 4). In this description of nursing, Henderson maintains a continuity with the past. Although *Notes on Nursing* (Nightingale, 1859a) guided people to take pains with basic human activity, it was written on the premise that performing that activity would prevent the spread of disease and comfort the patient so that nature could act upon him/her. Henderson saw similar basic human activity as the responsibility of the person and family and would nurse only when persons lacked strength, will or knowledge, and only until they could resume basic human activity. This would seem to limit the activities of the nurse to helping individuals or groups with specific, identifiable needs. Henderson believed that not until human beings are born, live, and die in an independent state—and not until the special knowledge and skill of the nurse becomes common knowledge and skill—can we abandon what we think of as basic nursing care (Henderson, 1960).

Henderson's definition contributed to establishing the phenomenon of nursing. In addition to identifying nursing functions as unique, Henderson's definition offered a rationale for nursing activities. Nursing activities are implemented when the individual lacks part or all of the necessary strength, will, or knowledge, and the activities are goal oriented to promote recovery, independence, or peaceful death.

She differentiated nursing from other disciplines, including medicine, on the basis of how knowledge is used. In her view, she was one of the first to use the phrase "nursing is both a unique science and an art." The nurse does not explicitly describe the bridge between content and action. It is implied that the nurse uses judgment founded on scientific knowledge and systematic evaluation of the individual to deliver care in a unique, artful, and competent way. Not until the 1960s, when Henderson's influence began to have an impact, were creativity, analytical thinking, and independent decision-making areas of reward for nurses (Fulton, 1987). Henderson also encouraged nurses not to be subservient to physicians (Clark, 1997). Nurses today can surely identify with this statement in an environment of managed care when they find themselves so burdened with heavy case loads and there seems to be little time to do much more than carry out doctors' orders.

The Harmer and Henderson (1939, 1955) textbook was used throughout nursing education as *the* fundamentals text. Nursing education in those days took place in hospital schools; in collegiate schools, nursing education was divided into college and hospital components. A fundamentals course was necessary to acquaint students rapidly with nursing procedures so they could assist in staffing the hospital wards. Although clinical skills were emphasized, Henderson placed procedures in the context in which nurses performed them, not because they were ordered to by physicians, but because persons would do the procedures themselves if only they had the strength, will, or knowledge. Henderson also articulated a rationale for all nursing activity—to *make the patient independent as quickly as possible.* Thus, skill performance was not an end in itself; rather, the aim of nursing activity was *patient independence.* A nurse could no longer "do everything" for a patient if that led to the patient's dependence on the nurse.

As further testament to the independence of nurses, the 1955 Harmer and Henderson text paid little attention to specific diseases and recommended nurses learn principles about illness, noting that diseases of similar origin are likely to be manifested by similar signs and symptoms. For example, diseases caused by microorganisms usually produce an increase in body temperature, an increased pulse rate, an increase in white blood cells, fatigue, and local signs of inflammation if the organisms are successful in attacking a part of the body where the reactions of the tissues can be observed (p. 13). Henderson recommended cooperation with physicians' therapeutic plans, recognizing that to do so requires nurses to have a body of knowledge that falls within the realm of medicine. Nursing, then, is neither the performance of procedures nor is it directed by physicians, although elements of both are incorporated into nursing care.

SCIENTIFIC EVIDENCE AND BASIC HUMAN NEEDS

When Henderson completed the 5th edition of her text, she was recruited to work with Leo Simmons (Simmons & Henderson, 1957, 1964) on a study of nursing research. She visited more than 20 states and a number of schools of nursing, and read master's theses and dissertations done by nurses. She and Simmons also reviewed the periodical literature and questioned nurses, teachers, administrators, and academic medical center leaders about nursing research. Henderson and Simmons concluded that much nursing research was about nurses but little research focused on patients and their needs. Henderson (1956) wrote an editorial for *Nursing Researcher* entitled, "Nursing Research—When?" that significantly influenced future nursing research.

Henderson, noting the difficulty in accessing the literature on nursing, applied for a U.S. Public Health Service grant to annotate, classify and index the nursing literature. The project lasted 12 years and produced a 4-volume *Nursing Studies Index* covering the English language literature published between 1900 and 1960. A direct outgrowth of the project was the joint *American Journal of Nursing,* National Library of Medicine *Cumulative Index of Nursing Literature*. Henderson referred to this as her greatest accomplishment. By any measure, this scientific project was immense, and although several librarians and nurses were involved in the project, the lion's share of the annotations were done by Henderson.

This exercise in gathering the writings of nurses convinced Henderson of the value to humanity of nursing services. During her research on the nursing literature, Henderson was asked by the International Council of Nurses, Nursing Service Committee, to write something that would express their belief that nursing principles exist that are applicable in any situation in which nursing is an essential part of treatment and are an aid to convalescence and rehabilitation. *Basic Principles of Nursing Care* (Henderson, 1960) was the result. Here, for the first time, Henderson articulated the components of basic nursing. They included assisting the patient with these functions or providing conditions that will enable him or her to:

1. Breathe normally
2. Eat and drink adequately
3. Eliminate by all avenues of elimination
4. Move and maintain desirable posture (walking, sitting, lying, and changing from one to the other)
5. Sleep and rest
6. Select suitable clothing, dress, and undress
7. Maintain body temperature within normal range by adjusting clothing and modifying the environment
8. Keep the body clean and well groomed and protect the integument
9. Avoid dangers in the environment and avoid injuring others
10. Communicate with others in expressing emotions, needs, fears, etc.
11. Worship according to his or her faith
12. Work at something that provides a sense of accomplishment

13. Play or participate in various forms of recreation
14. Learn, discover, or satisfy the curiosity that leads to "normal" health

Henderson then elaborated on circumstances that are always present that affect basic human needs and pathological states (as contrasted with specific diseases) that modify basic needs (p. 12). The following states were listed.

Conditions always present that affect basic needs:

1. Age: newborn, child, youth, adult, middle aged, aged, and dying
2. Temperament, emotional state, or passing mood:
    a) "normal"
    b) euphoric and hyperactive
    c) anxious, fearful, agitated, or hysterical, or
    d) depressed and hypoactive
3. Social or cultural status: A member of a family unit with friends and status, or a person relatively alone and/or maladjusted, destitute
4. Physical and intellectual capacity:
    a) normal weight
    b) underweight
    c) overweight
    d) normal mentality
    e) subnormal mentality
    f) gifted mentality
    g) normal sense of hearing, sight, equilibrium, and touch
    h) loss of special sense
    i) normal motor power
    j) loss of motor power

Pathological states that modify basic needs:

1. Marked disturbances of fluid and electrolyte balance including starvation states, pernicious vomiting, and diarrhea
2. Acute oxygen want
3. Shock (including collapse and hemorrhage)
4. Disturbances of consciousness: fainting, coma, delirium
5. Exposure to cold and heat causing markedly abnormal body temperatures
6. Acute febrile states (all causes)
7. A local injury, wound, and/or infection
8. A communicable condition
9. Preoperative state

10. Postoperative state
11. Immobilization from disease or prescribed as treatment
12. Persistent or intractable pain

(Henderson, 1960, pp. 12–13)

In explaining the complexity of nursing—after introducing her deceptively simple two-sentence description of nursing—Henderson said the nurse is temporarily the consciousness of the unconscious, the love of life for the suicidal, the leg of the amputee, the eyes of the newly blind, a means of locomotion for the infant, knowledge and confidence for the young mother, a voice for those too weak or withdrawn to speak, and so on (p. 5). No person had ever written so eloquently, some would say poetically (Fulton, 1987), about the potential of nurses' care. She did so because of her unwavering belief in the goodness and capabilities of nurses. She wrote a complementary volume, called *The Nature of Nursing* (Henderson, 1966), which expanded on her definition and its implications for practice, research, and education in nursing. By the time this work was prepared, Henderson had established herself as a scientist through her research on and categorization of the nursing literature. *Basic Principles of Nursing* and *The Nature of Nursing* were informed by science, just as *Notes on Nursing* (1859a) had been informed by the natural experiments conducted in the Crimean War and written about in pre-1860 publications (Nightingale, 1858a, 1858b, 1858c, 1859a, 1859b). These scholarly works deserve serious study by those who profess to understand contemporary nursing.

Henderson's writings on nursing research were well received at the Yale School of Nursing. Almost immediately after their publication, faculty and students there began a series of studies on the effects of nursing on patients. Among the faculty investigators were Ida Orlando and Ernestine Weidenbach, and students there included Rhetaugh Dumas and Jean Johnson (Orlando, 1961; Weidenbach, 1964; Dumas & Leonard, 1963). Early on, investigators at Yale stimulated the need for theory to guide research. The social scientists there, having the academic preparation for the conduct of research, influenced the direction of early nursing theory. The clinicians, however, insisted on theory that was practice based (Wald & Leonard, 1964).

THE PRINCIPLES AND PRACTICE OF NURSING

When the *Nursing Studies Index* was completed in 1972 and Henderson was in her 75th year, she began her most significant writing: a complete revision of her textbook. Completed in 1978, the *Principles and Practice of Nursing,* 6th ed. (Henderson & Nite) synthesized what is known about nursing into a single volume. Henderson, at this stage of her career, was an accomplished clinician, educator, scientist, and writer. The authority with which this volume is written cannot be overstated. Having reviewed and annotated nursing literature, and having authored a theory of nursing, Henderson set out to synthesize the two and, further, to link this monumental task to the past for the sake of continuity. Although the book had a coauthor and 17 contributors, Henderson wrote or cowrote 49 of its 50 chapters. Six years were spent on the project, which concluded in her 80th year of life. Henderson was not overwhelmed by the literature. Rather, she used it to make her point. In this volume's introduction to nursing, commonalties are emphasized. The great number and variety of sources cited (chapter 3 alone has more than 1,000 citations) are organized from oldest to most recent and from a universal to an individual perspective.

Like Nightingale's establishment of modern nursing, separate from and equal to the medical profession (Montiero, 1984), Henderson provided a compelling argument for the distinct nature of nursing, sometimes complementing and sometimes competing with modern medicine. Her emphasis on nurses providing strength, will, and knowledge (in conjunction with or in place of medicine, surgery, or institutionalization) to help others be independent is most timely in our era of an aging population, chronic diseases, high medical costs, and the marginal benefit of technology at life's end. That Henderson could so clearly convey the human need for nurses and nurses' potential to meet that need in our modern society is a tribute to her intellectual power as well as her tenacity. Much of what professional nursing organizations strive for today—autonomy and recognition for nurses—is offered to nurses in *Principles and Practice of Nursing* (Henderson & Nite, 1978). Autonomy and recognition, Henderson makes clear, comes through work with patients or clients.

The *Principles and Practice of Nursing* is a complete exposition of nursing. It is organized in five parts. The first section relates to the place of nursing in health services, and the second section is about the role of the nurse in health evaluation and planning patient care or meeting patients' health needs. The second section provides an extensive review of the health examination, a function that contemporary nurses tend to refer to as advanced practice (and is restricted to those nurses with master's degrees). Henderson forcefully argues that primary care is well within the domain of nurses and throughout the book teaches us how to provide primary care.

The last three sections of the *Principles and Practice of Nursing* are about basic needs, therapeutic measures, and common patient problems (or symptoms). These three sections are related to each other through complementary chapters on similar topics. For example, respiration, a basic human need, is covered in the first of these sections; in the next section there is a chapter on administration of oxygen and other gases and the use of ventilators, and the third section in this series of three has a chapter on marked disturbance of intake and output of gases, which is a pathological state, demanding medical attention or first aid. *Basic human needs* are the organizing theme for these three parts of the book. Although procedures and pathological states are covered in considerable detail, they are not the dominant theme in Henderson's view of nursing functions.

Basic human needs exist in all people, sick or well—a view that invites nurses to work with individuals who are not patients. In the opening parts of the *Principles and Practice of Nursing,* Henderson makes it clear that nurses have an important health role to play in schools, factories, prisons, homes, and public health agencies as well as where patients are found: hospices, nursing homes, and hospitals. Henderson was also a proponent of participation by nurses in primary care, the point of first contact by a person in search (or in need) of health service. The second part of the book specifies the role that nurses may play in primary care and details skills needed by nurses to perform primary care functions.

SELF-CARE

Just as Nightingale's *Notes on Nursing* was written for a general audience, Henderson also saw the best nursing as that which persons did for themselves. There are two dimensions of self-care written into the *Principles and Practice of Nursing:* the first, in the second sentence of the preface, addresses the use of the book by persons other than nurses. Henderson says it is a reference for those who want to guard their own or their family's health or take care of a sick relative or friend. She has made the book available to anyone by eliminating the need to understand jargon. Medical jargon is absent from the book and nursing jargon is explained in clear terms (only 1 of the 50 chapters escaped Henderson's coauthorship). The capability of making the most sophisticated text, drawn from thousands of citations to professional literature, readable to the nonprofessional is remarkable. Only internalizing her own description of nursing, in which ideal care is provided by oneself, could have produced such a document.

The second dimension of self-care relates to the danger of nurses considering it their responsibility to "do everything" for their patients. Many nurses in Henderson's era earned their living in private-duty care where successful nurses were required to ingratiate themselves to their patients. Some nurses caused their patients to be more dependent on them than was necessary if the goal of care was the person's independence. The secondary gain of income security for nurses who caused dependence in their patients prompted Henderson to incorporate the ideal of self-care into her definition of nursing. Her book also stressed rehabilitation, and she grieved over the expropriation of that term by medical and specialty hospitals. Henderson fervently believed that rehabilitation is the responsibility of every nurse.

HENDERSON AS THEORIST

Carper (1978) has identified four ways or patterns of knowing in nursing: empirics, ethics, personal, and aesthetics. Briefly, *empirical knowledge* is the science of nursing, the knowledge gained through empirical research; *ethical knowledge* describes, analyzes, and clarifies moral obligations and values in nursing; *personal knowledge* is gained through practicing nursing and interacting with patients, and through thinking, listening, and reflecting; and *aesthetic knowledge* is the art and act of nursing, and is gained through practice and critique (Fawcett, Watson, Neuman, Walker, & Fitzpatrick, 2001). Carper's work was significant in that it "not only highlighted the centrality of empirically derived theoretical knowledge, but also recognized with equal importance and weight, knowledge gained through clinical practice" (Stein, Corte, Colling, & Whall, 1998, p. 43).

A theory is defined as a way of seeing through "a set of relatively concrete and specific concepts and the propositions that describe or link those concepts" (Fawcett, 1999, p. 4). Theories of various phenomena are the lenses through which inquiry is conducted; each pattern of knowing may be regarded as a type of theory, subject to different types of inquiry (Fawcett et al., 2001). Therefore, although the emphasis in nursing research has been on testing empirical theories, there are equally valid ethical theories, personal theories, and aesthetic theories.

One could say that Henderson was an empirical theorist in that she synthesized the literature of nursing, including that of researchers, in her four-volume *Nursing Studies Index,* but others would argue that she never really conducted any research herself and was, therefore, not a theorist. She did, however, inspire nurses at Yale and elsewhere to conduct studies focused on patients and nursing care. For example, Henderson's description of nursing was explicitly examined in a study of cardiac patients authored by Nite and Wills (1964). In the introduction to the Nite and Wills (1964) volume, Henderson described her definition as a theory of nursing in need of testing in practice, which the authors performed (pp. vii, 273). Brooten and Naylor (1995) and their colleagues performed several examinations of Henderson's definition of nursing in their studies of very low birth weight infants, post-cesarean section women, and older sick, hospitalized adults with medical and surgical conditions. None of these studies made the theory testing explicit, although the results would have been strengthened by doing so. In addition, Schmieding (1990) proposed a theoretical framework for nursing practice and administration that integrated key concepts from the writings of Ida Orlando and Virginia Henderson.

Contemporary nursing literature, however, argues that evidence must extend beyond the current emphasis on empirical research and randomized clinical trials, to a broader view of evidence, including that of ethical, personal, and aesthetic theories (Mitchell, 1999). Whatever one's position on this issue, few would refute that Henderson was an ethical, personal, and aesthetic theorist of the first order. She practiced nursing for nearly 35 years before she began to define and describe the unique function of the nurse, and then she did so in eloquent style. Henderson sets the example for writing about ethical, personal, and aesthetic knowledge in nursing.

Although Henderson presented nursing as a systematic process involving analytical thinking and evaluation of patient needs, and therefore serving as the basis for the nursing process (Fulton, 1987), she did not subscribe to nursing being a process. She said that there is no such thing as *the* nursing process or even *a* nursing process because the word constrains the word *nursing*. Nurses around the world are being asked to limit the breadth and beauty incorporated into their writings about the very complex nursing profession and reduce it to nursing assessment, diagnosis, intervention, and outcome jargon. Nothing reflects her humanity as well as Henderson's (1955) admonition to "get inside the skin" of each patient to know not only what he or she wants but also what he or she needs to maintain life and regain health (Halloran, 1996).

Although Henderson's 6th edition of the *Principles and Practice of Nursing* contains what would be considered a set of nursing diagnoses similar to those set forth by the North American Nursing Diagnosis Association (NANDA), she refers to them as symptoms. In all their inelegant splendor, nursing diagnoses are located in chapter 5, the Health Examination, section 8, under the heading Diagnosis and Decision Making, Health Counseling.

Although the schema or organization of nursing interventions is different than what is found in the Nursing Interventions Classification (NIC) (McCloskey & Bulechek, 2000), nonetheless, the interventions used in 1976, which includes most used today, can be found in Henderson's text. Unlike outcomes as classified in the Nursing Outcomes Classification (NOC) (Johnson, Maas, & Moorhead, 2000), Henderson does not use the term *outcome* but refers to outcomes as evaluation. Henderson's criteria for evaluating care (1997) states simply, "The nurse's constant purpose should be kept in mind—to restore the patient's independence if this is possible, to help the patient live as effectively as feasible with the inescapable limitations, or to accept the inevitable end so that the patient can be said to have "died well." (p. 88). Henderson believed that professionals in health care should avoid the use of jargon and speak in plain language that most normally intelligent people would be able to understand and comprehend. Some of the terms used in both NIC and NOC are clearly nursing jargon, and classification schemas that separate nurses from all other health and illness management will isolate nurses from patient needs that they can reasonably manage.

CRITIQUE

It is arguable that reviewers should not subject works of the magnitude of *Principles and Practice of Nursing, Basic Principles of Nursing,* and *The Nature of Nursing* to critical analyses devised for nursing grand theories. The same, of course could be said for Nightingale's writings. Contemporary theory analysis in nursing could even be viewed as the latest in a long tradition of nursing's efforts to gain respectability as a profession.

Henderson's writings are suitable to bring to academic deliberations on their own merit. They inform, they are scholarly, and they continue in the tradition of science established by Nightingale. Unlike other academic writing, however, they are written for the world and they strive to share our knowledge with all who are interested in nurses and their patients. These works contain ideas that are similar to those of other nurses who have written about nursing (Flaskerud & Halloran, 1980), but they differ considerably in length, thoroughness, scholarship, and potential for practical application. That other academics have not availed themselves of Henderson's work (or Nightingale's, for that matter) seems odd in a world struggling to understand the quality and cost of health services.

When Virginia Henderson died in March of 1996, nursing journals were deluged with editorials and articles that reflected true adulation for her life and contributions to nursing (e.g., Bishop & Scudder, 1996; Jezierski, 1997; McCormick, 1996; O'Malley, 1996; Smith, 1997; and Anderson, 1999). She was proclaimed the "mother of modern nursing," "the 20th century Florence Nightingale," and a "modern legend." Her definition was likened to the "Apostles' Creed" of nursing. Many paid her tribute for her near century-long love and respect for nurses and what nurses do.

SUMMARY

Virginia Henderson wrote three texts that all contain a two-sentence description of nursing and a list of 14 basic human needs that concern all people: *Principles and Practice of Nursing* (5th and 6th eds.), *Basic Principles of Nursing,* and *The Nature of Nursing.* The three works should be read as a unit by those seeking an understanding of her ideas. Henderson's writings form the basis for a paradigm shift in nursing, away from the miasmic bases with nature, a healer upon which Nightingale oriented modern nursing (hygiene, comfort), toward helping people prevent illness and meet their universal health needs in a world where all individuals are healthy, acutely or chronically ill, or dying. Henderson's *Principles and Practice of Nursing* synthesizes previous editions of the text and her two essays on nursing, *Basic Principles of Nursing* and *The Nature of Nursing*, as well as relevant references from the *Nursing Studies Index* (Henderson & the Yale University School of Nursing Index Staff, 1963, 1966, 1970, 1972), and it is the most comprehensive exposition of nursing ever composed. It was written to help people, sick or well, in the performance of those activities contributing to health or its recovery (or to a peaceful death), that they would perform unaided if they had the necessary strength, will, or knowledge.

REFERENCES

Abel-Smith, B. (1964). *The hospitals, 1800–1948*. London: Heinemann.

Anderson, M. (1999). Virginia Avernal Henderson: A modern legend. *Wyoming Nurse, 12*(1), 9–10.

Bishop, A. H., & Scudder, J. R. (1996). "And Gina sews": A tribute to Virginia Henderson, 1898–1996. *Advances in Nursing Science, 19*(1), 1–2.

Brooten, D., & Naylor, M. D. (1995). Nurses' effect on changing patient outcomes. *Image: Journal of Nursing Scholarship, 27*(2), 95–99.

Carper, B. A. (1978). Fundamental patterns of knowing in nursing. *Advances in Nursing Science, 1*(1), 13–23.

Clark, D. J. (1997). The unique function of the nurse. *International Nursing Review, 44*(5), 144–152.

Dumas, R., & Leonard, R. C. (1963). The effect of nursing on the incidence of postoperative vomiting: A clinical experiment. *Nursing Research, 12,* 12–15.

Fawcett, J. (1999). *The relationship of theory and research* (3rd ed.). Philadelphia: F. A. Davis.

Fawcett, J., Watson, J., Neuman, B., Walker, P., & Fitzpatrick, J. (2001). On nursing theories and evidence. *Journal of Nursing Scholarship 33*(2), 115–119.

Flaskerud, J., & Halloran, E. (1980). Areas of agreement in nursing theory development, *Advances in Nursing Science, 3*(1), 1–7.

Fulton, J. S. (1987). Virginia Henderson: Theorist, prophet, poet. *Advances in Nursing Science, 10*(1), 1–9.

Halloran, E. J. (1996). Virginia Henderson and her timeless writings. *Journal of Advanced Nursing, 23*(1), 17–24.

Harmer, B. (1922, 1928, 1934). *The principles and practice of nursing* (1st, 2nd, 3rd eds.). New York: Collier Macmillan.

Harmer, B., & Henderson, V. (1939). *Textbook of the principles and practice of nursing* (4th ed.). New York: Collier Macmillan.

Harmer, B., & Henderson, V. (1955). *Textbook of the principles and practice of nursing* (5th ed.). New York: Collier Macmillan.

Henderson, V. (1955). Annie Warburton Goodrich. *American Journal of Nursing, 55,* 12.

Henderson, V. (1956). Nursing research—when? [editorial] *Nursing Research, 4*, February, 99.

Henderson, V. (1960). *Basic principles of nursing care.* Geneva: International Council of Nurses.

Henderson, V. (1997). *Basic principles of nursing care.* Geneva: International Council of Nurses.

Henderson, V. (1966). *The nature of nursing.* New York: Collier Macmillan.

Henderson, V. (1991). *The nature of nursing: Reflections after 25 years.* New York: National League for Nursing.

Henderson, V., & Nite, G. (1978). *Principles and practice of nursing* (6th ed.). New York: Collier Macmillan.

Henderson, V., & the Yale University School of Nursing Index Staff. (1963, 1966, 1970, 1972). *Nursing studies index* (4 Vols. I-1900–29, II-1930–49, III-1950–56, IV-1957–59). Philadelphia: J. B. Lippincott.

Jezierski, M. (1997). Virginia Henderson: Reflections on a twentieth century Florence Nightingale. *Journal of Emergency Nursing, 23*, 386–387.

Johnson, M., Maas, M., & Moorhead, S. (2000). *Nursing Outcomes Classification (NOC),* (2nd ed.). St. Louis: Mosby.

McCloskey, J. C., & Bulechek, G. M. (2000). *Nursing Interventions Classification (NIC)* (3rd ed.). St. Louis: Mosby.

McCormick, P. (1996). A tribute to Virginia Henderson. *Psychiatric Care, 3* (Suppl. 1), 47.

Mitchell, G. J. (1999). Evidence-based practice: Critique and alternative view. *Nursing Science Quarterly, 12*, 30–35.

Montiero, L. A. (1984). On separate roads: Florence Nightingale and Elizabeth Blackwell. *Signs, 9*(3), 520–533.

Nightingale, F. (1858a). *Notes on matters affecting the health, efficiency, and hospital administration of the British Army founded chiefly on the experience of the late war.* London: Harrison.

Nightingale, F. (1858b). *Subsidiary notes as to the introduction of female nursing into military hospitals in peace and war.* London: Harrison.

Nightingale, F. (1858c). *Mortality of the British Army, at home and abroad, and during the Russian War, as compared with the mortality of the civil population in England.* London: Harrison.

Nightingale, F. (1859a). *Notes on nursing: What it is and what it is not.* London: Harrison.

Nightingale, F. (1859b). *A contribution to the sanitary history of the British Army during the late war with Russia.* London: Harrison.

Nite, G., & Wills, F. (1964). *The coronary patient.* New York: Collier Macmillan.

O'Malley, J. (1996). A nursing legacy: Virginia Henderson. *Advanced Practice Nursing Quarterly, 2*(2), v.

Orlando, I. J. (1961). *The dynamic nurse-patient relationship,* New York: G. P. Putnam.

Schmieding, N. J. (1990). An integrative nursing theoretical framework. *Journal of Advanced Nursing, 15*, 463–467.

Simmons, L., & Henderson, V. (1957). A survey and assessment of research in nursing. In *The yearbook of modern nursing—1956.* New York: G. P. Putnam.

Simmons, L., & Henderson, V. (1964). *Nursing research: A survey and assessment.* New York: Appleton-Century-Crofts.

Smith, J. P. (1989). *Virginia Henderson: The first ninety years.* London: Scutari Press.

Smith, J. P. (1997). Virginia Avernal Henderson RN MA FAAN FRCN: 1897–1996. *Journal of Advanced Nursing, 25*(1), 1.

Southall, J. P. C. (1955). *Memoirs of the abbots of old Bellevue.* Charlottesville: The University of Virginia Press.

Stein, K. F., Corte, C., Colling K. B., & Whall, A. (1998). A theoretical analysis of Carper's ways of knowing using a model of social cognition. *Scholarly Inquiry for Nursing Practice, 12,* 43–60.

Thompson, J. D., & Goldin, G. (1975). *The hospital: A social and architectural history.* New Haven: Yale University Press.

Wald, F., & Leonard, R. C. (1964). Toward development of nursing practice theory, *Nursing Research, 13,* 309–313.

Weidenbach, E. (1964). *Clinical nursing—A helping art.* New York: Springer.

6

Johnson's Behavioral System Model

Sharon A. Wilkerson and Carol J. Loveland-Cherry

Dorothy Johnson received a BSN degree from Vanderbilt University School of Nursing and an MPH degree from Harvard University. Most of her career was spent as a professor of nursing in pediatrics at the University of California, Los Angeles. The foundations for Johnson's model are evident in her early publications, which focused on the role and functions of nurses (1959a), her philosophy of nursing (1959b), and the nature of nursing science (1968b). It was during her tenure as a faculty member and in her work with graduate students, however, that she formalized her work on her behavioral system model.

When Johnson began her teaching career in nursing, she was faced with two issues: (a) appropriate and necessary content for inclusion in a nursing curriculum, and (b) a method for organizing that material meaningfully (Johnson, 1981). Based on Nightingale's contention that nursing's appropriate goal is to assist individuals to prevent or recover from disease or injury, Johnson formulated a model for nursing. The development of the model was influenced further by Johnson's knowledge of sociological theory, particularly Talcott Parson's work, and intercultural theories of child-rearing practices. These two bodies of knowledge provided the basis for Johnson's conceptualization of a systems view of the individual in interaction with the environment (Johnson, 1981). Reflected in the development of the model are Johnson's beliefs that nursing as a professional discipline (a) is not dependent upon medical authority, (b) has a focus different from but complementary to medicine, and (c) has had available a body of relevant facts for nursing care but had not at that time developed a clear theoretical framework or conceptual basis to give direction to the development of the discipline (Johnson, 1961).

BASIC CONSIDERATIONS INCLUDED IN THE MODEL

In her writings, Johnson has stated that the development of a theory of nursing is not as important as the development of a conceptualization for nursing that provides direction for practice, education, and research (1968a). It is toward this end that she proposed a systems model of the individual that serves as the basis for nursing actions and outcomes (1978b). The conceptual model she proposed (1968a) would provide a focus for the science of nursing. This model consists of two major components: *nursing* and *person* (or *man* in her terminology). *Nursing* is defined by its actions and objectives and *person* is described as a behavioral system. The other traditional components of a nursing model, *environment* and *health,* are not directly defined, but rather are discussed in terms of their interaction with the behavioral system.

Definition of Nursing

Johnson views nursing as a professional discipline with a distinctive service to offer and encompassing both an art and a science component. A recurrent theme is the necessity to identify and develop the science of nursing based on a common objective. Nursing actions focus on the individual who is attempting to maintain or reestablish equilibrium (1961). Reduction of stress and tension promotes adaptation and stability. Within Johnson's model, nursing is defined as an *external regulatory force that assists the individual to achieve system balance and stability.* Therefore, nursing care is based on an understanding of person and human responses to change and stress (1959a, 1959b). Johnson (1968b) stated that, as contrasted with medicine, nursing is concerned with the behavior problems rather than biological functions. She emphasized, however, that nursing problems arise in the area of basic human needs, and the unique area of practice for nursing that is not shared with other health professionals involves such behaviors as feeding, bathing, and toileting (1959a, 1959b).

Description of Nursing Activity

When instability or disequilibrium is evident in the behavioral system, nursing as an external regulatory force acts to assist the person to regain stability or equilibrium. This is accomplished by imposing temporary regulatory or control mechanisms, attempting to change structural units in a desirable direction, or by providing resources to assist the person to meet the functional requirements of the subsystems.

Definition and Description of Person

The person (or man in Johnson's terminology) is defined as a *behavioral system,* which means that the individual is determined by actions and behaviors. These actions and behaviors are regulated and controlled by biological, psychological, and sociological factors (Johnson, 1968a, 1968b). As a behavioral system, the person is composed of interrelated subsystems. Each of these subsystems affects the way in which individuals will interact with the environment (1974). Thus, any change in one subsystem can directly or indirectly affect any other subsystem. The actions or behavioral patterns of the total system are efforts to maintain a behavioral system balance, whereas the environmental forces influence the system (1968b). Each person has a unique pattern of actions distinguishing him or her from other behavioral systems, namely other persons. Nursing is concerned with the person as a total entity, which would indicate an involvement with all the subsystems of the behavioral system.

Definition and Description of Environment

Although Johnson referred to internal and external environments in describing her model, neither was defined. The behavioral system functions to both maintain its own integrity and to manage the relationship to its environment. The implication in this instance is that the environment consists of that which is external to the behavioral system. Furthermore, the environment is ascertained to be a source of stimuli that can result in behavioral system imbalance as well as the supplies necessary for system nurturance.

Definition and Description of Health

Health was defined by Johnson (1978a) as an elusive state determined by psychological, social, and physiological factors that are held as a desired value by all the health professions. Based on the Nightingale model, the focus in nursing relative to health and illness is the person rather than illness itself. Illness is seen as a disrupting factor that disturbs the balance between the individual's subsystems. This is contrasted with the medical model, which focuses on disease as a biological system disorder (1968a). In her early work, Johnson (1959a, 1959b) pointed out that system equilibrium does not imply health, but rather a resting state for organizing resources for further movement. In later refinement of the model, however, health is described as a moving state of equilibrium (versus a static process), which occurs throughout the health change process (1961).

Interrelationship of Components

The interrelationship between person and environment is straightforward in Johnson's model. Environment is implied to consist of all factors not directly part of the individual behavioral system. These factors act on the behavioral system, which responds in an effort to maintain a balance. The pattern of behavior of an individual determines and limits the interactions between person and environment. Although the primary objective of the behavioral system is to achieve a balance, individuals may actively engage in new behaviors that at least temporarily disturb the system balance.

Health problems or lack of balance in the system are either structural or functional. They arise from the system itself or from environmental factors. The five major causes of instability or problems within the system are:

1. Inadequate or inappropriate development of the system or its parts.
2. Breakdown in internal regulatory or control mechanisms.
3. Exposure to noxious influences.
4. Inadequate stimulation of the system.
5. Lack of adequate environmental input

(Johnson, 1978b).

Identification of the source of problems in the behavioral system balance leads to appropriate nursing actions. These actions may include:

1. Repairing the structural unit through teaching or similar activities.
2. Temporarily imposing external regulatory or control measures such as limit setting.
3. Providing essential environmental conditions or resources in various situations. An example might be providing contact between mother and infant to facilitate bonding

(Johnson, 1978b).

These nursing actions contribute to the achievement of the nursing goal, which is to "maintain or restore a person's behavioral system balance and stability or help a person achieve a more optimal level of functioning (balance) with environmental interactions where possible or desirable" (Johnson, 1978b, p. 2).

An understanding of systems theory is helpful in evaluating Johnson's model of nursing. Johnson's definition of a system is based upon Rapoport's (1968) description of a system as being composed of interrelated subsystems or parts; it is the functioning of these parts together that determines the total system function. The more complex the system, the greater the number of subsystems that exist in the system. Subsystems are interrelated parts of a system that are linked and open (Johnson, 1980).

Johnson has identified seven subsystems of the behavioral system. These include the *attachment-affiliative,* the *aggressive,* the *dependency,* the *achievement,* the *ingestive,* the *eliminative,* and the *sexual* systems (1980).

The seven subsystems are open, linked, and interrelated. Motivational drives direct the activities of these subsystems, which are continually changing due to maturation, experience, or learning. The seven subsystems described appear to exist cross-culturally and are controlled by biological, psychological, and sociological factors. Each subsystem can be described and analyzed in terms of structure, function, and functional requirements. Four structural elements identified include (a) the drive or goal being sought; (b) the set, which the individual's predisposition for a pattern of action; (c) the choice, which is the group of alternatives for action; and (d) actions, which are the actual behavior of the individual (Johnson, 1980). Each subsystem has the same functional requirements: *protection, nurturance,* and *stimulation.* Although each subsystem has a specialized function, the system as a whole requires an integrated performance. The behavioral system (person) is, therefore, viewed as a totality of the subsystems. The attachment-affiliative subsystem is identified as the basis of social organization and is proposed to be the first subsystem to emerge developmentally. The general function of this system is security. Social inclusion, intimacy, and formation and maintenance of a strong social bond are the consequences of the system activities (Johnson, 1980).

The function of the aggressive subsystem is defined as self-protection and preservation. It is recognized that this function exists within the limits of protection and respect of others. In this context, aggression is not viewed as a learned, negative response (Johnson, 1980).

The dependency subsystem optimally evolves developmentally from total dependence on others to a large degree of independence with a component of interdependence. Succorance with an expected nurturance response is the general function of the dependency subsystem with consequences of approval, attention, or recognition and physical assistance (Johnson, 1980).

"Mastery or control of some aspect of the self or environment as measured against some standard of excellence" (Johnson, 1980, p. 213) was identified as the function of the achievement system. Proposed consequences include physical, creative, mechanical, and social skills.

Behavioral rather than biological aspects are the focus of the ingestive and eliminative subsystems. Therefore, appetite satisfaction per se is identified as the function of the ingestive subsystem and behavioral excretion of wastes as that of the eliminative subsystem. The emphasis is on when, where, how, what, how much, and under what conditions individuals eat and when, how, and under what conditions individuals eliminate wastes. Social and psychological factors are viewed as not only influencing the biological aspects of these systems, but also as being, occasionally, in conflict with or taking precedence over them (Johnson, 1980).

Procreation and gratification are the dual functions of the sexual subsystem. Cultural norms and values as well as biological sex influence the consequences of this subsystem. These consequences include gender identity, courting, and mating (Johnson, 1980).

In addition to the seven subsystems identified by Johnson, nurse clinicians suggested an eighth subsystem, the restorative that was defined by Grubbs (1980). The function of the restorative subsystem is to relieve fatigue or to redistribute energy to achieve a state of equilibrium.

Other concepts that are necessary for understanding the behavioral system model include *equilibrium, stability, instability, stressors,* and *tensions.* Equilibrium is defined as a "stabilized, but more or less transitory, resting state in which the individual is in harmony within himself and with his environment" (Johnson, 1961, p. 65). The system strives for a balance with the external influences, but this does not preclude occasional self-disturbances that result from learning experiences. The adjustments and adaptations in behavior must be useful to the maintenance of the system even if they are not considered to be within the norms for the individual's culture; all patterns of activity for the system or subsystem serve some purpose (Johnson, 1968b). Stability refers to the system state characterized by regularity and constancy in behavior. Stressors are stimuli from either internal or external sources, either positive or negative, which impinge upon a system and result in disruption of the stability of the system. Tension is defined as "a state of being stretched or strained and can be viewed as a product of disturbance in equilibrium" (Johnson, 1961, p. 65). Tension is a potential source of change. Disruption in the structure or function results in a system that needs outside intervention for restoration of balance. Nursing is one such outside intervention force that can help restore the behavioral system to an optimal level.

INTERNAL ANALYSIS

Internal analysis of theoretical models requires examination of both syntax (the logical relationships between units) and semantics (the meaning given to the units) (Hardy, 1974). Additional areas of concern in examining the internal analysis of theoretical models include logical adequacy, the ability to generalize, parsimony/simplicity, empirical precision, and clarity (Chinn

& Jacobs, 1983; Walker & Avant, 1983). Therefore, internal analysis of Johnson's model will be conducted along the following areas and criteria:

1. Statement of assumptions.
2. Clarity of definitions of units.
3. Consistency of use of units and relationships.
4. Efficiency of statements of interaction between units.
5. Clarity of values inherent in the model.
6. Adequacy, complexity, and scope of the model.

Underlying Assumptions

Assumptions constitute the foundational core of a theoretical model. Silva defines these as "statements of general truth that serve as essential premises for whatever is being investigated" (1977, p. 61). Assumptions can be either explicit or implicit. Johnson implies a number of assumptions regarding nursing and explicitly states others regarding man as a behavioral system. The assumptions made by Johnson derive from behavioral and systems theory and her philosophical view of nursing. They are consistent with her stated purpose of developing a model to provide direction for nursing practice, education, and research. The assumptions can be summarized as follows:

1. The knowledge required for practice in nursing consists of three types: (a) knowledge of order; (b) knowledge of disorder; and (c) knowledge of control (Johnson, 1968a).
2. The central concern of nursing is with man as an organized and integrated whole (Johnson, 1968a).
3. Man can be viewed as a behavioral system (Johnson, 1980).
4. The behavior of the system is characterized by organization, interaction, interdependency, and integration of the parts and elements (Johnson, 1980).
5. The interrelated parts are called subsystems of behavior (Johnson, 1980).
6. Man continually strives to maintain a behavioral system balance and steady state by more or less automatic adjustments and adaptations to the natural forces impinging upon him (Johnson, 1968c).
7. Man actively seeks new experiences that may disturb his balance and may require small or large behavior modifications to reestablish balance (Johnson, 1980).
8. Man requires a behavioral system characterized by some degree of regular and constant behavior (Johnson, 1980).

9. Balance in the behavioral system reflects adjustments and adaptations that are successful in some way and to some degree (Johnson, 1968c).
10. The integrity of a person is threatened by disturbance of behavioral system balance resulting from either extremely strong external forces or diminished resistance in ability to adjust to moderate disturbances (Johnson, 1968c).
11. Man expends extraordinary amounts of energy in attempting to maintain or reestablish behavioral system balance in response to imbalance caused by persistent excessive forces (Johnson, 1968c).
12. For any one individual, behavioral system balance results in a minimum demand for energy expenditure, which then frees more energy for maintaining biological processes and for recovery from illness (Johnson, 1968c).

Assumptions can be analyzed to determine if they are in conflict with each other and if they refer equally to all areas of the model, or are balanced (Chinn & Jacobs, 1983). The assumptions of the model do not compete with each other; they are compatible. The view of man as a behavioral system and the relationship to influences from the environment is consistently presented throughout the assumptions. Johnson's emphasis on man as a behavioral system is reflected in the predominance of explicit assumptions on this area of the model. Two implicit assumptions relate to nursing, and the environment and health are indirectly addressed in the assumptions related to the behavioral system. Although the assumptions are not balanced among the four metaparadigm concepts, the emphasis is appropriate and consistent with the focus of the model.

Central Components

According to Bush, "a model orders, clarifies and systematizes selected components of the phenomena it serves to depict" (1979, p. 16). Based on her belief that the patient is the proper focus of nursing action, Johnson presents two major units as basic components of the model: man as a behavioral system and nursing. The behavioral system is a complex unit derived from behavioral and systems theory with the following subunits.

Person: Behavioral system

1. Attachment-affiliative.
2. Dependency.
3. Achievement.
4. Aggressive.

5. Ingestive.
6. Eliminative.
7. Sexual.

Each subsystem has its own function with consequential behavior, four structural elements (drive, set, choice, and action), and the functional requirements of nurturance, projection, and stimulation.

The second major component, nursing, is also a complex unit identified by its goals and actions.

Nursing

1. Goal—achievement and maintenance of a stable state in behavioral system.
2. Actions (three intervention strategies):
   a) Change structural units.
   b) Impose temporary external regulatory or control measures.
   c) Provide essential environmental conditions or resources.

Analysis of Consistency

Definitions. The behavioral system is clearly defined. It is differentiated from the biological system that is considered the focus of medicine. The subunits of the complex unit, the seven subsystems, are clearly identified in terms of function and structure. The definitions are at an abstract level, but have been defined empirically by others (Auger & Dee, 1983; Derdiarian, 1983a, 1983b, 1990; Grubbs, 1980; Holaday, 1980; Rawls, 1980). Empirical indicators are easily extrapolated because the focus is on observable events, actions, or behaviors. For example, empirical indicators of the achievement subsystem could include age-appropriate developmental measures such as the activities of daily living. Johnson addressed the necessity of viewing man as a whole. Focused on the totality of the behavioral system, her definition of person is consistent with this contention. This is efficient, given that it clearly limits the domain of nursing's concern. It is consistent with Johnson's definition of nursing as a practice discipline focused on the unique aspect of behavior. Unless, however, the comprehensiveness of Johnson's definition of behavior is recognized, confusion may arise regarding the interaction and influence of physiological, psychological, and sociological factors.

Johnson defines nursing as an external regulatory force. The objective of nursing is clearly defined and limited. The three intervention strategies emphasized are consistent with the goal of nursing as defined by Johnson and with the view of man as a behavioral system. The model focuses on the person in potential or actual illness situations. Although Johnson states that a nursing role exists related to optimizing behavioral system functioning, the nursing actions that are identified focus on individuals who experience either a threat of illness or who are ill. The role of nursing in relation to health maintenance and promotion is not clearly defined. Johnson alludes to the latter two situations in the presentation of her model, but does not develop or explicate a nursing role.

Both the behavioral system and nursing are major components in Johnson's model; nevertheless, the behavioral system is given primary emphasis. This unit is defined in more specific detail and serves as the focal point of the model. Nursing is discussed in terms of the behavioral system, not the reverse. Nursing's objectives and actions are predicated upon and defined in terms of the behavioral system. Unless there is instability or less than optimal functioning in the behavioral system, nursing has no identified goal. The philosophical foundation of critical theory as expressed by Stevens (1979), who states, "nursing is an enhancement used to improve the quality of the patient's existence" (p. 240), is consistent with Johnson's components of nursing and her assumptions of nursing's concerns.

Relationships. Dubin (1978) contended that specifying the interactions between units is an indispensable step in developing a scientific model. Johnson's model indicates that the state of the behavioral system determines the type and amount of nursing actions necessary. Generally, living systems, including the behavioral system, must maintain both balance and a certain level of stability internally and in interactions with the environment to function efficiently and effectively. Imbalance and/or instability in the system may arise from five sources: (a) inadequate or inappropriate development of the system or its parts; (b) breakdown in internal regulatory or control mechanisms; (c) exposure to noxious influences; (d) inadequate stimulation of the system; or (e) lack of adequate environmental input (Johnson, 1978b). When a state of imbalance or instability occurs relative to preventing or coping with illness, nursing input is necessitated to maintain or restore equilibrium. This is accomplished via the nursing actions defined in the model. In the latter instance, little information is available regarding the type of role played by the patient. The question can be raised as to whether the relationship between the behavioral system and nursing is interactive or reactive.

Applying the principles of Dubin's (1978) work, the relationships between the two major units in this model can be stated as follows: A state of imbalance or instability in the behavioral system results in the need for nursing actions; appropriate nursing actions result in the maintenance or restoration of behavioral system balance and stability. Using Dubin's (1978) system of evaluating relationships between units, two sequential laws of interaction are proposed by the model. That is, a state of imbalance or instability must exist before nursing actions are necessary, and appropriate nursing actions must be implemented to restore balance and stability in the system. According to Dubin, a sequential law of interaction is one employing a time dimension to order relationships among units. Furthermore, these statements identify a positive associational relationship between nursing and behavioral system balance and between behavioral system imbalance and the need for nursing. Derdiarian (1990) has expanded the investigation of relationships among the subsystems of the behavioral system model and has demonstrated the scientific relevance of the subsystems as well as their application to practice.

Internal consistency. The units and relationships between units are consistently defined and used, except in the instance that the behavioral system is open and has the ability to initiate action. Although Johnson implied that the behavioral system is an open, active one in interaction with the environment, the relationships identified between the behavioral system and the environment, including nursing, suggest only that the behavioral system reacts and adapts. Nursing is defined as acting on the behavioral system; less consideration is evident about the individual's role in the process of preventing and coping with disturbances or in initiating change or growth. The model does not explicate the potential for active decision making on the part of the individual. Man is defined as an active, open system but in terms or nursing intervention becomes, at least temporarily, passive.

The units identified by the model and their definitions are consonant with Johnson's beliefs about the appropriate focus for nursing. The relationships stated are consistent with the assumptions specified. In addition, the model consistently reflects Johnson's belief that health is not the sole or major concern of nursing. The definition of nursing's objective is clearly compatible with an illness model, but less so with a health-promotion model. This, however, does not present difficulties in terms of internal consistency; rather, it is a concern in terms of scope, which will be addressed in a later section.

Johnson clearly explicates her value for developing a model for nursing practice, education, and research. The model is in consonance with and reflective of this value. The three types of knowledge required for nursing practice, as she states (Johnson, 1968a), are also addressed by the model.

Analysis of Adequacy

The adequacy of Johnson's model will be addressed using criteria suggested by Walker and Avant (1983), Ellis (1968), Jacox (1974), and Hardy (1974). Jacox identifies three levels of theory development: "(1) a period of specifying, defining, and classifying the concepts used in describing the phenomena of the field; (2) developing statements or propositions which propose how two or more concepts are related; and (3) specifying how all the propositions are related to each other in a systematic way" (p. 5). Johnson's model evidences the criteria for the first two levels. The units of behavioral system and nursing are delimited and defined, and statements are developed regarding the relationship among them. The statements of relationship are developed at a general level and are not sufficiently specified or systematized to satisfy the third level of development. The model does, however, suggest opportunities for this to be done.

Johnson's definition of nursing in terms of the patient is consistent with Ellis' contention that "nursing . . . cannot be defined apart from the patient, the definition centers on functions for the patient" (1968, p. 21). Scope is a second criterion identified as important to the significance of a theory by Ellis: ". . . [those] most important for nursing would be those that encompass both biological and behavioral observations, and have the potential for explaining their relationships" (1968, p. 219). Johnson's model focuses on behavioral aspects but does imply the impact of biological factors. The goal of nursing is clearly defined and delimited, but presents some concern in terms of scope. Although prevention is incorporated in the definition of nursing's goal, promotion and maintenance are not. Because the emphasis on promotion and maintenance of health as appropriate foci for nursing has evolved subsequent to Johnson's development of the model, inclusion of these concepts cannot be reasonably expected. Moreover, the model primarily addresses the individual as the patient. Groups such as families are alluded to but not specifically identified as recipients of nursing care. Johnson does not state that her purpose is to include groups, such as families; nevertheless, the model does not preclude this being done in a future development of the model. Some restriction of the types of nursing actions taken and the overall context of the model (namely, illness-related situations), may, however, provide limited opportunity for further development. Given that the scope or the width of the focus is related to the theoretical model's ability to be generalized (Walker & Avant, 1983), the application of the model in its present form may be limited.

A third characteristic of significant theories is complexity (Ellis, 1968). Either multiple variable relationships are included, or a limited number of variables are viewed in great complexity. The variables in Johnson's model are few and the range of meaning of the variables is somewhat restricted. The behavioral system is, however, treated in detail and complexity with the explication of the subsystems and their functional and structural properties. The second major unit in the model, nursing, is treated fully. The nursing actions identified reflect the complexity of the behavioral system unit. The syntax of the model is somewhat limited in complexity, dealing primarily with reactive relationships within an illness focus.

Ellis identified a fourth criterion of usefulness as an essential characteristic of significant theories for nursing. Theoretical models are not significant if they do not provide guidance for practice. Johnson's behavioral model clearly provides this guidance in illness-related situations. The role of nursing to nonillness situations is not as clearly defined. This can, however, be understood in terms of the era in which the model was first explicated.

In summary, using criteria identified by Walker and Avant (1983), Ellis (1968), Jacox (1974), and Hardy (1974), the internal analysis of Johnson's model leads to several conclusions. It is a model developed for nursing practice with the two major units—behavioral system and nursing—clearly and consistently defined and used. The scope of the model is largely confined to the behavioral aspects of the individual in illness-related situations; this is consistent with Johnson's values and philosophy. It is concluded that Johnson's model is overall, clearly defined and meets the criteria of identifying and defining phenomena and relationships.

EXTERNAL ANALYSIS

Relationship to Nursing Research

Research in nursing has been used to verify conceptual models and has led toward the goals of establishing the scientific base of nursing. Johnson (1974) stated that nursing in the past was not based upon a scientific foundation, and this situation allows the nurse researcher many choices that are not available to researchers in other fields. It is the nurse-researcher who will influence the development of both the scientific discipline and the professional practice of nursing. By choosing one of the nursing models for the basis of research, the researchers not only influence the profession, but also determine the direction of their own research. The behavioral system model leads the researcher in at least two directions. One person might choose to concentrate on the basic sciences, which are investigating the functioning of the subsystems as well as the functioning of the whole behavioral system. Another researcher may choose instead to investigate problems related to the behavioral system and methods of solving those problems. The area of applied research that deals with identification and solution of problems would be more closely linked to the practice of nursing as stated by Johnson (1959a, 1959b). Nurse researchers have demonstrated the usefulness of Johnson's model in clinical practice in a variety of ways. The nursing process and assessment have been studied in relation to the behavioral system model. When using the Johnson model, nursing assessments are based on the patterns that individuals have for meeting their needs. This requires that nurses determine patterns that the clients have rather than merely basing assessment of needs on the diagnosis (Crawford, 1982). Fawz (1979) employed Johnson's model to examine the behavioral characteristics of patients in isolation and found it useful. Damus (1980) developed a classification system for nursing diagnosis based on behavioral subsystems and effectively tested the model with serum hepatitis patients. In 1980, Grubbs also developed a patient assessment tool and described how the Johnson model is congruent with nursing process. Based on the Johnson model, a patient classification system was developed by Auger and Dee (1983). In the psychiatric setting, this patient classification system was found to increase communication as well as help nurses identify their role. Their classification system was found to be applicable to most clinical settings and to all ages (Auger & Dee, 1983; Poster & Beliz, 1992; Poster, Dee, & Randell, 1997).

Johnson's behavioral system model also has been used as a framework for nursing intervention. Norris (1970) developed a framework that is compatible with the behavioral system approach and adapts itself to the individual patterns of the client, thus allowing "personalization" of nursing intervention. A combination of the behavioral system model and body image theory was found effective in providing nursing care to an amputee patient (Rawls, 1980). Broncatello (1980) applied Auger's (1975) expanded version of Johnson's behavioral system model to the care of patients receiving hemodialysis. She found that this model permitted the personalization of care and also provided the basis of support for adaptive behavior while identifying maladaptive behavior. Derdiarian (1983a) investigated cancer patients' behavioral changes in relation to Johnson's behavioral system model. She developed an instrument to measure behavioral changes (Derdiarian, 1983b), and her research supported the contention that behavioral instability results from illness. In recent work, Derdiarian (1990) analyzed further Johnson's premise of open and interactive subsystems in cancer patients. Derdiarian concluded that although all of the subsystems should be considered, changes in the aggressive-protective subsystem may be the more important indicator for early intervention needs in cancer patients. On the other side of the issue, Reynolds and Cormack (1991) report that nursing practice in their institution is based on Johnson's model, and it has been found to be very useful in making nursing diagnoses but can only provide "hints rather than specifics" about nursing interventions.

Johnson's model also has been researched in the nursing care of children and their families. Holaday (1974) compared the achievement behavior of chronically ill and healthy children. The achievement subsystem of the behavioral system model was used as a framework for this study. She used Johnson's concept of "behavioral set" to help ascertain how mothers of chronically ill infants develop responses to their children's crying (Holaday, 1981a, 1981b, 1982, 1997; Holaday et al., 1996). Skolny and Riehl (1974) found the model useful in developing a plan of action to help the mother of a dying young man maintain hope. Johnson's model was used to explain the findings of a study of handicapped preschool children whose body image and spatial awareness was compared with those of normal children (Small, 1980). An assessment tool of family functioning based on the behavioral system model was developed by Lovejoy (1983) and was evaluated in a study of leukemic children. She found that these children were affected by their perceptions of family behavioral disturbances that demonstrated an interaction between systems. Following the description of Campbell and Bunting (1991) of research in the study of emancipation, Cox (1994) based her work on Johnson's model and did not use "triangulation" just as a methodological technique but as an attempt to identify the client system interdependence in her study of mothers and their newborns. All of these research studies have tested the behavioral model system and have increased nursing's body of knowledge.

Relationship to Nursing Education

Nursing education based on the behavioral system model would have definite goals, and course planning would be relatively straightforward. A background in biological, psychological, and sociological fields would be necessary for complete understanding of the behavioral system. The primary focus of nursing education would be the study of the person as a behavioral system. Behavioral subsystems could be identified as areas for nursing specialization (Rogers, 1978). Also included would be the study of behavioral system problems that would require the use of the nursing process in relation to disruptions in behavioral system functioning. Johnson stated that the study of behavioral system problems presents difficulties for curriculum content development because "the knowledge base tends to be disorganized and more intuitive and speculative than scientific" (Johnson, 1980, p. 215). Given the scientific study of the model, results and methodologies can be incorporated into education as a basis for practice.

Relationship to Professional Nursing Practice

Nursing practice is operationalized by its definition in the behavioral system model. The model itself states the "end product," which is the goal of nursing practice (Johnson, 1968c). Nursing's objective is to maintain or restore the person's behavioral system balance and stability or to help the person achieve a more optimum level of function. Change of any magnitude toward recovery from illness or toward more desirable health practices depends upon the periodic achievement and maintenance, perhaps for only a short time, of this stable state.

An example of practice based on Johnson's model would be preoperative teaching. By giving patients information regarding their surgery and what they can expect to have happen both preoperatively and postoperatively, and by providing support by listening to their concerns and questions, their tension, anxiety, and fatigue would be reduced. This reduction would help them to develop attitudes and behaviors leading to the achievement of equilibrium. Assessment of the effectiveness of preoperative teaching would be included in the nursing process.

With the goal of maintaining or restoring balance to an individual's behavioral system clearly stated, nursing can develop precise measurements for evaluating the efficacy of nursing action. Patient indicators of nursing care based on Johnson's model were developed by Majesky, Brester, and Nishio (1978) and tested with a number of patients with a variety of diagnoses. This tool is considered one measure of quality nursing care. Glennin (1980) specifically classified standards of nursing practice with the concepts of Johnson's model and found the classification useful. Holaday (1981b) also wrote of the use of this model as a measure of quality health care. Using the operational indices of behavior developed by Auger and Dee (1983) from Johnson's model, nurses in a California neuropsychiatric hospital have been able to evaluate actively the outcomes of nursing interventions (Reynolds & Cormack, 1991). In addition to this application of the behavioral system model as a measure of quality, numerous research studies have demonstrated the usefulness of this model in nursing practice in a variety of settings. These include the community, hospice, long-term care facilities and acute-care facilities. Specific interventions have been identified with cancer patients, those with acquired immunodeficiency syndrome (AIDS), Alzheimer's disease, and a variety of chronic conditions as well as a variety of psychiatric diagnoses (Auger & Dee, 1983; Broncatello, 1980; Damus, 1980; Derdiarian, 1983a, 1990; Fruehwirth, 1989; Holaday, 1974; Lovejoy, 1983; Raudonis & Acton, 1997; Rawls, 1980; Stuifbergen, Becker, Rogers, Timmerman, & Kullberg, 1999).

Nursing Diagnosis and the Model

Johnson's model is well suited to the identification of nursing diagnoses. Disruptions in subsystems can be identified using the five causes of instability or difficulty (inadequate system, internal regulatory breakdown, exposure to noxious influences, inadequate stimulation, and lack of environmental input) identified by Johnson (1978b). This identification of problems can then be linked to the eight subsystems and nursing diagnoses can be made from the problem assessments. Based on the diagnosis made from the identified disruption of the subsystem, nursing actions can be planned in terms of teaching, external control, or providing resources needed by the client.

Using the North American Nursing Diagnosis Association (NANDA) Taxonomy I Revised (1986), the patterns can be identified with specific subsystems, as shown in Table 6–1. A large proportion of the NANDA diagnoses can be identified under the aggressive-protective subsystem. Derdiarian (1990) reported most diagnoses related to needs of cancer patients also fell in this subsystem. However, not all diagnoses can be placed under one subsystem without thought for other subsystems and other factors. Given that Johnson's model is based on system's theory, there is a need to identify environmental regulators that influence the subsystems when making diagnoses. In addition, the interactions of the subsystems must be considered. For instance, the diagnosis "high risk for fluid value deficit" is obviously an elimination issue but it also places the client at risk biophysically, so the diagnosis is also related to the aggressive-protective subsystem. By considering the effects of the problem on the two subsystems together, nursing interventions can be more individualized for the client. Based on a parent-child interaction focus, some of the diagnoses such as parental role conflict and caregiver role strain might be classified in different behavioral subsystems depending on which person is the primary client. For the parent, the subsystem may be achievement, whereas for the child, the appropriate subsystem may be dependence. Because the two individuals influence each other, the nursing diagnosis is still meaningful— it is just the classification within Johnson's model that becomes complex.

It should be noted that the NANDA diagnosis of sensory-perceptual alteration would need to be identified for a specific sensory modality to place the diagnosis in the appropriate behavioral subsystem. The NANDA taxonomy, spiritual distress, was the one diagnosis that was difficulty to categorize as relating to a specific subsystem as described by Johnson. Depending on the individual assessment, this diagnosis may relate to the aggressive-protective subsystem with regard to psychosocial needs, but it might also relate to the dependence subsystem as a need for fulfillment and nurturance from others, or perhaps even the affiliative subsystem. No subsystem was without NANDA diagnoses that could be related to them, which indicates that Johnson's model is relevant to clinical nursing practice.

Relationship to Theory-Driven, Evidence-Based Practice

Based on Carper's (1978) four fundamental patterns of knowing, Johnson's behavioral system theory can be described. Using the patterns of knowing identified by Fawcett, Watson, Neuman, Walker, and Fitzpatrick (2001), the evidence for Johnson's model is presented in Table 6–1.

TABLE 6–1 Behavioral Subsystems and NANDA Diagnoses

Aggressive-protective	Achievement	Dependency	Eliminative
1.2.1.1–	3.2.1	3.2.1.1.1[a]–	1.3.1.1–
1.2.3.1[a]	3.2.1.1.1[a]–	3.2.1.1.2	1.5.1.3.2
1.6.1–	3.2.1.1.2	6.5.1–	
1.6.2.1.2.2	5.1.1.1–	6.5.1.4	
	5.4	7.2.1.1	
6.1.1.1–	6.4.1.1–		
6.1.1.1.1	6.4.2		
	6.5.2–		
	6.5.7		
8.1.1	7.1.1–		
8.3	7.1.3		
9.1.1–	7.3.1–		
9.3.2	7.3.2		
	9.1.1–		
	9.3.2		

[a]Patterns that can be identified in two or more subsystems simultaneously. NANDA, North American Nursing Diagnosis Association.

Empiric and ethical patterns of knowing are well defined for Johnson's model. Person and aesthetical patterns of knowing are less clear and should be the focus of future studies.

SUMMARY

Johnson's model for nursing focuses on the person as a behavioral system composed of seven interrelated subsystems. The goal of the behavioral system is to achieve and/or maintain equilibrium. When the behavioral system is in a state of imbalance or instability, nursing activity as an external regulatory force assists the person to regain equilibrium.

The two major components in the model, behavioral system and nursing, are clearly and consistently defined and used. The model as presented emphasizes the individual in a context of threatened or actual illness. Nursing's role in health promotion and maintenance is alluded to but is not as clearly developed. Johnson's model provides direction for nursing education, research, and practice.

REFERENCES

Auger, J. A. (1975). *Behavioral systems and nursing*. Englewood Cliffs, NJ: Princeton-Hall.
Auger, J. A., & Dee, V. (1983). A patient classification system based on the behavioral system model of nursing: Part 1. *The Journal of Nursing Administration, 13,* 38–43.

TABLE 6-1   *Continued*

Ingestive	Attachment-affiliative	Restorative	Sexual
1.1.2.1–	2.1.1.1	6.1.1.2.1–	3.2.1.2.1
1.1.2.3	3.1.1–	6.3.1.1	3.3
1.2.3.1	3.1.2		
6.5.1–	3.2.2–		
6.5.1.4	3.2.3.1		

Broncatello, K. F. (1980). Auger in action: Application of the model. *Advances in Nursing Science, 2*(2), 13–24.

Bush, H. A. (1979). Models for nursing. *Advances in Nursing Science, 1,* 13–20.

Campbell, J., & Bunting, S. (1991). Voices and paradigms: Perspectives on critical and feminist theory in nursing. *Advances in Nursing Science, 13*(3), 1–15.

Carper, B.A. (1978). Fundamental patterns of knowing in nursing. *Advances in Nursing Science, 1*(1), 13–23.

Chinn, P. L., & Jacobs, M. K. (1983). *Theory and nursing: A systematic approach.* St. Louis: Mosby.

Cox, M. (1994). *Statistical analysis triangulation of infant outcomes of a nurse managed obstetrical clinic.* Paper presented at the Texas Medical Center National Nursing Research Conference, Houston, TX.

Crawford, G. (1982). The concept of patterns in nursing: Conceptual development and measurement. *Advances in Nursing Science, 5,* 1–6.

Damus, K. (1980). An application of the Johnson behavioral system model for nursing practice. In J. P. Riehl & S. C. Roy (Eds.). *Conceptual models for nursing practice* (2nd ed.). New York: Appleton-Century-Crofts.

Derdiarian, A. K. (1983a). An instrument for theory and research development using the behavioral system model for nursing: The cancer patient: Part 1. *Nursing Research, 32*(4), 196–201.

Derdiarian, A. K. (1983b). An instrument for theory and research development using the behavioral system model for nursing: The cancer patient: Part 2. *Nursing Research, 32*(5), 260–266.

Derdiarian, A. K. (1990). The relationships among the subsystems of Johnson's behavioral system model. *IMAGE: Journal of Nursing Scholarship, 22*(4), 219–225.

Dubin, R. (1978). *Theory building.* New York: The Free Press.

Ellis, R. (1968). Characteristics of significant theories. *Nursing Research, 17,* 217–222.

Fawcett, J., Watson, J., Neuman, B., Walker, P. H., & Fitzpatrick, J. J. (2001). On nursing theories and evidence. *Journal of Nursing Scholarship 33*(2), 115–119.

Fawz, N. W. (1979). Development of methodology and examination of characteristics of isolation patients utilizing the Johnson model. Unpublished master's thesis, University of California.

Fruehwirth, S. E. S. (1989). An application of Johnson's behavioral model: A case study. *Journal of Community Health Nursing, 6*(2), 61–71.

Glennin, C. (1980). Formulation of standards of nursing practice using a nursing model. In J. P. Riehl & S. C. Roy (Eds.). *Conceptual models for nursing practice* (2nd ed.). New York: Appleton-Century-Crofts.

Grubbs, J. (1980). An interpretation of the Johnson model for nursing practice. In J. P. Riehl & S. C. Roy (Eds.). *Conceptual models for nursing practice* (2nd ed.). New York: Appleton-Century-Crofts.

Hardy, M. E. (1974). Theories: Components, development, evaluation. *Nursing Research, 23*, 199–206.

Holaday, B. (1974). Achievement behavior in chronically ill children. *Nursing Research, 23*, 25–30.

Holaday, B. (1980). Implementing the Johnson model for nursing practice. In J. P. Riehl & S. C. Roy (Eds.). *Conceptual models for nursing practice* (2nd ed.). New York: Appleton-Century-Crofts.

Holaday, B. (1981a). Maternal response to their chronically ill infants' attachment behavior of crying. *Nursing Research, 30*, 343–348.

Holaday, B. (1981b). The Johnson behavioral system model for nursing and the pursuit of quality health care. In G. E. Lasker (Ed.). *Applied systems and cybernetics* (Vol. 4), *Systems research in health care, biocybernetics and ecology.* New York: Pergamon.

Holaday, B. (1982). Maternal conceptual set development: Identifying patterns of maternal response to chronically ill infant crying. *Maternal-Child Nursing Journal, 11*, 47–59.

Holaday, B. (1997). Johnson's behavioral system model in nursing practice. In Alligood, M. et al., (Eds.), *Nursing theory: Utilization and application* (pp. 49–70). St. Louis, MO: Mosby-Year Book.

Holaday, B., Turner-Henson, A., & Swan, J. (1996). The Johnson Behavioral System Model: Explaining activities of chronically ill children. In Newman, B. & P. H. Walker, (Eds.), *Blueprint for use of nursing models: Education, research, practice and administration* (pp. 33–63). NY: National League for Nursing. NLN Publication No.14-2696.

Jacox, A. (1974). Theory construction in nursing: An overview. *Nursing Research, 23*, 4–13.

Johnson, D. E. (1959a). A philosophy of nursing. *Nursing Outlook, 7*, 198–200.

Johnson, D. E. (1959b). The nature of a science of nursing. *Nursing Outlook, 7*, 291–294.

Johnson, D. E. (1961). The significance of nursing care. *American Journal of Nursing, 61*(11), 63–66.

Johnson, D. E. (1968a). Theory in nursing: Borrowed and unique. *Nursing Research, 17*(3), 206–209.

Johnson, D. E. (1968b). Toward a science of nursing. *Southern Medical Bulletin, 56*(4), 13–23.

Johnson, D. E. (1968c). *One conceptual model or nursing.* Paper presented at Vanderbilt University, Nashville, TN.

Johnson, D. E. (1974). Development of theory: A requisite for nursing as a primary health profession. *Nursing Research, 23*(5), 372–377.

Johnson, D. E. (1978a). State of the art of theory development in nursing. In *Theory development: What, why, how?* New York: National League for Nursing.

Johnson, D. E. (1978b). *Behavioral system model for nursing.* Paper presented at the 2nd Annual Nurse Educator Conference, New York, NY.

Johnson, D. E. (1980). The behavioral system model for nursing. In J. P. Riehl & S. C. Roy (Eds.), *Conceptual models for nursing practice* (2nd ed.). New York: Appleton-Century-Crofts.

Johnson, D. E. (1981). Private communication.

Lovejoy, N. (1983). The leukemic child's perceptions of family behaviors. *Oncology Nursing Forum, 10*(4), 20–25.

Majesky, S. J., Brester, M. H., & Nishio, K. T. (1978). Development of a research tool: Patient indicators of nursing care. *Nursing Research, 27*(6), 365–371.

Norris, C. M. (1970). The professional nurse and body image. In C. E. Carlson (Ed.), *Behavioral concepts and nursing intervention.* Philadelphia: J. B. Lippincott.

North American Nursing Diagnosis Association (1986). *NANDA nursing diagnosis taxonomy I.* St. Louis: North American Nursing Diagnosis Association, St. Louis University School of Nursing.

Poster, E. C., & Beliz, L. (1992) The use of the Johnson Behavioral System Model to measure changes during adolescent hospitalization. *International Journal of Adolescence and Youth, 4,* 73–84.

Poster, E. C., Dee, V., & Randell, B. P. (1997). The Johnson Behavioral Systems Model as a framework for patient outcome evaluation. *Journal of the American Psychiatric Nurses Association, 3*(3), 73–80.

Rapoport, A. (1968). Foreword. In W. Buckley (Ed.), *Modern systems research for the behavioral scientist.* Chicago: Aldine.

Raudonis, B. M., & Acton, G. J. (1997). Theory-based nursing practice. *Journal of Advanced Nursing, 26*(1), 138–145.

Rawls, A. C. (1980). Evaluation of the Johnson behavioral model for clinical practice. Report on a test and evaluation of the Johnson theory. *IMAGE: Journal of Nursing Scholarship, 12*(1), 13–16.

Reynolds, W., & Cormack, D. (1991). An evaluation of the Johnson Behavioral System Model of nursing. *Journal of Advanced Nursing, 16,* 1122–1130.

Rogers, C. G. (1978). Conceptual models as guides to clinical nursing specialization. *The Journal of Nursing Education, 12,* 2–6.

Silva, M. C. (1977). Philosophy, science, theory: Interrelationships and implications for nursing research. *Image, 9,* 59–63.

Skolny, M. A., & Riehl, J. P. (1974). Hope: Solving patient and family problems by using a theoretical framework. In J. P. Riehl & S. C. Roy (Eds.), *Conceptual models for nursing practice.* New York: Appleton-Century-Crofts.

Small, B. (1980). Nursing visually impaired children with Johnson's model as a conceptual framework. In J. P. Riehl & S. C. Roy (Eds.), *Conceptual models for nursing practice.* New York: Appleton-Century-Crofts.

Stevens, B. (1979). *Nursing theory: Analysis, applications, evaluation.* Boston: Little Brown.

Stuifbergen, A., Becker, H., Rogers, S., Timmerman, G., & Kullberg, V. (1999). Promoting wellness for women with multiple sclerosis. *Journal of Neuroscience Nursing, 31*(2), 73–79.

Walker, L. O., & Avant, K. C. (1983). *Strategies for theory construction in nursing.* East Norwalk: CT. Appleton-Century-Crofts.

7

Orem's Model of Self-Care

Original Chapter by Hertha L. Gast
Updated by Kristen S. Montgomery

In the late 1950s, Dorothea Orem originated the self-care model of nursing as a way to define "nursing's domain and boundaries," and to articulate a "field of knowledge" for nursing commensurate with nursing as a "field of practice" (Orem, 1991, p. v). Her interest in clarifying the domain of nursing and systematically developing nursing knowledge arose, in part, because she was asked to design curricula for nurses at various educational levels. To that end she posed the question, "What is the proper object of nursing?" Reportedly, the answer came to her in the form of an insight, which was that nursing is needed when persons are unable to provide for themselves the amount and quality of self-care needed to regulate their own functioning and development because of personal health problems. This insight closely parallels the definition of nursing proposed by Henderson during the same time period, namely, that the nurse functions "to assist the individual, sick or well, in the performance of those activities . . . that he/she would perform unaided if he/she had the necessary strength, will or knowledge" (Harmer, 1955, p. 4). Orem acknowledged this parallel, but, according to her claim, was not directly influenced by Henderson.

The self-care theory of nursing was developed over a period of several years in collaboration with a group of scholars known as the Nursing Development Conference Group. This development can be traced in six editions of a basic text written by Orem: *Nursing: Concepts of Practice*

(1971, 1980, 1985, 1991, 1995, 2001) and two editions of a book edited by Orem, but based on the work of the Nursing Development Conference Group: *Concept Formalization in Nursing: Process and Product* (1973, 1979). The 1991 edition of the basic text incorporates the work of the Nursing Development Conference Group because this group disbanded and the book they produced is out of print.

The primary theory development strategy used both by Orem and the Nursing Development Conference Group was induction from practice. Orem claimed that "formulation and expression of a general theory of nursing proceeds as a creative synthesis of the conceptualized recurring dominant features of nursing situations and the relationships among them" (Orem, 1991, p. 58). Induction from practice is clearly evident in Orem's detailed accounts of how concepts in the theory were determined and defined based on "experiences in concrete nursing practice situations or results of analyses of nursing case materials" (Orem 1991, p.148). Of interest in this regard is the relative inattention given to literature in and outside of nursing as a source for theory development. Orem did, however, read widely and identified some of the major influences on her thinking, suggesting that there was an element of deduction in her work. Sources of influence include Kotarbinski's (1965) notions about praxiology, ideas about deliberate human action and motivation advanced by Arnold (1960), Parsons' (1937, 1951) ideas about units of action, and the notions of levels of good and desirable ends put forth by Lonergan (1972).

With regard to theory development for the discipline of nursing, Orem (1988, 1991) proposed a five-stage model in which knowledge becomes increasingly complex and integrated. Accordingly, in stage 1, concepts relevant to persons are delineated; in stage 2, variations in the qualitative and quantitative features of persons are described; in stage 3, description expands to the nursing care situation; in stage 4, nursing knowledge encompasses the entire nursing system; and stage 5 describes nursing systems for population groups. These stages parallel, to some extent, the four theory levels proposed by Dickoff, James, and Wiedenbach, (1968): factor isolating, factor relating, situation relating, and situation producing. Using her own classification scheme, Orem asserted that her work represents theory development at stages 1 to 3.

Epistemologically, according to her own claim, Orem embraced "a philosophical system of moderate realism" (Orem, 1991, p. 87). The self-care theory, thus, is in the tradition of logical positivism and the received view of the nature of knowledge. Further evidence for this is the lack of attention given to the influence of context in shaping the self-care theory; for example, to observer biases or historical context. In addition, an unspoken assumption underlying this work is that the conceptualization proposed is a product of objective observations of the practice field. Moreover, Orem explicitly contended that the theory is ". . . descriptively explanatory of the lawlike relationships or universal conditions implicit in [her] premises . . . " (Orem, 1991, p. 67).

Orem's position on the nature of science in nursing is similar to that held by Dickoff et al. (1968), who argued the case for nursing as practice discipline; her arguments in this regard are, however, unique. First is her portrayal of nursing as deliberate action; that is, action to affect certain results. Using her words: "Nursing in every instance of its practice is action deliberately performed by some members of a social group to bring about events and results that benefit others in specified ways" (Orem, 1991, p. 79; 1997). Second is her characterization of nursing as a practical science. Her sources of authority in arriving at this designation are Wallace (1983) and Maritain (1959), who differentiated practical sciences concerned with the principles and courses of things to be done from theoretical sciences concerned with things that are knowable about a subject of investigation. As a practical science, nursing is made up of two types of knowledge: speculatively practical and practically practical. The difference between speculatively and practically practical knowledge seems to pertain to a level of generality and abstraction. For example, concepts in the self-care theory are designated speculatively practical knowledge, whereas knowledge about self-care as it relates to a specific health condition would be designated practically practical knowledge. In addition, knowledge immediately transferable to (or abstracted from) practice would be practically practical. Of interest is the somewhat excessive use of the word *practical* in this discussion, to the point of awkwardness, which probably reflects the strength of Orem's position about the role of nursing knowledge in solving practice problems. A third type of knowledge in nursing is applied knowledge from other fields; this is not the same as the practical science of nursing.

The six editions of Orem's basic text give witness to her dedication in developing the self-care theory and her central position in this endeavor. Nevertheless, the theory has a relatively wide constituency that includes an international group of nursing scholars and scientists. Among the supports for the efforts of these scholars are the International Orem Society for Nursing Science and Scholarship, the annual International Conference on Self-Care Deficit Nursing Theory sponsored by the University of Missouri, and the Pre- and Postdoctoral Training Program in Self-Care Nursing at Wayne State University. There is a large body of literature pertaining to the theory, both in clinical articles and reports of research.

The popularity of the self-care theory is attributable to a number of reasons beyond those intended by Orem. Among them are consumerism and the self-help movement in health care, the fact that many contemporary health problems are related to lifestyle, and the shift to home health care as an alternative to hospitalization and as a way to control healthcare costs. It bears mentioning that, for the most part, Orem was not influenced by these developments in the healthcare scene. Her interest was not in self-care as a way to empower the consumer, affect healthy lifestyles, increase competence in home-based care, or control healthcare costs. In contrast, for her, self-care is the *sine qua non* of nursing; that is, the answer to the question, "What is the proper object of nursing?"

BASIC ELEMENTS IN THE MODEL

Orem presented her conceptualization in the form of a conceptual framework consisting of four concepts about persons and two about nursing, and three theories derived from this model: the *self-care deficit theory,* the *theory of self-care,* and the *theory of nursing system.* Structurally, each theory is presented as a set of assumptions or, to use her language, presuppositions, and a set of propositions. Concepts in the model are *self-care, self-care agency, self-care demand, self-care deficit, nursing agency,* and *nursing system.* An additional concept, *basic conditioning factors,* although not usually included as part of the model, is described in text, appears in some propositions, and contributes importantly to the explanatory power of the theory.

Definition of Nursing

Orem portrayed nursing as a unique field of knowledge and an action system; that is, as professional practice. As noted previously, nursing knowledge can be classified in terms of two levels of abstraction: speculatively practical and practically practical; both are aspects of nursing as a practical science. In this scheme, the self-care model is a contribution to the evolution of nursing as a practical science and an instance of speculatively practical knowledge. One of the noteworthy contributions of Orem, indeed an unequivocal impetus for her work, is the clarification of a distinctive focus for nursing knowledge and practice. For Orem, nursing is defined by its unique focus, or, using her words, by its proper object, that which legitimates nursing, or "criteria that members of the society use in determining whether a particular human service can or should be used" (Orem, 1991, p. 41). Nursing, when defined in terms of focus (for knowledge and practice), is a specialized health service necessitated by an adult's inability to maintain the amount and quality of self-care that is therapeutic in sustaining life and health, in recovering from disease or injury, or in coping with their effects.

Although nursing is a unique field of knowledge, it also is a complex action system (nursing as practice) that is goal oriented or results seeking.

This action system can be analyzed in terms of discrete units of action and, more generally, in terms of two phases or types of action also known as operations: *estimative* and *productive*. Estimative operations entail investigation, reflection, and judgments about the patient, including how the patient's situation can be improved and decisions about desired ends and means to achieve these improvements. Based on decisions about desired ends and means, productive operations entail planning and carrying out actions (means), and evaluating them in terms of the goal to be attained (desired ends). Although this language of operations is idiosyncratic to Orem, in effect, it is another way of describing what is more commonly known as the nursing process; the parallel to estimative operations being assessment, diagnosis, and planning, and the parallel to productive operations being intervention and evaluation. Language somewhat more consistent with traditional descriptions of nursing process appears in the 1985 edition of Orem's text; however, this is less so in the 1991 and more recent editions. In the 1985 text, three steps of the nursing process are described: diagnosis and prescription, design and planning, and production and control. A straightforward case application of these steps that also incorporates the language of estimative and productive operations was provided by Taylor (1988), a major interpreter of Orem's work. In this application, Taylor designated all steps of the nursing process as operations, and equated estimative operations with diagnosis, and productive operations with intervention (production and control in Orem's 1985 characterization of nursing process). Thus, although it is not clear whether estimative and productive operations subsume the steps of the nursing process (as seems to be the case in Orem's description of the two operations) or whether the steps of the nursing process subsume these operations (as seems to be the case in Taylor's interpretation), the phenomena being described in either case are the same.

Performing the operations of nursing or engaging in the nursing process constitutes the professional-technological dimension of nursing practice that is embedded in the interpersonal and social dimensions. The social dimension refers to the laws and standards that govern nursing practice and the social structures in which nursing is practiced. The interpersonal dimension refers to relationships among the nurse, the patient, and the family. Important in this regard is that the needs of the patient are determined, and decisions about role arrangements among the nurse, the patient, and the family are made in the context of the interpersonal dimension of practice.

Orem proposed two concepts to depict nursing: nursing agency and nursing systems. Nursing agency is the complex property of persons trained as nurses that enables them to help others with respect to their self-care or in the care of others. Nursing agency is a corollary to another concept in the theory, self-care agency, which depicts the abilities that enable the patient to perform self-care. Indeed, Orem portrayed the nurse as ". . . 'another self,' in a figurative sense, for the person under nursing care" (Orem, 1991, p. 61). The abilities of the nurse (nursing agency) are acquired through formal education and training and are in that respect specialized and unique to nursing. Moreover, the abilities of the nurse are used in the service of the patient—more specifically, toward helping the patient with self-care issues. The term *agency* depicts abilities as well as the reflection and deliberation needed to perform the estimative and productive operations of nursing practice.

Nurses "exercise" their nursing agency through operations (estimative and productive) in the context of their interpersonal relationships with patients to create nursing systems. A nursing system coordinates the role relationship between the nurse and the patient and consists of the action sequences of the nurse and the patient in the interest of accomplishing the patient's requirements for self-care. Orem proposed three types of nursing system that vary in terms of the degree to which the patient is able to accomplish self-care requirements. In a wholly compensatory nursing system, the nurse takes over all self-care functions for the patient who is completely unable to act on his or her own behalf; in a partly compensatory nursing system, the nurse performs some self-care measures for the patient whose ability to act on his or her own behalf is limited; in a supportive-educative nursing system, the nurse provides education and support for the patient so that he or she will be able to successfully meet his- or herself-care requirements. Nursing systems are helping systems in which the method of helping is determined by the degree to which the patient is able to accomplish his-or herself-care requirements. As with nursing systems, methods of helping can be classified in terms of the extensiveness of help provided: (a) doing for another; (b) guiding and directing another; (c) providing physical support; (d) providing psychological support; (e) providing a supportive environment; and (f) teaching.

Definition of Person

Orem described the person as able to appraise situations, reflect upon them, and reason and understand them. Based on this description, the person deliberately chooses to perform specific actions, something he or she can do even in the face of internal and external pressures to the contrary. Moreover, actions are goal directed; that is, undertaken to achieve valued outcomes (Orem, 1997). This view of the person as self-determined, action oriented, and goal directed is captured in Orem's portrayal of the person as agent or as having agency. In putting forth this view, Orem challenged, to some extent, the more prevalent view in nursing that the person is an adaptive system and can be understood as adapting to his or her environment.

Although difficult to trace, the use of the terms *agent* and *agency* seems to have some connection to the notion of self-as-agent advanced in the field of philosophy by Macmurray (1957).

Four concepts in the self-care theory derive from this general view of person and are descriptive of the person in the context of nursing: self-care agency, self-care, therapeutic self-demand, and self-care deficit. In a general sense, the term *agency* refers to the capacity of the person to voluntarily and deliberately engage in goal-achieving actions. A part of this is the capacity to engage in actions directed toward one's own health and well being. Orem labeled this more specific capacity self-care agency. More formally defined, self-care agency is the complex acquired ability to meet one's continuous requirements for care that regulates life processes, maintains structural and functional integrity, and promotes development and well-being. Extensive descriptions of this complex ability (self-care agency) come from the work of Orem and the Nursing Development Conference Group. In these descriptions, self-care agency is depicted as consisting of three types of abilities: (a) general abilities of the person that are not specific to engagement in self-care, which are called foundational capabilities and dispositions; (b) abilities that generally enable one to engage in self-care operations, referred to as the power components (from the notion of power to perform self-care); and (c) abilities that relate directly to performing the operations of self-care.

Backsheider, a member of the Nursing Development Conference Group (1973, 1979), is credited with explicating the foundational capabilities and dispositions of self-care agency. According to her analysis, these abilities include fundamental functions such as sensation, perception, and memory; rational and intellectual abilities; self-understanding; and abilities pertaining to orientation and organization. The notion of foundational capabilities and dispositions is exceedingly broad, something that is all the more evident in the research literature emanating from this theory in which concepts as varied as ego development (Gast, 1984), sense of coherence (Baker, 1992), coping dispositions (Haas, 1990), and depression (West, 1993) are viewed as foundational abilities.

Abilities of the second type in the self-care agency concept are more specific to self-care and were labeled power components. Ten such abilities were proposed, all in the context of performing self-care: (a) attention; (b) physical energy; (c) mobility; (d) reasoning; (e) motivation; (f) decision making; (g) use of technical knowledge; (h) repertoire of skills; (i) organization and coordination; and (j) integration of self-care with other aspects of life. These abilities enable one to engage in three types of self-care operations: estimative, transitional, and productive. Although not clear in Orem's writings, abilities of the third type in the self-care agency concept are specific abilities to perform these operations. In the case of estimative operations, this would mean ability to assess oneself with regard to needs for self-care. For transitional operations, abilities would pertain to deciding on a course of action, and for productive operations, abilities would pertain to preparing for, performing, and monitoring self-care actions.

Persons develop the abilities that constitute self-care agency over time and in the context of various social structures. Self-care agency can therefore be assessed with regard to how developed it is. In addition, self-care agency can be assessed for how operable it is at a given time, indicating that abilities, even when developed, may not always be operable. An example of this would be the self-care abilities of a person immediately after receiving anesthesia. Finally, self-care agency can be assessed for adequacy by determining whether abilities for self-care are commensurate with the need for self-care.

To the extent that persons have abilities for self-care (self-care agency), they can perform self-care. Orem (1991) defined self-care as "activities that individuals initiate and perform on their own behalf in maintaining life, health, and well-being" (p. 117). As such, self-care consists of behaviors, or actions, that persons perform in the interest of their health and well-being. Additional descriptors for these behaviors are that they are learned, deliberately chosen, and intentional, and that they may or may not have a desired salutary effect. In addition, these behaviors can be oriented toward changing internal aspects of the self, such as thoughts and feelings, or toward moderating external realities, such as aspects of the environment. As action, self-care proceeds through three phases or the three sequential operations described previously: estimative, transitional, and productive. In other words, in a self-care event the person assesses the need for self-care, decides on a course of action, and then plans, executes, and evaluates the course of action.

The concept, therapeutic self-care demand, describes a typology of necessary self-care actions. Therapeutic self-care demand stands for the sum of the self-care measures required to meet the specific self-care requisites of a person at a point in time. Generally, self-care requisites are necessary and purposeful actions of three types: *universal, developmental,* and *health deviation.* Overall, the purpose achieved by these actions is to support life processes, maintain structural and functional integrity, and promote development and well-being; this explains the use of the adjective *therapeutic* in describing the self-care demand. Universal requisites are actions that all persons need to take and are described as (a) maintaining a sufficient intake of air, water, and food; (b) managing elimination processes; (c) maintaining a balance between activity and rest; (d) maintaining a balance between solitude and social interaction; (e) preventing hazards to life, health, and well-being; and (f) promoting normalcy. Developmental requisites are actions that support normal development or are needed at certain developmental stages. Health-deviation requisites are actions occasioned by health problems and treatment regimens. At a given time the therapeutic self-care demand for a person is calculated by evaluating the need for specific actions in these areas.

To determine a need for nursing, the nurse considers whether the abilities (self-care agency) of the person are adequate for accomplishing the self-care demand. If the self-care demand exceeds self-care agency (i.e., when there is a limitation in self-care agency), a self-care deficit is said to exist and a need for nursing is established. In the theory, a self-care deficit is defined as a relationship between self-care agency and the therapeutic self-care demand in which self-care agency is not equal to some or all components of the therapeutic self-care demand. Orem specifically qualified the self-care deficit as a relationship and not a disorder of the person. Deficits can be complete or partial and as such indicate whether a wholly or partially compensatory nursing system is needed to accomplish the self-care demand. Although Orem delineated types of limitations in abilities for self-care, this is necessarily redundant with the notion that abilities described as the complex components of self-care agency can be judged with regard to their development, operability, and adequacy. The important aspect of the self-care deficit concept is that it identifies the need for nursing; nursing is needed only in the case of an existing or potential self-care deficit. In the case of a potential self-care deficit, a supportive educative nursing system would be appropriate.

Although Orem presented her theory assuming the individual to be the unit of service, she also considered the possibility of other units of service. These are described as multiperson units and include caregivers, families, residential groups, and groups that meet for specific health-related purposes. Among these, caregivers are the only unit to receive any formal attention in the theory in the form of the concepts of dependent-care agency and dependent care. These concepts are analogous to the concepts of self-care agency and self-care except that, in the case of the caregiver, the care needs addressed are those of a child or dependent adult. Definitions are provided for the concepts of dependent-care agency and dependent care; nevertheless, these concepts are less fully developed than those pertaining to the individual. For example, there is little to describe the abilities that constitute dependent-care agency or dependent-care requirements. Other multiperson units, while acknowledged, are given even less systematic attention in Orem's writings. Orem, did, however, endorse Taylor's (1989) interpretation of family in the context of the self-care theory (Orem, 1991, p. 296).

Definition of Health

According to Orem, nursing is one of a family of healthcare services. The unique focus in nursing is the potential or actual self-care deficits of patients that can be addressed through nursing systems. When self-care deficits are addressed, self-care requisites are met, meaning that actions that persons need to take on their own behalf in the interest of supporting life processes, maintaining structural and functional integrity, and promoting development and well-being are accomplished. Important in this regard is that these actions, whether taken by the patient or the nurse (on behalf of the patient), in and of themselves do not determine health and well-being outcomes even though they are directed toward that end. Stated otherwise, self-care (the focus of nursing) is a necessary but not sufficient predictor of health and well-being.

Orem described health as the state of being sound and whole, *sound* meaning strength, vigor and the absence of disease, and *whole* meaning that nothing is missing or diminished. Repeated in her discussion of health is the notion of structural and functional integrity, which suggests that health pertains not only to one's bodily state but also to how one functions in everyday living. Progressive development, that is, movement toward higher and higher levels of integration, also is an aspect of health. Physical, psychological, interpersonal, and social aspects of health are considered to be inseparable based on a unitary view of human beings that rejects the duality of mind and body. In a healthcare context, judgments about health are made by professionals based on systematic data collection and a complex set of norms.

Although health is a state of the person as determined by a set of norms, well-being relates to the person's perceived state of being. Well-being is the experience of contentment, pleasure, and happiness; it may entail spiritual experiences; it is evident in movement toward fulfilling ideals and continuing personalization; and it is associated with success in personal endeavors and sufficient resources. Importantly, persons can experience well-being even under conditions of adversity and in the absence of structural and functional integrity. As with health, well-being is, in part, an outcome of self-care; however, self-care is not a sufficient condition for well-being.

It adds to the complexity of Orem's conceptualization that health is presented as an outcome of self-care *and* as one of numerous factors that influence self-care agency and self-care demand. To clarify, a person in a poor state of health is likely to have diminished self-care agency; moreover, a poor state of health is likely to occasion health-deviation requisites that add to the person's self-care demand. It follows that a person in a poor state of health is likely to experience a self-care deficit.

Definition of Environment

There is little explicit attention to the concept of environment in Orem's writings. The claim is made that person and environment are a functional unit in which exchanges are reciprocal and influence is mutual. In that regard, Orem contended that person and environment are separate entities only "in our thought processes" and that it requires considerable sophistication to conceptualize them as a single unit (Orem, 1991, p. 143). In addition, persons are viewed as existing in their environments and never isolated from them. Features of the environment can be described and evaluated for their impact on the health and well-being of the person and the family; some of these features also can be regulated to effect better outcomes for the person. Orem listed numerous environmental features and claimed that they can be generally classified in four types: physical, chemical, biologic, and social.

The concept of basic conditioning factors, although peripheral in the theory, applies directly to the environment, albeit only in part. This concept is described in greater detail in a subsequent section; however, briefly stated, basic conditioning factors are human and environmental properties that affect the person's self-care agency and therapeutic self-care demand. Although there are inconsistencies in Orem's analysis of this concept, basic conditioning factors can be classified into three types: one of them being "factors that relate persons within family constellations and sociocultural groups," and a second being "factors that describe individuals in their worlds of existence" (Orem, 1991, p. 237). Basic conditioning factors of the first type include the person's family system and sociocultural orientation; factors of the second type include patterns of living of the person, environmental factors, healthcare system factors, and resource availability and adequacy. One can conclude from this analysis that environment, as conceptualized in this theory, is a wide spectrum of contextual factors that influence the abilities of the person for self-care (self-care agency) and the need for self-care (therapeutic self-care demand).

INTERRELATIONSHIPS AMONG CONCEPTS OF NURSING, PERSON, HEALTH, AND ENVIRONMENT

In Orem's model, relationships are further described in the form of three sets of propositions that make up the theory of self-care, the theory of self-care deficit, and the theory of nursing system. It is difficult to arrive at a straightforward specification of relationships among the seven concepts in the theory from these sets of propositions because several propositions are existence statements or definitional statements and most propositions are constructed using language other than the formal language of the theory. Nevertheless, one can conclude that (a) basic conditioning factors influence the self-care agency and therapeutic self-care demand of the person; (b) self-care agency enables the person to perform self-care; (c) self-care is directed toward accomplishing the self-care demand; (d) a self-care deficit exists when the self-care demand of a person exceeds his or her self-care agency; and (e) nursing agency enables the nurse to assess potential or actual self-care deficits of a person and construct a nursing system to address these deficits.

Orem's most recent work (2001) is the 6th edition of her text, *Nursing: Concepts of Practice.* New to this text is the chapter entitled "The Practical Science of Nursing," in which she describes three practice sciences: (a) wholly compensatory nursing science, (b) partly compensatory nursing science, and (c) supportive-developmental nursing science. These are identified as the way the nurse practices and are similar to medicine's practice sciences (e.g., internal medicine, surgery) (Fawcett, 2001; Orem, 2001). These practice sciences are related to her "foundational sciences" that are now called "the science of self-care, the science of the development and exercise of self-care agency, and the science of human assistance for persons with health-associated self-care deficits" (Fawcett, 2001, p. 35). Each of the practice sciences (wholly compensatory, partly compensatory, supportive-developmental) has cases, models, and rules of practice for types of cases. Orem (2001) provides a beginning foundation that needs to be further developed into content, the operations of nursing practice (or nursing process), to ensure that the theory is relevant to practice.

Descriptions of Other Concepts in the Model

As noted earlier, a peripheral concept in the theory is basic conditioning factors, which denotes aspects of the person and the environment that influence self-care agency and self-care demand. Orem (1991) proposed the following list of 10 basic conditioning factors, but with the caveat that this list may need to be amended: (a) age, (b) gender, (c) developmental level, (d) health state, (e) sociocultural orientation, (f) healthcare system, (g) family system, (h) patterns of living, (i) environmental factors, and (j) resource availability and adequacy. Included in her analysis are two sets of general categories for classifying these factors; however, no explanation is provided for why two sets are needed and how they relate to one another. One set, which seems to have been derived inductively from descriptions of cases provided by a group of clinical nurse specialists, depicts basic conditioning factors as they pertain to various characteristics of the patient, the patterns of living of the patient, the patient's health state and healthcare regimen, and the developmental state of the patient. The other set seems to have been proposed primarily as a scheme for classifying the 10 basic conditioning factors. As such, age, gender, and developmental state are factors descriptive of individuals; family system and sociocultural orientation are factors that locate persons within families and sociocultural groups; and health state, healthcare system, pattern of living, environment, and resource availability and adequacy are factors that describe individuals in their worlds of existence. Clearly, the concept of basic conditioning factors is very broad; as indicated earlier, this concept adds substantially to the explanatory power of the theory.

INTERNAL ANALYSIS AND EVALUATION

Underlying Assumptions

Orem clarified two sets of assumptions about human beings, several premises about human beings, and three sets of presuppositions corresponding to the three theories that make up the self-care theory. These were considered to be different types of statements in that premises were viewed as "true and not merely assumed" (Orem, 1991, p. 67) and presuppositions were presented as immediate precursors to the propositions of the theory. The assumptions about human beings were derived from Arnold's (1960) ideas about human action and motivation and are a late addition to Orem's work, appearing for the first time in the 1991 edition of her text. In the first set of assumptions, human beings are said to (a) know and appraise situations in terms of their effects on ends being sought; (b) know directly by sensing, but also through reflection, reasoning, and understanding; (c) be capable of self-determined action even when faced with an emotional pull in the opposite direction; (d) be able to prolong reflection indefinitely in deliberating about what action to take by raising questions and attending to different aspects of a situation and different possibilities for action; (e) be able to concentrate on a suitable course of action and exclude other courses of action; (f) engage in purposeful actions; and (g) act deliberately to attain goals (Orem, 1991, pp. 80–81). The second set of assumptions about conditions necessary for human action can be summarized as (a) persons need time and knowledge to clarify desired goals, and review and decide on actions to attain them; and (b) persons incorporate deliberations and choices about goals and actions into their self-image (Orem, 1991, p. 81).

In contrast to assumptions, premises about human beings were viewed as true and universally applicable statements. The following premises were proposed: (a) to stay alive and function, human beings must continuously and deliberately perform self- and environmentally directed actions; (b) human beings have agency, which is the power to act deliberately in identifying a need for action and in performing self- and environmentally directed actions; (c) human beings can experience limitations in their agency; (d) human agency also entails the power to help another person identify a need for action and perform self- or environmentally directed actions; and (e) human beings can work together in structured groups to help other persons identify the need for action and perform self- and environmentally directed actions.

Presuppositions are the third type of statement presented and accompany the propositions for each of the three theories that constitute the self-care theory. The first of the three theories, the theory of self-care, has seven propositions consisting of descriptive statements about self-care and relational statements that link self-care and self-care requisites. These propositions rest on the following presuppositions: (a) human beings can develop the skills essential to performing self-care; (b) means used to meet self-care requisites vary for persons in different cultural and social groups; (c) self-care as deliberate action is determined, in part, by the action repertoire of the person and the person's predilection for action at a point in time; and (d) when persons have recurring self-care requisites and establish consistent means to meet them, they form self-care habits.

The second theory, the theory of self-care deficit, has six propositions that posit relationships between self-care agency and self-care demand, nursing and the presence of a self-care deficit, and basic conditioning factors and self-care agency. Nine presuppositions arranged into two sets were viewed as foundational to these propositions. The first set pertains to the influence of environmental change, values, culture, and social context on self-care abilities and self-care. Presuppositions in the second set, summarized as follows, are that (a) societies institute ways to aid persons who are socially dependent; (b) social dependence can be age-related or health-related; and (c) in Western civilization nursing is regarded as one of a family of health services.

The third theory, the theory of nursing system, has eight propositions that pertain to relationships between nursing and self-care deficits, and describe the estimative and productive operations of nursing, the complementary roles of nurse and patient, and the nursing system. These propositions rest on the presuppositions that (a) nursing as a practical endeavor can be located in time and space; and (b) the "proper object" of nursing delimits the boundaries and unique domain of nursing as an institutionalized health service.

By way of evaluation, several conclusions can be drawn from the analysis. It is clear that Orem gave a lot of attention to the task of specifying underlying beliefs and relating them to theory propositions. The assumptions derived from Arnold (1960) are particularly helpful in clarifying beliefs about human beings that shaped the theory. The premises and pre-suppositions are somewhat problematic because, in many cases, they are similar to, even indistinguishable from, the propositions of the theory ex-cept that they have been rephrased. In a critique of the self-care theory, Smith (1987) argued that the premises and presuppositions in this theory are at a concrete, empirical level of discourse and "do not express a singu-lar belief in a clear way at either the philosophical or more general level of discourse" (p. 93). Typically, theories are constructed so that induction and deduction occur across three levels of discourse: general philosophical statements, a given conceptualization, and empirical statements. In Orem's work, there is little movement across these levels of discourse, given that most statements (premises, presuppositions, and propositions) are rela-tively concrete; redundancies apparent across statements are a conse-quence of this.

RELATIVE IMPORTANCE OF BASIC CONCEPTS AND OTHER COMPONENTS OF THE THEORY

The relative popularity and widespread adoption of the self-care theory in nursing attests to its importance as a conceptualization. Meleis (1997) attrib-uted this to the language of the theory, which corresponds to traditional lan-guage in nursing about human needs and functions, and also to the fact that this language necessitates only a gentle and gradual shift from the medical model and is not alien to the medical model. One could argue that this theory is appealing because it is relatively concrete, was derived inductively from practice, and was envisioned by Orem as contributing to the practical science of nursing; it is thus close to practice and comprehensible even for the aver-age practitioner. Another reason for its popularity is the contemporary em-phasis on self-care in health care in general. Finally, it accomplishes to some extent what Orem intended; that is, it delineates a unique focus for nursing, and thus serves to circumscribe nursing as a discipline and practice domain.

The concepts of basic conditioning factors, self-care agency, and self-care are particularly noteworthy for their contribution to nursing knowledge; all are richly descriptive and extensively developed. Basic conditioning fac-tors are 10 types of environmental or personal factors that influence abilities and demand for self-care; of these, six are broad contextual factors, such as the family system of the person and the person's cultural affiliation. Although the analysis of this concept was considered to be incomplete, contextual fac-tors identified to date contribute significantly to our capacity to explain self-care. The concept of self-care agency contributes importantly to the extent that it conveys a nonmechanistic view of the person as agent. It also focuses attention on health-related abilities of persons, not just actions, and amply describes these abilities at three levels, including 10 types of abilities specific to self-care known as the power components. In the concept of self-care demand, the extensive descriptions of three types of self-care requisites, in effect, constitute a typology of self-care actions that persons need to perform in the interest of their health and well-being. Although this typology is clearly useful, it is worth noting that self-care requisites actually are self-care norms and thus not concrete phenomena that can be examined empirically.

Although less extensively developed, the concept of nursing systems as three types of nurse-patient configurations (wholly and partly compensatory and educative-supportive) also contributes to the descriptiveness of the theory. This is less the case for the concepts of self-care and self-care deficit. Presumably, a systematic description of normative self-care would be redundant with the three types of self-care requisites because requisites are actions persons need to perform in the interest of their health and well-being. Self-care deficit seems to be a derivative concept with no actual concrete referent because it refers to the particular relationship between self-care agency and self-care demand in which demand exceeds agency. It bears mentioning that Orem viewed this concept as important because it identifies *the* condition that occasions the need for nursing.

IMPORTANCE OF RELATIONSHIPS BETWEEN BASIC CONCEPTS AND OTHER COMPONENTS OF THE THEORY

Among the relationships posited in this theory, the relationships between basic conditioning factors and self-care agency or self-care demand, and between self-care agency and self-care are the most straightforward. Arguably, the agency-action relationship is important because it focuses attention on complex intrapersonal reasons for the health-related behaviors of patients. The same can be said for the relationship between basic conditioning factors and self-care agency, which focuses attention on numerous factors that explain variance in abilities for self-care and self-care needs. Other relationships are less clear. For example, a relationship is stated between self-care agency and self-care demand in which demand can be equal to or greater than agency. However, given that self-care demand is actually a set of normative expectations, a rephrasing of this statement would be that the adequacy of a person's self-care agency is determined based on a set of norms about what a person ought to do in the interest of his or her health and well-being. Curiously, Orem claimed that the nurse assesses the relationship between demand and ability (agency), *not* demand and action (self-care), to assess the presence of a self-care deficit. The relationship posited between nursing systems and actual or potential self-care deficits also is more complicated than it seems: First, because a nursing system coordinates nurse and patient abilities and actions; and second, because the nurse can influence the deficit indirectly through her impact on the self-care agency of the person or directly by performing actions the patient ordinarily would perform for himself.

As noted earlier, health and well-being are not the explicit dependent variables in this theory as one might expect. Indeed, health state as a conditioning factor is an independent variable that predicts, in part, abilities and needs for self-care and, thus, whether a self-care deficit is likely. In other words, the person in a poor state of health is likely to have a diminished capacity for self-care and an increased demand for self-care and, thus, experience a self-care deficit. The explicit outcome variable in this theory would seem to be potential or actual self-care deficits. One can, however, imply that a lessening of the deficit leads to improved health or well-being because, by definition, self-care is directed toward that end. Health and well-being have been viewed as self-care outcomes in some of the studies emanating from this theory. A notable example is a study reported by Denyes (1988) using an aggregate sample from five previous studies of well adolescents. Support was found for the following sequence of relationships: health problem as a basic conditioning factor→ self-care agency→ self-care→ health as a general state.

Analysis of Internal Consistency

Orem provided formal definitions for all concepts in the self-care theory and, for the most part, these definitions are used consistently throughout her writings. As indicated above, the concepts of basic conditioning factors, self-care agency, self-care demand, and nursing systems received extensive analyses but this is less the case for self-care, self-care deficit, and nursing agency. There are several inconsistencies across analyses that in some instances seem to be a consequence of Orem's attempt to bring together her analyses and those undertaken by the Nursing Development Conference Group. Logical problems that relate to the concepts in this theory include the unclear boundaries between certain concepts and the use of concepts with no referents, or concepts that are in effect criteria for evaluating the substantive concepts. For example, what is the logical argument for viewing some broad person characteristics as basic conditioning factors and others as foundational capabilities and dispositions of self-care agency? Similarly, what are the boundaries between foundational capabilities, power components, and abilities specific to performing self-care operations in the concept of self-care agency? As previously noted, the self-care deficit concept has no concrete referent; rather, it designates an evaluation made about the adequacy of self-care abilities. The self-care requisites that constitute the self-care demand also have no concrete referents but describe norms for self-care actions that can be used to classify or evaluate actual self-care or to determine the adequacy of self-care abilities. In support of this analysis is the one offered by Smith (1987), who argued that the concepts of self-care agency, self-care, self-care deficit, and self-care demand are so closely tied to each other that it might be more logically coherent to view them as points of elaboration for a single concept—self-care.

Logical problems also are apparent in the relational aspects of this theory. First, the use of three theories with separate sets of assumptions and propositions lacks logical defense. The various formal statements in these theories also are inherently problematic. As already stated, there is little in the way of logical deduction from assumptions to propositions because all statements are at the concrete empirical level of discourse. Second, several propositions are existence or definitional statements. Interestingly, Orem used terms that define concepts instead of the concepts per se in constructing the formal statements of the theory, resulting in language that is excessive and ultimately obfuscating. Smith (1987) attributed this to the concreteness of the conceptualization and to Orem's tendency to attempt clarification primarily through restatement or further elaboration.

Analysis of External Consistency

One can infer external consistency from the widespread adoption of the self-care theory. Even so, worthwhile criticisms pertaining to external consistency are that (a) the theory is primarily illness focused and does not support health promotion as a nursing function; (b) the theory is culturally biased; (c) the theory leads to an overemphasis on competence and independence in self-care; (d) personal characteristics are given too central a position among the possible predictors of health outcomes; and (e) eventually this theory could serve to increase the medicalization of personal health-related activities and, therefore, could paradoxically serve to foster dependence with regard to health care.

Melnyk (1983), among others, claimed that the self-care theory excludes a health-promotion focus given its emphasis on self-care deficits that result from health problems. Although understandable, this criticism is not entirely justified. It is true that, more often than not, Orem characterized nursing as a service to people who, because they are in a poor state of health, are unable to perform some or all of their self-care. Yet, in the formal conceptualization, health state is merely a *possible* factor among numerous basic conditioning factors that influence self-care abilities, indicating that the presence of a health problem is not assumed. Moreover, as a service nursing can also address potential self-care deficits, primarily in the form of supportive educative nursing systems. Interestingly, the clinical and research literature coming from this theory has many health-promotion applications. Good examples are Hartweg's (1993) study of well-being-related self-care actions of healthy middle-aged women, Moore's (1987a, 1987b, 1993) studies of self-care agency in school-aged children, and Cretain's (1989) studies of breast self-examination.

Several scholars have argued that the self-care theory is not appropriate for group-oriented cultures because it rests on an ideology of individualism in which autonomy, self-determinism, and self-reliance are highly valued (Anna, Christensen, Hohon, Ord, & Wells, 1978; Leininger, 1993). To counter this, proponents of the Orem theory have argued that cultural determinants of personal healthcare practices are accounted for in the notion of culture as a basic conditioning factor that influences self-care agency and demand. The cultural criticism seems somewhat hard to sustain given the widespread adoption of this theory outside the North American culture, including in Australia (Avery, 1992), in Brazil (Beckman, 1987), in England (Clark & Bishop, 1988; Dyer, 1990; Hunter, 1992), in Germany (Whetstone, 1987), with Navajo Indians (Hammons, 1985), in the Netherlands and Scandinavia (Lorenson, Holter, Evers, Isenberg, & van Acterberg, 1993; van Acterberg et al., 1991; Whetstone & Hansson, 1989), in New Zealand (Finnegan, 1986), with Puerto Ricans (Chamorro, 1985), in Thailand (Dier, 1987; Hanucharurnkul, 1989; Hanucharurnkul & Vinyanguag, 1991), and with Vietnamese (Hautman, 1987).

In a critical theory context, one can argue that this theory neglects or gives insufficient attention to important contextual and environmental factors that influence health outcomes (for example, poverty, racism, and environmental pollution). To the degree that self-care theory directs the patient and the nurse to target their efforts on improving self-care, it may divert attention from unhealthful social and environmental structures even when they are robust predictors of health outcomes. In defense of the theory is the argument that contextual and environmental influences are addressed in the concept of basic conditioning factors; moreover, self-care includes actions of the patient or the nurse (on behalf of the patient) directed at environmental changes that improve the patient's health and well-being. In a critique of self-care ideology, Northrup (1993) acknowledged that "self-care can become a process of empowerment and a vehicle for social transformation" (p. 65). She warned, however, that "the empowering process that engages people in critical analysis of root causes as the basis of social action differs from the emphasis on achievement of attainable goals," (p. 65) and questioned whether the self-care ideology currently being articulated in nursing concurs with the tenet's critical scholarship.

In a somewhat different vein, Northrup (1993) claimed that greater dependence in health care could be a paradoxical outcome of the widespread adoption of the self-care ideology in nursing. Using a line of reasoning similar to that advanced by Illich (1976), one could anticipate that increasingly institutionalized nursing claims to self-care expertise would likely serve to erode lay confidence in self-care. In effect, if self-care were increasingly medicalized, nursing self-care expertise would increasingly become a commodity in the marketplace, and patients would experience ever-growing needs to purchase self-care expertise. In that regard, Northrup noted that "contemporary proponents of self-care have a tendency to confuse self-determination with the exercise of consumer choice" (p. 62). Leininger's (1988) theory, which directs attention to two systems of health care, professional and folk, is instructive in this regard.

Analysis of Pragmatic Adequacy

The literature describes many applications of the self-care theory in practice. Arguably, the pragmatic appeal of this theory is a function of its relative concreteness and its success in delineating a discrete focus for nursing assessment and intervention. Some concepts and relationships have proven to be more helpful in guiding practice than others. The concept of self-care as actions, behaviors, or practices of a person has had particular appeal, all the more so because required self-care is systematically and richly described in the concept of self-care requisites. A noteworthy example of how this concept has been used in practice is the set of universal self-care assessment protocols for psychiatric patients emanating from the work of Underwood (1979, 1980; Morrison, Fisber, Wilson, & Underwood, 1985; Ringerman & Luz, 1990). The concept of self-care agency also is highly descriptive, but exceedingly complex, which probably detracts from its practical utility. Although presented as a single concept depicting abilities for self-care and implying self-determinism, self-care agency encompasses a wide spectrum of general and specific attributes as disparate as personality traits, physical energy, mobility, motivation, knowledge, and skill. Among the relationships posited in the theory, the relationships among basic conditioning factors, self-care agency, and self-care are particularly useful in practice because they lead the clinician to consider complex contextual and personal factors that explain self-care behaviors. Finally, the concept of nursing systems aptly describes types of nurse-patient configurations in practice.

Analysis of Empirical Adequacy

The self-care theory has generated a relatively large body of research, however, only a portion of this meets Silva's (1986) criteria for theory testing research. Germane to evaluating the empirical adequacy of Orem's theory are various attempts to operationalize major concepts of the theory: self-care agency, self-care, and nursing systems, and studies of relationships stated in the theory propositions. Operational measures of self-care agency using paper and pencil self-report questionnaires have received the most attention and there now are five measures of this concept at various stages of development. Of these, four were compared in terms of their conceptual structure in a review article by a group of Orem scholars at Wayne State University (Gast et al., 1989); three were compared in an empirical study by McBride (1991); and one postdates either of these reviews (Geden & Taylor, 1991). Briefly, these instruments are (a) the Exercise of Self-Care Agency Scale developed by Kearney and Fleischer (1979), factor analyzed by Reisch and Hauck (1988), and studied for psychometric properties by McBride (1987); (b) the Denyes Self-Care Agency Instrument developed by Denyes (1982) for adolescents but used subsequently for adults as well; (c) the Perception of Self-Care Agency Questionnaire developed by Hanson and Bickel (1985), subsequently analyzed by Weaver (1987), and critiqued by Cleveland (1989); (d) the Appraisal of Self-Care Agency Scale developed and tested cross-culturally by a group of Dutch and American researchers (van Acterberg et al., 1991; Lorsenson et al., 1993); and (e) the Self-As-Carer Inventory developed by Geden and Taylor (1991) as a revision of the Perception of Self-Care Agency Questionnaire. A newer related article examines measurement issues for the concept of self-care agency (Carter, 1998). Carter identified that one of the main difficulties of comparing research that measures self-care agency is the varying conceptual definition and instruments used. She notes that researchers need to examine carefully whether they wish to measure an individual's personal abilities for self-care or the actions that will be taken by the individual for self-care, and then choose the appropriate instrument to achieve this goal.

For the most part, these instruments operationalize the power components of self-care agency; in each case the power component analysis was used to inform construction of the questionnaire and/or was partially confirmed by factor analytic studies of the questionnaire. Two instruments purportedly measure power components as they relate to the operational aspects of self-care agency: the Appraisal of Self Care Agency Scale is said to measure the power to perform the productive operations, and the Self-As-Carer Inventory is said to measure the power components as they relate to estimative operations (phase I) and productive operations (phase II). Several problems are apparent in all of these efforts to operationalize the power components and operations of self-care agency. First, the notion of 10 power components gains only partial support in the factor or principal component analysis of these instruments, even in instances for which this notion was used to inform instrument construction. This raises questions about the use of a single instrument to assess such a wide array of abilities as opposed to the use of various independent operationalizations for each, or at least some, of the power components. It bears mentioning that the literature reports several studies of more discrete power components even though they may not be designated as power components. Examples are (a) motivation for self-care (Urbanic, 1992); (b) self-care knowledge (Allan, 1988; Dodd, 1984b, 1987, 1988a; Malik, 1992); (c) mobility (Baulch, Larson, Dodd, & Dietrich, 1992); and (d) energy (Rhodes, Watson, & Hanson, 1988). The Appraisal of Self-Care Agency Scale, although built on the power component analysis, has only one general factor, and thus can be said to operationalize self-care agency in a global or general sense. This also raises questions, in this case, about the meaning of a general sense of power to perform the productive operations, especially in clinical practice.

Foundational capabilities and dispositions of self-care agency also have been studied empirically. As indicated in an earlier section of this chapter, a formal analysis of this aspect of agency was advanced by Backsheider through the Nursing Development Conference Group work (1979) and endorsed by Orem. In contrast to that for the power components, this analysis has had only a global influence on efforts to measure foundational capabilities or dispositions; in other words, there is little in the way of direct correspondence between the Backsheider analysis and various operationalizations proposed for this concept. For the most part, researchers have studied single broad personal characteristics or attributes for their influence on more specific aspects of self-care agency (power components or operations), self-care, or health and well-being, using existing instruments. In addition to that noted previously, characteristics that have been studied include (a) mental status (Hamilton & Creason, 1992), (b) learned helplessness (McDermott, 1993), (c) autonomy (Monsen, 1992; Moore, 1987a, 1987b), (d) visual acuity and tactile sensitivity (Baulch et al., 1992), (e) locus of control (Lakin, 1988; Moore, 1987a; Rew, 1987a), (f) and self-concept (Saucier, 1984; Smits & Kee, 1992).

A number of strategies have been used to operationalize the concept of self-care which, by and large, can be classified along the lines of (a) informed versus not informed by Orem's conceptualization of self-care requisites, (b) general self-care versus self-care specific to a health condition, and (c) actual self-care versus self-care evaluated on the basis of some norms. For example, the Denyes Self-Care Practice Instrument (Denyes, 1982) and the Children's Self-Care Performance Questionnaire (Moore, 1993) are used to assess general self-care practices of adolescents based on norms derived from Orem's description of self-care requisites. Similarly, Underwood's (1979, 1980) protocols provide norms for evaluating universal self-care at four levels of competence in adults with severe and persistent mental illnesses. Harris (1990; Harris & Williams, 1991), in contrast, described actual universal self-care in homeless elderly men and adults with schizophrenia in a set of qualitative studies. The actual versus normative distinction clearly is evident in studies by Hanucharurnkul (1989) and Hagopian (1990), and later studies by Dodd and Dibble (1993) in which self-care for radiation side effects was assessed using questionnaires constructed around normative self-care for this health condition, and earlier studies by Dodd (1984a) in which patients were asked to list actual self-care practices to manage postradiotherapy side effects and evaluate their effectiveness. Empirical studies of self-care specific to a health condition (health-deviation self-care) predominate the literature and include, in addition to those already mentioned, studies of self-care for weight control (Allan, 1988), colds and influenza (Conn, 1991), diabetes (Frey & Denyes, 1989; Frey & Fox, 1990; Germaine & Nemchik, 1989; Saucier, 1984), breast cancer (Dodd, 1988b), side effects of chemotherapy (Dodd, 1982, 1983), contraception (Oakley, Denyes, & O'Connor, 1989), cystic fibrosis (Baker, 1992), respiratory illnesses (Hautman, 1987), urinary incontinence (Dowd, 1991; Klemm & Creason, 1991), perimenstrual syndrome (Kirkpatrick, Brewer, & Stocks, 1990), spinal cord injury (McFarland, Sasser, Boss, Dickerson, & Stelling, 1992), and asthma (Rew, 1987b). More recently, Anderson (2001), Denyes, Orem and Bekel (2001), Söderhamn and Cliffordson (2001), and Taylor, Renpenning, Geden, Neuman, and Hart (2001) worked to further develop the structure of self-care agency.

Orem (1991) viewed nursing systems as being of three types: wholly and partially compensatory and supportive educative, and described them in terms of various methods of helping. By far, most of the research on nursing systems is concerned with supportive educative nursing systems, although not always explicitly designated as such. Within that category, studies of educative nursing systems designed to increase self-care knowledge or skills predominate. Examples are studies of informational interventions for cancer patients undergoing radiotherapy or chemotherapy (Dodd, 1987, 1988a, 1988b; Hagopian, 1991; Hagopian & Rubenstein, 1990), nursing preparation of stoma patients (Ewing, 1989), teaching diabetes (Frey & Fox, 1990), preparation for pulmonary surgery (Goodwin, 1979), instructions for asthmatics (Huss, Salerno, & Huss, 1991), aerobic interval training (MacVicar, Winningham, & Nickel, 1989), teaching for tonsillectomies (McCord, 1990), assertion training and first aid instruction for children (Moore, 1987b), information on hormone replacement therapy (Rothert et al., 1990), social skills training for chronically mentally ill (Whetstone, 1986), and preparation for mastectomy (Williams, et al.,

1988). It is reasonable to ask why so few studies to date are of wholly or partially compensatory nursing systems considering that these systems employ a great deal of nursing time and energy. One possible explanation is that this reflects an undue alignment between self-care theory in nursing and the contemporary emphasis on self-help and self-reliance in health care. Another possible explanation is that wholly and partially compensatory nursing systems are more difficult to study. There are, nevertheless, a few studies about how the respective contributions of patient and nurse to meeting the patient's self-care deficit are determined (Krouse & Roberts, 1989; Sandman, Norberg, Adolfsson, Axelsson, & Hedley, 1986). In a study by Denyes, Neuman, & Villarruel (1991), Orem's typology of methods of helping was used to classify various strategies employed by nurses to alleviate pain in hospitalized children.

The empirical adequacy of the relationships claimed in the formal propositions of the self-care theory has been examined in a number of studies, including some of those cited above. One could classify these studies broadly as examining (a) the influence of selected basic conditioning factors on self-care agency or self-care; (b) the influence of various foundational dispositions on power components of self-care agency, and self-care; (c) the contribution of self-care to health and well-being; and (d) and the impact of nursing systems on self-care agency, self-care, and/or well-being. At least four studies have been submitted as tests of the theory per se. One is the study by Denyes (1988) described in a previous section of this chapter in which the basic conditioning factor of health state, self-care agency, and self-care were found to account for 41% of the variance in health as a general state. The second is a study by Frey and Denyes (1989) in which a basic conditioning factor (health state) and universal self-care accounted for 64% of the variance in overall health of insulin-dependent diabetic adolescents, and self-care specific to diabetes explained 21% of the variance in control over diabetes (glycosylated hemoglobin). A third study by Dodd and Dibble (1993) examined the influence of various basic conditioning factors and power components of self-care agency on self-care for chemotherapy side effects in cancer patients. Support for the theory was equivocal in this study; the basic conditioning factors of health state, family system, and education accounted for 38% of the variance in self-care, but only one of several dimensions (anxiety) of self-care agency studied added explanation, and that in the opposite direction expected. In a fourth study reported by Moore (1993), basic conditioning factors (age, gender, socioeconomic status, living situation, ethnic group, and health state) and self-care agency accounted for 36% of the variance in self-care behaviors of healthy school-aged children.

EXTERNAL ANALYSIS

Nursing Research on the Model

A review of the research literature on the self-care theory is beyond the scope of this chapter (200 articles, more than 130 doctoral dissertations, and more than 120 master's theses are cited [Fawcett, 2000, pp. 345–355]). It should be said that such reviews definitely are needed to support the ongoing development of this theory. Several observations can be made about this body of research. First, studies from this theory can be described using all three categories of theory testing research proposed by Silva (1986). In one group are studies, such as those proposed by Allan (1988) and Hamera, Peterson, Young, and Schammloffel (1992), in which the theory is acknowledged but used only minimally, if at all, in guiding the research. In a second group are studies such as those by Chang, Uman, Linn, Ware, and Kane (1984) and Sandman et al. (1986) in which the theory is assumed to be correct and is used primarily to organize the research. In a third group are studies that are put forth as explicit tests of the theory, or operationalize and test theory concepts and relationships; among them are studies by Denyes (1988), Villarruel and Denyes (1991, 1997), Hanucharurnkul (1989), and Humphreys (1991). A fourth group, which could be added to the category containing Silva's study, are studies of midrange theories derived from the self-care theory (Campbell, 1989; Campbell & Weber, 2000; Ulbrich, 1999; Zehnder, 1996).

In addition to these uses of Orem's theory, the theory has been used in combination with other theoretical perspectives to develop new theoretical models. For example, Wang (2001) used major concepts from Orem's self-care model (1995), Pender's health promotion model (1987), and the ideas of other scholars (Hartweg, 1990; Simmons, 1990) to propose a theoretical model of health-promoting lifestyle. Similarly, Porter (1998) used Rogers' science of unitary human beings, Orem's self-care theory, and Rosenstack's health belief model to develop a family-focused, school-based family planning program. Taylor et al. (2001) described development of the Theory of Dependent Care, which they identified as a corollary theory.

A second observation about self-care research to date is that both qualitative and quantitative methodologies have been used. Although most of the research is quantitative, examples of qualitative studies include Baird and Pierce's (2001) study of men's adherence to cardiac therapy, Hungelmann's (1984) study of self-care abilities of older persons with chronic disease, Harris' (1990; Harris & Williams, 1991) studies of universal requisites of elderly homeless men and persons with persistent mental illnesses, Hartweg's (1993) study of health promotion self-care in middle-aged women, and Dowd's (1991) study of self-care needs of women with urinary incontinence. Silva (2001) conducted a qualitative study to develop an instrument that characterized the therapeutic self-care needs of individuals who receive bone marrow transplantation. Participants reflected on the discharge planning activities of the nurse based on Orem's model.

In 1998, Banfield concluded that the empiricist research paradigm is most consistent with Orem's work. She identified descriptive, descriptive-correlational, case study, and quasi-experimental designs as most in concert with Orem's self-care deficit theory of nursing. Phenomenological, ethnographic, and grounded theory research methods were identified as possibly in concert with Orem's theory. Methods associated with the critical theory research paradigm were identified as having limited usefulness given that Orem has not addressed the major concepts inherent in the philosophy (Banfield, 1998). Finally, Banfield noted that instruments used for data collection in research guided by Orem's theory should be consistent with or directly derived from the theory.

A third observation is that the research to date has addressed all concepts and relationships in the theory but certain concepts and relationships have received more attention than others; the previous section on empirical adequacy supports this observation. Considerable research attention has been given to relationships between various basic conditioning factors and self-care agency or self-care; to exploring foundational aspects of self-care agency; to operationalizing self-care agency and examining predictors of, or consequence of, self-care agency; and to identifying self-care requisites particular to certain health conditions, and age or developmental groups. There also are many studies of nursing interventions, most of which would be classified as supportive-educative nursing systems. The concept of nursing agency and the subconcepts of fully or partially compensatory nursing systems have received the least attention.

A fourth observation is that the research literature demonstrates applications of the self-care theory to a wide range of populations. With regard to age groups, although studies of adults predominate, there are numerous studies of children, including studies of preschoolers (Arneson & Triplett, 1990; Villarruel & Denyes, 1991), school-age children (Alexander, Younger, Cohen, & Crawford, 1988; Blazek & McClellen, 1983; Carlisle et al., 1993; Dashiff, 1992; Humphreys, 1991; Moore, 1987a, 1987b, 1993; Mosher & Moore, 1998; Rew, 1987a, 1987b; Saucier, 1984; Wanich, Sullivan-Marx, Gottlieb, & Johnson, 1992), and adolescents (Degenhart-Leskosky, 1989; Denyes, 1982; Denyes et al., 1991; Frey & Fox, 1990; Gaut & Kieckhefer, 1988; McCaleb & Cull, 2000; Monsen, 1992; Slusher, 1999). Studies of elderly persons also are numerous (Biggs, 1990; Brock & O'Sullivan, 1985;

Chang et al., 1984, 1985; Conn, Taylor, & Kelley, 1991; Harper, 1984; Harris, 1990; Harris & Williams, 1991; Jirovec & Kasno, 1990, 1993; Jopp, Carroll, & Waters, 1993; Karl, 1982; Kerkstra, Castelein, & Phillipsen, 1991; Sandman et al., 1986; Smits & Key, 1992; Wanich et al., 1992; Weinrich, 1990).

In addition to research applications across age groups are studies that span the spectrum of health promotion, illness prevention, and illness care. The categories of health promotion and illness prevention include studies of (a) general health promotion (Hartweg, 1993; Moore, 1993); (b) health promotion related to specific issues such as weight control (Allan, 1988) and breast self-examination (Baulch et al., 1992; Edgar, Shamian, & Patterson, 1984; Malik, 1992); and (c) developmental issues such as menarche and menstruation (Dashiff, 1992; Kirkpatrick et al., 1990; Patterson & Hale, 1985; Seideman, 1990; Woods, Taylor, Mitchell, & Lentz, 1992; Zehnder, 1996), pregnancy and childbirth (Bliss-Holtz, 1988, 1991; Cooksey-James, 1999; Hart & Foster, 1998; Renker, 1999), and menopause (McElmurry & Huddleston, 1991; Rothert et al., 1990).

Studies of self-care for specific health deviations pertain to (a) asthma (Alexander et al., 1988; Huss et al., 1991; Rew, 1987a, 1987b); (b) cardiac conditions (Baird & Pierce, 2001; Toth, 1980; Utz, Hammer, Whitmire, & Grass, 1990; Utz & Ramos, 1993); (c) cystic fibrosis (Kruger, Shawver, & Jones, 1980); (d) diabetes (Frey & Fox, 1990; Miller, 1982; Saucier, 1984); (e) cancer (Dodd, 1982, 1983, 1984a, 1984b, 1987, 1988a, 1988b; Dodd & Dibble, 1993; Gammon, 1991; Hagopian, 1990, 1991; Hagopian & Rubenstein, 1990; Hanucharurnkul, 1989; Hiromoto & Dungan, 1991; Kubricht, 1984; MacVicar, Winningham, & Nickel, 1989; Mosher & Moore, 1998; Nambayan, 1997; Oberst, Hugest, Chang, & McCubbin, 1991; Palmer & Meyers, 1990; Richardson, 1992; Weintraub & Hagopian, 1990; Williams et al., 1988); (f) multiple sclerosis (Gulick, 1987, 1988, 1989a, 1989b); (g) mental illness (Crockett, 1982; Hamera et al., 1992; Harris, 1990; Whetstone, 1986; Youssef, 1987); (h) physical abuse (Campbell, 1986, 1989; Campbell & Weber, 2000; Humphreys, 1991; Renker, 1999); (i) respiratory illnesses (Hautman, 1987); (j) suicide (Palikkathayil & Morgan, 1988); (k) renal transplant (Hayward et al., 1989); (l) spinal cord injury (McFarland et al., 1992); (m) spina bifida (Monsen, 1992); (n) pain (Denyes et al., 1991; Villarruel & Denyes, 1991); (o) fatigue (Rhodes, Watson, & Hanson, 1988; Robinson & Posner, 1992); and (p) urinary incontinence (Dowd, 1991; Klemm & Creason, 1991).

Nursing Education Based on the Theory

Orem developed the self-care theory of nursing, at least in part, in response to questions prevalent in the late 1950s and 1960s about the character and organization of essential content in nursing curricula. Thus, like many of the theories of its time, the self-care theory has had a strong association with nursing education from the outset. Over time it has become one of the more ubiquitous theories in nursing education; it is widely recognized and taught to some extent in many nursing curricula. One of the most consistent and well-developed applications is at the University of Missouri, where much of the curriculum development work has been done in consultation with Orem and the theory has been used over a number of years to inform both undergraduate and graduate programs. There are other noteworthy educational applications of the self-care theory that have stood the test of time; for example, at the Medical College of Ohio and Illinois Wesleyan University, and many schools that adopted the self-care theory during the years when the National League for Nursing viewed nursing conceptualization as criteria for accreditation.

The literature on educational applications of the self-care theory, although relatively limited, has some particularly noteworthy entries. Among them is the anthology edited by Riehl-Sisca (1985a), which has a number of chapters that describe curricular applications for preservice students (Taylor, 1985a), RN-BSN students (Farnham & Fowler, 1985), and undergraduate and graduate students (Riehl-Sisca, 1985b; Taylor, 1985b). Aids to teaching the self-care theory have been proposed; for example, model assessment and care plan forms designed to help students learn to apply the theory in practice were described by Lashinger (1990). Ankele, Lohner, and Masiulaniec (2001) describe a nursing resource center that is consistent with Orem's work. The literature also reports a few studies of the impact of the theory on educational parameters. Hartweg and Metcalfe (1986) found significantly greater improvements in attitudes toward self-care in baccalaureate nursing students who completed a self-care nursing curriculum as compared with nonnursing undergraduate students. Berbiglia (1991) examined implementation of the self-care theory among administrators, faculty, and students in a small baccalaureate program using an "ideal perspective" as the criterion measure. Findings were that the perspectives of students and faculty were similar, and were closer to the ideal than were those of administrators. Satisfaction with the theory was associated with faculty-related difficulties (e.g., turnover) for faculty and familiarity with the theory for administrators; student dissatisfaction was associated with difficult terminology in the theory. Although these examples exist in the professional literature, it is important to note that even though Orem describes the self-care deficit theory of nursing as useful in all levels of education, she cautions that one needs to examine both the students' backgrounds and the educational outcomes that are sought from a program to best determine the portion(s) of her work that are most relevant (Fawcett, 2001).

Applications of the theory to staff and continuing education also are described in the literature. Examples include two articles (Harman et al., 1989; Reid, Allen, Gauthier, & Campbell, 1989) that describe various educational strategies used to prepare staff to implement the self-care model at the Toronto General Hospital; one strategy was a very innovative multimedia exhibit based on the theory. Another example is an 8-day course in gerontological nursing based on self-care theory described by Langland and Farrah (1990), which at 6 to 9 months posttest had a significant impact on participants' ability to maintain a strong nursing perspective.

Nursing Practice Based on the Theory

There is a large and varied literature on the self-care theory in practice. Fawcett (2000) identified more than 200 articles or chapters on practice applications and another 90 articles on administration. Among these are applications to children, adolescents, adults, the elderly, parents, and families; a wide variety of health conditions across the health-illness continuum; diverse practice settings; and different ethnic groups. As a way to demonstrate practice relevance, the theory has been placed in the context of the nursing process. An example is the article by Taylor (1988) cited previously, which describes how the theory can be applied to all steps of the nursing process using a case vignette. A good example of how the theory informs assessment was provided by Underwood (1980) and her colleagues (Morrison, Fisber, Wilson, & Underwood, 1985), who established protocols for assessing universal self-care of psychiatric patients, or for determining acuity ratings (Ringerman & Luz, 1990). More recently, Cooksey-James (1999) identified Orem's model as a way to improve prenatal care comprehensively with a specific focus on interventions to address identified self-care deficits (Cooksey-James, 1999), and Burks (1999) developed a nursing practice model for chronic illness based on Orem's model. Phillips and Morrow (1998) addressed the use of Orem's model as a frame of reference for nursing care for human immunodeficiency virus (HIV) patients. Taylor (2001), building on previous work, described ways that Orem's theory enhances nursing care to families, and Geden, Isaramalai, and Taylor (2001) identified ways to enhance primary-care practice by nurse practitioners with the use of Orem's theory. Some of the excellent literature on nursing diagnosis and the self-care theory will be reviewed in the next section of this chapter.

Compelling evidence for the applicability of this theory in practice is found in the fact that it serves as the model of practice in a number of health-care institutions. As documented in a number of articles (Allison, McLaughlin, & Walker, 1991; Del Togno-Armanasco, Olivas, & Harter, 1989; Fernandez, Brennan, Alvarez, & Duffy, 1990; Holzmer, 1992; Sella & MacLeod, 1991; Titus & Porter, 1989), the processes used to accomplish this often extend over a period of a year or more and typically include efforts to gain sufficient administrative support, extensive initial and on-going staff education, revision of assessment instruments and documentation forms to reflect the theory, and evaluation. By way of evaluation is a study reported by Faucett, Ellis, Underwood, Naqvi, & Wilson (1990), which demonstrated that nurses in a long-term care setting who were taught to use the self-care theory engaged in more comprehensive assessments about personal capabilities of patients and articulated more specific and varied roles for patients' participation in care, when compared with those who were not taught to use the theory. A study reported by Rossow-Sebring, Carrieri, & Seward (1992) showed that nurses on three medical-surgical units of an acute-care hospital where the self-care theory had been introduced over a period of a year expressed greater satisfaction with the nursing role and greater value for patient teaching.

The self-care theory is being used to develop a computerized nursing information system. This work is being done in three hospitals in New Jersey (Bliss-Holtz, McLaughlin, & Taylor, 1992; McLaughlin, Taylor, Bliss-Holtz, Sayers, & Nickle, 1990). An initial system reportedly is in place and has been validated using postpartum patients (Bliss-Holtz, McLaughlin, & Taylor, 1990).

NURSING DIAGNOSIS AND THE THEORY

Nursing Diagnoses Derived from Practice
Discussion Found in the Theory

There is relatively little attention to nursing diagnosis in Orem's writings, although a distinction between diagnosis as process and outcome, or content, clearly is evident. As process, diagnosis is one of the estimative operations of the nurse, and as outcome, a diagnosis is a statement about the relationship between the patient's self-care demand and self-care agency. A noteworthy addition to this is Taylor's (1991) interpretation and elaboration of Orem's position on nursing diagnosis. Like Orem, Taylor portrayed nursing diagnosis as part of the nursing process and, thus, as an aspect of the professional-technological dimension of nursing practice. Diagnosis entails the operations of "(a) calculating the therapeutic self-care demand, (b) estimating self-care agency, and (c) determining the existence or potential for self-care deficits" (Taylor, 1991, p. 25).

Congruence Between Model-Derived Nursing
Diagnoses and North American Nursing Diagnosis
Association (NANDA) Diagnoses

In contrast to Taylor's position is Jenny's (1989, 1991) effort to align self-care theory and the NANDA taxonomy, undertaken, in part, as a way to improve the latter. Jenny criticized the NANDA Taxonomy I on the grounds that (a) it lacks a "principle of order that will pinpoint groups eligible for inclusion in the system" (p. 84); and (b) the language of the nine human response categories used to classify diagnoses is ambiguous and unfamiliar. Nevertheless, she argued against discarding the NANDA system because it represents more than 15 years of work and is widely used; moreover, the introduction of another system might "simply add to the confusion" (p. 84). To resolve the first criticism, the case was made for self-care as a concept that could serve as an organizing principle for a diagnostic taxonomy. To address the second criticism, a hierarchical classification scheme was proposed for organizing self-care diagnoses using the categories of physiological homeostasis, bodily care, ego integrity, social interaction, health protection, health restoration, and environmental management. Her claims were that "Although [these] taxonomic categories are different from the self-care requisites specific to self-care deficit theory, they accommodate all of the concepts in the domains of universal, developmental, and health deviation self-care requisites" (p. 85). In addition, with only a few revisions, most NANDA diagnoses can be classified using these categories.

Relationship of the Model to Other Nursing Classification Systems

It is likely that Orem's model could be used relatively easily in conjunction with a number of the other types of nursing classification systems. However, some work would be required to ensure congruence among systems, particularly in terms of language. For example, the self-care deficit theory of nursing could inform and guide organization and further development of the Nursing Intervention Classification (NIC) (McCloskey & Bulecheck, 2000); however, because NIC was not developed specifically using Orem's theory as a guide, considerable rework would be needed to do this. In addition, the Nursing Outcomes Classification (NOC) (Johnson, Maas, & Moorehead, 2000) could be structured in a way that was consistent with Orem's model; however, again, language changes would be needed. Other classification systems based on NANDA terminology (e.g., Home Health Care Classification [HHCC] [Saba, 1997], the Patient Care Data Set [PCDS] [Ozbolt, 1997], Omaha System [Martin & Scheet, 1992], and the Perioperative Nursing Data Set [PNDS] [Kleinbeck, 1996]) would be compatible with Orem's model following reorganization as discussed above.

Relationship of the Model to Theory-Driven, Evidence-Based Practice, and Knowledge Development

Orem's model has contributed to knowledge development during the last 30 years as it has evolved and been revised over time as more knowledge has been gained regarding health and illness experiences, self-care, and nursing outcomes. As previously mentioned, Orem's model is well liked among nurses in the clinical area, particularly because of the language of her theories and its direct applicability to nursing practice. Nurses at the bedside can easily relate to the model and understand its concepts without extensive theoretical training. Thus, Orem's model is well suited to guide evidence-based practice for nursing. Orem's model has had much support and has been used frequently to guide research; it is a logical transition to build on this past enterprise to implement theory-driven, evidence-based practice according to the principles set forth by Orem and discussed in this chapter. Orem's model is comprehensive and addresses a variety of topics, making it applicable to both wellness and disease situations.

SUMMARY

Orem's Self-Care Model focuses on assisting an individual to improve care of the self. This theoretical perspective was derived via induction from practice. Three propositions are included in Orem's Self-Care Model: The Theory of Self-Care, The Theory of Self-Care Deficit, and The Theory of Nursing System. The Model also includes 10 basic conditioning factors, which may influence Self-Care Agency and Self-Care Demand. Orem's Self-Care Model is useful in understanding a wide variety of patient care situations and has been used extensively in research.

REFERENCES

Alexander, F. S., Younger, R. E., Cohen, R. M., & Crawford, L. V. (1988). Effectiveness of a nurse-managed program for children with chronic asthma. *Journal of Pediatric Nursing, 3,* 312–317.

Allan, J. D. (1988). Knowing what to weigh: Women's self-care activities related to weight. *Advances in Nursing Science, 11*(1), 47–60.

Allison, S. E., McLaughlin, K., & Walker, D. (1991). Nursing theory: A tool to put nursing back into nursing administration. *Nursing Administration Quarterly, 15*(3), 72–78.

Anderson, J. A. (2001). Understanding homeless adults by testing the theory of self-care. *Nursing Science Quarterly, 14,* 59–67.

Ankele, R., Lohner, L., & Masiulaniec, B. A. S. (2001). Innovative teaching within the nursing resource center: A blueprint for student success. *Journal of Multicultural Nursing and Health, 7*(3), 6–9.

Anna, D. J., Christensen, D. G., Hohon, S. A., Ord, L., & Wells, S. R. (1978). Implementing Orem's conceptual framework. *Journal of Nursing Administration, 8*(11), 8–11.

Arneson, S. W., & Triplett, J. O. (1990). Riding with Bucklebear: An automobile safety program for preschoolers. *Journal of Pediatric Nursing, 5,* 115–122.

Arnold, M. B. (1960). Deliberate action. In *Emotion and personality* (Vol. 11). *Neurological and physiological aspects* (pp. 193–204). New York: Columbia University Press.

Avery, P. (1992). Self-care in the hospital setting: The Prince Henry Hospital experience. *Lamp, 492,* 26–28.

Baird, K. K., & Pierce, L. L. (2001). Adherence to cardiac therapy for men with coronary artery disease. *Rehabilitation Nursing, 26,* 233–237.

Baker, L. K. (1992). Predictors of self-care in adolescents with cystic fibrosis: A test and explication of Orem's theories of self-care and self-care deficit. *Dissertation Abstracts International, 53,* 1290B.

Banfield, B. E. (1998). A philosophical inquiry of Orem's self-care deficit nursing theory. *Dissertation Abstracts International, 58,* 5885B.

Baulch, Y. S., Larson, P. J., Dodd, M. J., & Dietrich, C. (1992). The relationship of visual acuity, tactile sensitivity and mobility of the upper extremities to proficient breast self-examination in women 65 and older. *Oncology Nursing Forum, 19,* 1367–1372.

Beckman, C. A. (1987). Maternal-child health in Brazil. *Journal of Obstetric, Gynecologic, and Neonatal Nursing, 16,* 238–241.

Berbiglia, V. A. (1991). A case study: Perspectives on a self-care deficit nursing theory-based curriculum. *Journal of Advanced Nursing, 16,* 1158–1163.

Biggs, A. J. (1990). Family care-giver versus nursing assessments of elderly self-care abilities. *Journal of Gerontological Nursing, 16*(8), 11–16.

Blazek, B., & McClellen, M. (1983). The effects of self-care instruction on locus of control in children. *Journal of School Health, 53,* 554–556.

Bliss-Holtz, V. J. (1988). Primiparas' prenatal concern for learning infant care. *Nursing Research, 37,* 20–24.

Bliss-Holtz, V. J. (1991). Developmental tasks of pregnancy and parental education. *International Journal of Childbirth Education, 6*(1), 29–31.

Bliss-Holtz, J., McLaughlin, K., & Taylor, S. G. (1990). Validating nursing theory for use within a computerized nursing information system. *Advances in Nursing Science, 13*(2), 46–52.

Brock, A. M., & O'Sullivan, P. (1985). A study to determine what variables predict institutionalization of elderly people. *Journal of Advanced Nursing, 10,* 533–537.

Burks, K. J. (1999). A nursing practice model for chronic illness. *Rehabilitation Nursing, 24,* 197–200.

Campbell, J. C. (1986). Nursing assessment for risk of homicide with battered women. *Advances in Nursing Science, 8*(4), 36–51.

Campbell, J. C. (1989). A test of two explanatory models of women's responses to battering. *Nursing Research, 38,* 18–24.

Campbell, J. C., & Weber, N. (2000). An empirical test of a self-care model of women's responses to battering. *Nursing Science Quarterly, 13*(1), 45–53.

Carlisle, J. B., Corser, N., Cull, V., Dimicco, W., Luther, L., McCaleb, A., et al. (1993). Cardiovascular risk factors in young children. *Journal of Community Health Nursing, 10,* 1–9.

Carter, P. A. (1998). Self-care agency: The concept and how it is measured. *Journal of Nursing Measurement, 6,* 195–207.

Chamorro, L. C. (1985). Self-care in the Puerto Rican Community. In J. Riehl-Sisca (Ed.), *The science and art of self-care* (pp. 189–195). Norwalk, CT: Appleton-Century-Crofts.

Chang, B., Uman, G., Linn, L., Ware, J., & Kane, R. (1984). The effect of systematically varying components of nursing care on satisfaction in elderly ambulatory women. *Western Journal of Nursing Research, 6,* 367–386.

Chang, B., Uman, G., Linn, L., Ware, J., & Kane, R. (1985). Adherence to health care regimens among elderly women. *Nursing Research, 34,* 27–31.

Clark, J., & Bishop, J. (1988). Model-making. *Nursing Times, 84*(27), 37–40.

Cleveland, S. A. (1989). Re: Perceived self-care agency: A LISREL factor analysis of Bickel and Hanson's questionnaire [Letter to the editor]. *Nursing Research, 38,* 59.

Conn, V. (1991). Self-care actions taken by older adults for influenza and colds. *Nursing Research, 40,* 176–181.

Conn, V. S., Taylor, S. G., & Kelley, S. (1991). Medication regimen complexity and adherence among older adults. *IMAGE: Journal of Nursing Scholarship, 23,* 231–235.

Cooksey-James, T. (1999). Utilization of prenatal care by women of St. Thomas, United States Virgin Islands: A descriptive study. Unpublished doctoral dissertation, University of Miami, FL.

Cretain, G. K. (1989). Motivational factors in breast self-examination: Implications for nurses. *Cancer Nursing, 12,* 250–256.

Crockett, M. S. (1982). Self-reported coping histories of adult psychiatric and nonpsychiatric subjects and controls [Abstract]. *Nursing Research, 31,* 122.

Dashiff, C. J. (1992). Self-care capabilities in black girls in anticipation of menarche. *Health Care for Women International, 13,* 67–76.

Degenhart-Leskosky, S. M. (1989). Health education needs of adolescent and nonadolescent mothers. *Journal of Obstetric, Gynecologic and Neonatal Nursing, 18,* 238–244.

Del Togno-Armanasco, V. Olivas, G. S., & Harter, S. (1989). Developing an integrated nursing care management model. *Nursing Management, 20*(10), 26–29.

Denyes, M. J. (1982). Development of an instrument to measure self-care agency in adolescents. *Dissertation Abstracts International, 49,* 3102B.

Denyes, M. J. (1988). Orem's model used for health promotion: Directions from research. *Advances in Nursing Science, 11*(1), 13–21.

Denyes, M. J., Neuman, B. M., & Villarruel, A. M. (1991). Nursing actions to prevent and alleviate pain in hospitalized children. *Issues in Comprehensive Pediatric Nursing, 14,* 31–48.

Denyes, M. J., Orem, D. E., & Bekel, G. (2001). Self-care: A foundational science. *Nursing Science Quarterly, 14,* 48–54.

Dier, K. A. (1987). A model for collaboration in nursing practice: Thailand and Canada. In K. F. Hannah, M. Reimer, W. C. Mills, & S. Letourneau (Eds.), *Clinical judgment and decision making: The future with nursing diagnosis* (pp. 323–327). New York: John Wiley & Sons.

Dickoff, J., James, P., & Wiedenbach, E. (1968). Theory in practice disciplines. Part I: Practice oriented theory. *Nursing Research, 17*(5), 415–435.

Dodd, M. J. (1982). Assessing patient self-care for side effects of cancer chemotherapy—Part 1. *Cancer Nursing, 5,* 447–451.

Dodd, M. J. (1983). Self-care for side effects in cancer chemotherapy: An assessment of nursing interventions—Part 2. *Cancer Nursing, 6,* 63–67.

Dodd, M. J. (1984a). Patterns of self-care in cancer patients receiving radiation therapy. *Oncology Nursing Forum, 11,* 23–27.

Dodd, M. J. (1984b). Measuring informational intervention for chemotherapy knowledge and self-care behaviors. *Research in Nursing and Health, 7,* 43–50.

Dodd, M. J. (1987). Efficacy of proactive information on self-care in radiation therapy patients. *Heart and Lung, 16,* 538–544.

Dodd, M. J. (1988a). Efficacy of proactive information on self-care in chemotherapy patients. *Patient Education and Counseling, 11,* 215–225.

Dodd, M. J. (1988b). Patterns of self-care in patients with breast cancer. *Western Journal of Nursing Research, 10,* 7–24.

Dodd, M. J., & Dibble, S. L. (1993). Predictors of self-care: A test of Orem's model. *Oncology Nursing Forum, 20,* 895–901.

Dowd, T. (1991). Discovering older women's experience of urinary incontinence. *Research in Nursing and Health, 14,* 179–186.

Dyer, S. (1990). Team work for personal patient care. *Nursing the Elderly, 3*(7), 28–30.

Edgar, L., Shamian, J., & Patterson, C. (1984). Factor affecting the nurse as a teacher and practicer of breast self-examination. *International Journal of Nursing Studies, 21,* 255–265.

Ewing, G. (1989). The nursing preparation of stoma patients for self-care. *Journal of Advanced Nursing, 14,* 411–420.

Farnham, S., & Fowler, M. (1985). Demedicalization, bilingualization, and reconceptualization: Teaching Orem's self-care model to the RN-BSN student. In J. Riehl-Sisca, *The science and art of self-care* (pp. 35–40). Norwalk, CT: Appleton-Century-Crofts.

Faucett, J., Ellis, V., Underwood, P., Naqvi, A., & Wilson, D. (1990). The effect of Orem's self-care model on nursing care in a nursing home setting. *Journal of Advanced Nursing, 15,* 659–666.

Fawcett, J. (2000). *Analysis and evaluation of contemporary nursing knowledge.* Philadelphia: F. A. Davis.

Fawcett, J. (2001). The nurse theorists: 21st-century updates—Dorothea E. Orem. *Nursing Science Quarterly, 14,* 34–38.

Fernandez, R., Brennan, M. L., Alvarez, A. R., & Duffy, M. A. (1990). Theory-based practice: A model for nurse retention. *Nursing Administration Quarterly, 14*(4), 47–53.

Finnegan, T. (1986). Self-care and the elderly. *New Zealand Nursing Journal, 79*(4), 10–13.

Frey, M. A., & Denyes, M. J. (1989). Health and illness self-care in adolescents with IDDM: A test of Orem's theory. *Advances in Nursing Science, 12*(1), 67–75.

Frey, M. A., & Fox, M. A. (1990). Assessing and teaching self-care to youths with diabetes mellitus. *Pediatric Nursing, 16,* 597–800.

Gammon, J. (1991). Coping with cancer: The role of self-care. *Nursing Practice, 4*(3), 11–15.

Gast, H. L. (1984). The relationship between stages of ego development and developmental stages of health self-care operations. *Dissertations Abstracts International, 44,* 3039B.

Gast, H. L., Denyes, M. J., Campbell, J. C., Hartweg, D. L., Schott-Baer, D., & Isenberg, M. (1989). Self-care agency: Conceptualizations and operationalizations. *Advances in Nursing Science, 12*(1), 26–38.

Gaut, D. A., & Kieckhefer, G. M. (1988). Assessment of self-care agency in chronically ill adolescents. *Journal of Adolescent Health Care, 9,* 55–60.

Geden, E. A., Isaramalai, S., & Taylor, S. G. (2001). Self-Care Deficit Nursing Theory and the nurse practitioner's practice in primary care settings. *Nursing Science Quarterly, 14,* 29–33.

Geden, E., & Taylor, S. (1991). Construct and empirical validity of the Self-As-Carer Inventory. *Nursing Research, 40*(1), 47–50.

Germaine, C. P., & Nemchik, R. M. (1989). Diabetes self-management and hospitalization. *IMAGE: Journal of Nursing Scholarship, 20,* 74–78.

Goodwin, J. O. (1979). Programmed instruction for self-care following pulmonary surgery. *International Journal of Nursing Studies, 16,* 29–40.

Gulick, E. E. (1987). Parsimony and model confirmation of the ADL self-care scale for multiple sclerosis persons. *Nursing Research, 36,* 278–283.

Gulick, E. E. (1988). The self-administered ADL scale for persons with multiple sclerosis. In C. F. Waltz & O. L. Strickland (Eds.), *Measurement of nursing outcomes* (Vol. 1). *Measuring client outcomes* (pp. 128–159). New York: Springer.

Gulick, E. E. (1989a). Model confirmation of the MS-related symptom checklist. *Nursing Research, 38,* 147–153.

Gulick, E. E. (1989b). Work performance by persons with multiple sclerosis: Conditions that impede or enable the performance of work. *International Journal of Nursing Studies, 26,* 301–311.

Haas, D. (1990). *The relationship between coping dispositions and power components of dependent-care agency in parents of children with special health care needs.* Unpublished doctoral dissertation, Wayne State University, Detroit, MI.

Hagopian, G. (1990). The measurement of self-care strategies of patients in radiation therapy, In O. L. Strickland & C. F. Waltz (Eds.), *Measurement of nursing outcomes* (Vol. 4). *Measuring client self-care and coping skills* (pp. 475–570). New York: Springer.

Hagopian, G. A. (1991). The effects of a weekly radiation therapy newsletter on patients. *Oncology Nursing Forum, 18,* 1199–1203.

Hagopian, G. A., & Rubenstein, J. H. (1990). Effects of telephone call interventions on patients' well-being in a radiation therapy department. *Cancer Nursing, 13,* 339–344.

Hamera, E. K., Peterson, K. A., Young, L. M., & Schammloffel, M. M. (1992). Symptom monitoring in schizophrenia: Potential for enhancing self-care. *Archives of Psychiatric Nursing, 6,* 324–330.

Hamilton, L. W., & Creason, N. S. (1992). Mental status and functional abilities: Change in institutionalized elderly women. *Nursing Diagnosis, 3,* 81–86.

Hammons, T. A. (1985). Self-care practices of Navajo Indians. In J. Riehl-Sisca (Ed.), *The science and art of self-care* (pp. 171–180). Norwalk, CT: Appleton-Century-Crofts.

Hanson, B. R., & Bickel, L. (1985). Development and testing of the questionnaire on perception of self-care agency. In J. Riehl-Sisca (Ed.), *The science and art of self-care* (pp. 271–278). Norwalk, CT: Appleton-Century-Crofts.

Hanucharurnkul, S. (1989). Predictors of self-care in cancer patients receiving radiotherapy. *Cancer Nursing, 12,* 21–27.

Hanucharurnkul, S., & Vinya-nguag, P. (1991). Effects of promoting patients' participation in self-care on postoperative recovery and satisfaction with care. *Nursing Science Quarterly, 4,* 14–20.

Harman, L., Wabin, D., MacInnis, L., Baird, D., Mattiuzzi, D., & Savage, P. (1989). Developing clinical decision-making skills in staff nurses: An educational program. *Journal of Continuing Education in Nursing, 20,* 102–106.

Harmer, B. (1955). *Textbook of the principles and practice of nursing* (4th ed.). New York: Collier McMillan.

Harper, D. (1984). Application of Orem's theoretical constructs to self-care medication behaviors in the elderly. *Advances in Nursing Science, 6*(3), 39–43.

Harris, J. L. (1990). Self-care of chronic schizophrenics associated with meeting solitude and social interaction requisites. *Archives of Psychiatric Nursing, 4*(5), 293–307.

Harris, J. L., & Williams, L. K. (1991). Universal self-care requisites as identified by homeless elderly men. *Journal of Gerontological Nursing, 19*(6), 39–43.

Hart, M. A., & Foster, S. N. (1998). Self-care agency in two groups of pregnant women. *Nursing Science Quarterly, 11,* 167–171.

Hartweg, D. L. (1990). Health promotion self-care within Orem's general theory of nursing. *Journal of Advanced Nursing, 15,* 35–41.

Hartweg, D. L. (1993). Self-care actions of healthy middle-aged women to promote well-being. *Nursing Research, 42*(4), 221–227.

Hartweg, D. L., & Metcalfe, S. A. (1986). Self-care attitude changes of nursing students enrolled in a self-care curriculum: A longitudinal study. *Research in Nursing and Health, 9,* 347–353.

Hautman, M. A. (1987). Self-care responses to respiratory illnesses among Vietnamese. *Western Journal of Nursing Research, 9,* 223–243.

Hayward, M. B., Kish, J. P., Jr., Frey, G. M., Kirchner, J. M. Carr, L. S., & Wolfe, C. M. (1989). An instrument to identify stressors in renal transplant recipients. *Journal of the American Nephrology Nurses Association, 16,* 81–84.

Holzmer, W. L. (1992). Linking primary health care and self-care through case management. *International Nursing Review, 39,* 83–89.

Hiromoto, B. M., & Dungan, J. (1991). Contract learning for self-care activities: A protocol study among chemotherapy outpatients. *Cancer Nursing, 14,* 148–154.

Humphreys, J. (1991). Children of battered women: Worries about their mothers. *Pediatric Nursing, 17,* 342–345, 354.

Hungelmann, J. A. (1984). Components of self-care ability of older persons with chronic disease. Doctoral dissertation, Rush University, Chicago, IL.

Hunter, L. (1992). Applying Orem to skin. *Nursing (London), 5*(4), 16–18.

Huss, K., Salerno, M., & Huss, R. W. (1991). Computer-assisted reinforcement of instruction: Effects on adherence in adult atopic asthmatics. *Research in Nursing and Health, 13,* 259–267.

Illich, I. (1976). *Medical nemesis: The expropriation of health.* New York: Pantheon Books.

Jenny, J. (1989). Classifying nursing diagnoses: A self-care approach. *Nursing and Health Care, 10*(2), 83–89.

Jenny, J. (1991). Self-care deficit theory and nursing diagnoses: A test of conceptual fit. *Journal of Nursing Education, 30,* 227–232.

Jirovec, M. M., & Kasno, J. (1990). Self-care agency as a function of patient-environmental factors among nursing home residents. *Research in Nursing and Health, 13,* 303–309.

Jirovec, M. M., & Kasno, J. (1993). Predictors of self-care abilities among the institutionalized elderly. *Western Journal of Nursing Research, 15,* 314–324.

Johnson, M., Maas, M., & Moorehead, S. (2000). *Nursing outcomes classification* (2nd ed.). St. Louis: Mosby.

Jopp, M., Carroll, M. C., & Waters, L. (1993). Using self-care theory to guide nursing management of the older adult after hospitalization. *Rehabilitation Nursing, 18,* 91–94.

Karl, C. (1982). The effect of an exercise program on self-care activities for the institutionalized elderly. *Journal of Gerontological Nursing, 8,* 282–285.

Kearney, B. Y., & Fleischer, B. J. (1979). Development of an instrument to measure exercise of self-care agency. *Research in Nursing and Health, 2,* 35–44.

Kerkstra, A., Castelein, E., & Phillipsen, H. (1991). Preventive home visits to elderly people by community nurses in the Netherlands. *Journal of Advanced Nursing, 16,* 631–637.

Kirkpatrick, M. K., Brewer, J. A., & Stocks, B. (1990). Efficacy of self-care measures for perimenstrual syndrome (PMS). *Journal of Advanced Nursing, 15,* 281–285.

Kleinbeck, S. V. (1996). In search of perioperative nursing data elements. *Association of Operating Room Nursing (AORN), 63,* 926–931.

Klemm, L. W., & Creason, N. S. (1991). Self-care practices of women with urinary incontinence—A preliminary study. *Health Care for Women International, 12,* 199–209

Kotarbinski, T. (1965). *Praxiology: An introduction to the sciences of efficient action* (O. Wojtasiewicz, Trans.). New York: Pergamon Press.

Krouse, H. J., & Roberts, S. J. (1989). Nurse-patient interactive styles: Power, control and satisfaction. *Western Journal of Nursing Research, 11,* 717–725.

Kruger, S., Shawver, M., & Jones, L. (1980). Reactions of families to the child with cystic fibrosis. *IMAGE: Journal of Nursing Scholarship, 12,* 67a–72.

Kubricht, D. (1984). Therapeutic self-care demands expressed by outpatients receiving external radiation therapy. *Cancer Nursing, 7,* 43–52.

Lakin, J. A. (1988). Self-care, health locus of control, and health value among faculty women. *Public Health Nursing, 5,* 37–44.

Langland, R. M., & Farrah, S. J. (1990). Using a self-care framework for continuing education in gerontological nursing. *Journal of Continuing Education in Nursing, 21,* 267–270.

Lashinger, H. S. (1990). Helping students apply a nursing conceptual framework in the clinical setting. *Nurse Educator, 15*(3), 20–24.

Leininger, M. M. (1988). Leininger's theory of nursing: Cultural care diversity and universality. *Nursing Science Quarterly, 1*(4), 152–160.

Leininger, M. M. (1993). Self-care ideology and cultural incongruities: Some critical issues. *Journal of Transcultural Nursing, 4*(1), 2–4.

Lonergan, B. J. F. (1972). *Method in theology.* Minneapolis: Seabury Press.

Lorenson, M., Holter, I. M., Evers, G. C., Isenberg, M. A., & van Acterberg, T. (1993). Cross-cultural testing of the appraisal of self-care agency: ASA scale in Norway. *International Journal of Nursing Studies, 30,* 15–23.

Macmurray, J. (1957). *The self as agent.* London: Faber and Faber.

MacVicar, M. G., Winningham, M. L., & Nickel, J. L. (1989). Effects of aerobic interval training on cancer patients' functional capacity. *Nursing Research, 38,* 348–351.

Malik, U. (1992). Women's knowledge beliefs and health practices about breast cancer and breast self-examination. *Nursing Journal of India, 83,* 186–190.

Maritain, J. (1959). *The degrees of knowledge* (G. B. Phelan, Trans.). New York: Scribners.

Martin, K. S., & Scheet, N. I. (1992). *The Omaha System: Applications for community health nursing.* Philadelphia: W. B. Saunders.

McBride, S. H. (1987). Validation of an instrument to measure exercise of self-care agency. *Research in Nursing and Health, 10,* 311–316.

McBride, S. H. (1991). Comparative analysis of three instruments designed to measure self-care agency. *Nursing Research, 40,* 12–16.

McCaleb, A., & Cull, V. V. (2000). Sociocultural influences and self-care practices of middle adolescents. *Journal of Pediatric Nursing, 15*(1), 30–35.

McCloskey, J. C., & Bulecheck, G. M. (Eds.). (2000). *Nursing intervention classification* (3rd ed.). St. Louis: Mosby.

McCord, A. S. (1990). Teaching for tonsillectomies: Details mean better compliance. *Today's OR Nurse, 126,* 11–14.

McDermott, M. A. N. (1993). Learned helplessness as an interacting variable with self-care agency: Testing a theoretical model. *Nursing Science Quarterly, 6,* 28–38.

McElmurry, B. J., & Huddleston, D. L. (1991). Self-care and menopause: Critical review of research. *Health Care for Women International, 12,* 15–26.

McFarland, S. M., Sasser, L., Boss, B. J., Dickerson, J. L., & Stelling, F. D. (1992). Self-Care Assessment Tool for spinal cord injured person. *SCI Nursing, 9,* 111–116.

McLaughlin, K., Taylor, S. G., Bliss-Holtz, J., Sayers, P., & Nickle, L. (1990). Shaping the future: The marriage of nursing theory and informatics. *Computers in Nursing, 8,* 174–179.

Meleis, A. I. (1997). *Theoretical nursing: Development and progress* (3rd ed.). Philadelphia: J. B. Lippincott.

Melnyk, K. A. M. (1983). The process of theory analysis: An examination of the nursing theory of Dorothea E. Orem. *Nursing Research, 32*(3), 170–178.

Miller, J. F. (1982). Categories of self-care needs of ambulatory patients with diabetes. *Journal of Advanced Nursing, 7,* 25–31.

Monsen, R. B. (1992). Autonomy, coping and self-care agency in healthy adolescents and in adolescents with spina bifida. *Journal of Pediatric Nursing, 7,* 9–13.

Moore, J. B. (1987a). Determining the relationship of autonomy to self-care agency or locus of control in school-aged children. *Maternal Child Nursing Journal, 16*(1) 47–60.

Moore, J. B. (1987b). Effects of assertion training and first aid instruction on children's autonomy and self-care agency. *Research in Nursing and Health, 10,* 101–109.

Moore, J. B. (1993). Predictors of children's self-care performance: Testing the theory of self-care deficit. *Scholarly Inquiry for Nursing Practice, 7,* 199–212.

Morrison, E., Fisber, L., Wilson, H., & Underwood, P. (1985). NSGAE: Nursing adaptation evaluation. *Journal of Psychosocial Nursing, 23,* 10–13.

Mosher, R. B., & Moore, J. B. (1998). The relationship of self-concept and self-care in children with cancer. *Nursing Science Quarterly, 11,* 116–122.

Nambayan, A. G. (1997). The effects of collaborative nursing care delivery on the self-care behaviors and coping patterns of rural cancer patients. Unpublished doctoral dissertation, University of Alabama at Birmingham, AL.

Northrup, D. T. (1993). Self-care myth reconsidered. *Advances in Nursing Science, 15*(3), 59–66.

Nursing Development Conference Group. (1973). *Concept formalization in nursing: Process and product.* Boston: Little Brown.

Nursing Development Conference Group. (1979). *Concept formalization in nursing: Process and product* (2nd ed.). Boston: Little Brown.

Oakley, D., Denyes, M. J., & O'Connor, N. (1989). Expanded nursing care for contraceptive use. *Applied Nursing Research, 3,* 121–127.

Oberst, M. T., Hugest, S. H., Chang, A. S., & McCubbin, M. A. (1991). Self-care burden, stress appraisal and mood among persons receiving radiotherapy. *Cancer Nursing, 14,* 7–78.

Orem, D. E. (1971). *Nursing: Concepts of practice.* New York: McGraw-Hill.

Orem, D. E. (1980). *Nursing: Concepts of practice* (2nd ed.). New York: McGraw-Hill.

Orem, D. E. (1985). *Nursing: Concepts of practice* (3rd ed.). New York: McGraw-Hill.

Orem, D. E. (1988). The form of nursing science. *Nursing Science Quarterly, 1*(2), 75–79.

Orem, D. E. (1991). *Nursing: Concepts of practice* (4th ed.) St. Louis: Mosby-Year Book.

Orem, D. E. (1995). *Nursing: Concepts of practice* (5th ed.). St. Louis: Mosby.

Orem, D. E. (1997). Views of human beings specific to nursing. *Nursing Science Quarterly, 10,* 26–31.

Orem, D. E. (2001). *Nursing: Concepts of practice* (6th ed.). St. Louis: Mosby.

Ozbolt, J. G. (1997). From minimum data to maximum impact. Using clinical data to strengthen patient care. *MD Computing, 14,* 195–301.

Palikkathayil, L., & Morgan, S. A. (1988). Emergency department nurses' encounters with suicide attempters: A qualitative investigation. *Scholarly Inquiry for Nursing Practice, 2,* 237–253.

Palmer, P., & Meyers, F. J. (1990). An outpatient approach to the delivery of intensive consolidation chemotherapy to adults with acute lymphoblastic leukemia. *Oncology Nursing Forum, 17,* 553–558.

Parsons, T. (1937). *The structure of social action.* New York: McGraw-Hill.

Parsons, T. (1951). *The social system.* New York: The Free Press.

Patterson, E., & Hale, E. (1985). Making sure: Integrating menstrual care practices into activities of daily living. *Advances in Nursing Science, 7*(3), 18–31.

Pender, N. J. (1987). *Health promotion nursing practice* (2nd ed.). Norwalk, CT: Appleton & Lange.

Phillips, K. D., & Morrow, J. H. (1998). Nursing management of anxiety in HIV infection. *Issues in Mental Health Nursing, 19,* 375–397.

Porter, L. S. (1998). Reducing teenage and unintended pregnancies through client-centered and family-focused school-based family planning programs. *Journal of Pediatric Nursing, 13,* 158–163.

Reid, B., Allen, A. F., Gauthier, T., & Campbell, H. (1989). Solving the Orem mystery: An educational strategy. *Journal of Continuing Education in Nursing, 20,* 108–110.

Reisch, S. K., & Hauck, M. R. (1988). The Exercise of Self-Care Agency: An analysis of construct and discriminant validity. *Research in Nursing and Health, 11,* 245–255.

Renker, P. R. (1999). Physical abuse, social support, self-care, and pregnancy outcomes of older adolescents. *Journal of Obstetric and Neonatal Nursing, 28,* 377–388.

Rew, L. (1987a). Children with asthma: The relationship between illness behaviors and health locus of control. *Western Journal of Nursing Research, 9,* 465–483.

Rew, L. (1987b). The relationship between self-care behaviors and selected psychosocial variables in children with asthma. *Journal of Pediatric Nursing, 2,* 333–341.

Rhodes, V. A., Watson, P. M., & Hanson, B. M. (1988). Patients' descriptions of the influence of tiredness and weakness on self-care abilities. *Cancer Nursing, 11,* 186–194.

Richardson, A. (1992). Studies exploring self-care for the person coping with cancer treatment: A review. *International Journal of Nursing Studies, 29,* 191–204.

Riehl-Sisca, J. (1985a). *The science and art of self-care.* Norwalk, CT: Appleton-Century-Crofts.

Riehl-Sisca, J. (1985b). Determining criteria for graduate and undergraduate self-care curriculums. In J. Riehl-Sisca (Ed)., *The science and art of self-care* (pp. 307–309). Norwalk, CT: Appleton-Century-Crofts.

Ringerman, E., & Luz, S. (1990). A psychiatric patient classification system. *Nursing Management, 21*(10), 66–71.

Robinson, K. D., & Posner, J. D. (1992). Patterns of self-care needs and interventions related to biologic response modifier therapy: Fatigue as a model. *Seminars in Oncology Nursing, 8*(4, Suppl. 1), 17–22.

Rossow-Sebring, J., Carrieri, V., & Seward, H. (1992). Effect of Orem's model on nurse attitudes and charting behavior. *Journal of Staff Development, 8,* 207–212.

Rothert, M., Rovner, D., Holmes, M., et al. (1990). Women's use of information regarding hormone replacement therapy. *Research in Nursing and Health, 13,* 355–366.

Saba, V. K. (1997). Why the Home Care Classification is a recognized nomenclature. *Computers in Nursing, 15,* 567–573.

Sandman, P. O., Norberg, A., Adolfsson, R., Axelsson, K., & Hedley, V. (1986). Morning care of patients with Alzheimer-type dementia: A theoretical model based on direct observation. *Journal of Advanced Nursing, 11,* 369–378.

Saucier, C. (1984). Self-concept and self-care management in school-age children with diabetes. *Pediatric Nursing, 10,* 135–138.

Seideman, R. Y. (1990). Effects of a premenstrual syndrome education program on premenstrual symptomatology. *Health Care for Women International, 11,* 491–501.

Sella, S., & MacLeod, J. A. (1991). One year later: Evaluating a changing delivery system. *Nursing Forum, 26*(2), 5–11.

Silva, L. M. G. (2001). A brief reflection on self-care in hospital discharge planning after a bone marrow transplantation (BMT): A case report [Abstract]. *Revista Latino-Americana de Enfermagem, 9*(4), 75–82.

Silva, M. C. (1986). Research testing nursing theory: State of the art. *Advances in Nursing Science, 9*(1), 1–11.

Simmons, S. J. (1990). The health-promotion self-care system model: Directions for nursing research and practice. *Journal of Advanced Nursing, 15,* 1162–1166.

Slusher, I. L. (1999). Self-care agency and self-care practice of adolescents. *Issues in Comprehensive Pediatric Nursing, 22*(1), 49–58.

Smith, M. J. (1987). Critique of Orem's theory. In R. Parse (Ed.), *Nursing science: Major paradigms, theories and critiques* (pp. 91–105). Philadelphia: W. B. Saunders.

Smits, J., & Kee, C. C. (1992). Correlates of self-care among the independent elderly: Self-concept affects well-being. *Journal of Gerontological Nursing, 18*(9), 13–18.

Söderhamn, O., & Cliffordson, C. (2001). The structure of self-care in a group of elderly people. *Nursing Science Quarterly, 14,* 55–58.

Taylor, S. G. (1985a). Curriculum development for preservice programs using Orem's theory of nursing. In J. Riehl-Sisca (Ed.), *The science and art of self-care* (pp. 25–32). Norwalk, CT: Appleton-Century-Crofts.

Taylor, S. G. (1985b). Teaching self-care deficit theory to generic students. In J. Riehl-Sisca (Ed.), *The science and art of self-care* (pp. 41–46). Norwalk, CT: Appleton-Century-Crofts.

Taylor, S. G. (1988). Nursing theory and nursing process: Orem's theory in practice. *Nursing Science Quarterly, 1,* 111–119.

Taylor, S. G. (1989). An interpretation of family within Orem's general theory of nursing. *Nursing Science Quarterly, 2,* 131–137.

Taylor, S. G. (1991). The structure of nursing diagnosis from Orem's theory. *Nursing Science Quarterly, 4,* 24–32.

Taylor, S. G. (2001). Orem's General Theory of Nursing and families. *Nursing Science Quarterly, 14,* 7–9.

Taylor, S. G., Renpenning, K. E., Geden, E. A., Neuman, B. M., & Hart, M. A. (2001). A Theory of Dependent Care: A corollary theory to Orem's Theory of Self-Care. *Nursing Science Quarterly, 14,* 39–47.

Titus, S., & Porter, P. (1989). Orem's theory applied to pediatric residential treatment. *Pediatric Nursing, 15,* 465–468, 556.

Toth, J. C. (1980). Effect of structured preparation for transfer on patient anxiety leaving coronary care unit. *Nursing Research, 29,* 28–34.

Ulbrich, S. L. (1999). Theory. Nursing practice theory of exercise as self-care. *IMAGE: Journal of Nursing Scholarship, 31,* 65–70.

Underwood, P. (1979). Nursing care as a determinant in the development of self-care behavior by hospitalized adult schizophrenics. *Dissertation Abstracts International, 40,* 679B.

Underwood, P. (1980). Facilitating self-care. In P. C. Pothier (Ed), *Psychiatric nursing: A basic text* (pp. 115–135). Boston: Little Brown.

Urbanic, J (1992). Incest trauma resolution in adult female survivors. Unpublished doctoral dissertation. Wayne State University, Detroit, MI.

Utz, S. W., Hammer, J., Whitmire, V. M., & Grass, S. (1990). Perceptions of body image and health status in persons with mitral valve prolapse. *IMAGE: Journal of Nursing Scholarship, 22,* 18–22.

Utz, S. W., & Ramos, M. C. (1993). Mitral valve prolapse and its effects: A programme of inquiry within Orem's self-care deficit theory of nursing. *Journal of Advanced Nursing, 18,* 742–751.

van Acterberg, T., Lorensen, M., Isenberg, M. A., Evers, G. C. M., Levin E., & Phillipsen, H. (1991). The Norwegian, Danish and Dutch versions of the Appraisal of Self-Care Agency Scale: Comparing reliability aspects. *Scandinavian Journal of Caring Sciences, 5,* 101–108.

Villarruel, A. M., & Denyes, M. J. (1991). Pain assessment in children: Theoretical and empirical validity. *Advances in Nursing Science, 14*(2), 32–41.

Villarruel, A. M., & Denyes, M. J. (1997). International scholarship. Testing Orem's theory with Mexican Americans. *IMAGE: Journal of Nursing Scholarship, 29,* 283–288.

Wallace, W. A. (1983). Being scientific in a practice discipline. In *From a realist point of view: Essays on the philosophy of science* (pp. 273–293). Washington, DC: University Press of America.

Wang, H. (2001). A comparison of two models of health promoting lifestyle in rural elderly Taiwanese women. *Public Health Nursing, 18,* 204–211.

Wanich, C. K., Sullivan-Marx, E. M., Gottlieb, G. L., & Johnson, J. C. (1992). Functional status outcomes of nursing intervention in hospitalized elderly. *IMAGE: Journal of Nursing Scholarship, 24,* 201–207.

Weaver, M. T. (1987). Perceived self-care agency: A LISREL factor analysis of Bickel and Hanson's questionnaire. *Nursing Research, 36,* 381–387.

Weinrich, S. P. (1990). Predictors of older adults, participation in fecal occult blood screening. *Oncology Nursing Forum, 17,* 715–720.

Weintraub, F. N., & Hagopian, G. A. (1990). The effect of nursing consultation on anxiety, side effects and self-care of patient receiving radiation therapy. *Oncology Nursing Forum, 17*(3, Suppl.), 31–36.

West, P. (1993). *The relationship between depression and self-care agency in young adult women.* Unpublished doctoral dissertation, Wayne State University, Detroit, MI.

Whetstone, W. R. (1986). Social dramatics: Social skills development for the chronically mentally ill. *Journal of Advanced Nursing, 11,* 67–74.

Whetstone, W. R. (1987). Perceptions of self-care in East Germany: A cross-cultural empirical investigation. *Journal of Advanced Nursing, 12,* 167–176.

Whetstone, W. R., & Hansson, A. M. O. (1989). Perceptions of self-care in Sweden: A cross-cultural empirical investigation. *Journal of Advanced Nursing, 14,* 962–969.

Williams, P. D., Valderrama, D. M., Gloria, M. D., Pascoguin, L. G., Saavedra, L. D., De La Rama, D. T., et al. (1988). Effects of preparation for mastectomy/hysterectomy on women's post-operative self-care behaviors. *International Journal of Nursing Studies, 25,* 191–206.

Woods, N. F., Taylor, D., Mitchell, E. S., & Lentz, M. J. (1992). Perimenstrual symptoms and health-seeking behavior. *Western Journal of Nursing Research, 14,* 418–443.

Youssef, F. A. (1987). Discharge planning for psychiatric patients: The effects of a family-patient teaching programme. *Journal of Advanced Nursing, 12,* 611–616.

Zehnder, N. R. (1996). The influence of basic conditioning factors on menopausal self-care agency and menopausal self-care in midlife women. Unpublished doctoral dissertation. Wayne State University, Detroit, MI.

8

Roy's Adaptation Model

Mary E. Tiedeman

Sister Callista Roy received a bachelor's degree in nursing in 1963 from Mount Saint Mary's College. She received a master's degree in pediatric nursing in 1966, a master's degree in sociology in 1975, and a doctorate in sociology in 1977, all from the University of California, Los Angeles. In 1985, she completed a 2-year postdoctoral fellowship in neuroscience nursing at the University of California, San Francisco, and she spent an additional 2 years doing clinical research with patients who had neurological deficits. Roy's professional career has included positions in both clinical and educational settings. Her major professional positions have been in educational settings; she is currently a professor at the School of Nursing, Boston College. She also is an active member of the Sisters of Saint Joseph of Carondolet and a Fellow of the American Academy of Nursing (Roy, personal communication, March 6, 1986; Roy, 1983; 1997; Roy & Andrews, 1991, 1999).

According to Roy (personal communication, March 6, 1986), her major professional interest is the development of nursing as a scientific and humanistic discipline with an articulated and tested theory base that directs nursing practice and nursing education. Her clinical and research interests focus on neuroscience nursing and are aimed at understanding basic human cognitive processes, particularly cognitive recovery in persons with head injury.

The development of the adaptation model for nursing has been influenced by Roy's personal and professional background. She is committed to philosophical assumptions characterized by the general principles of humanism, veritivity, and cosmic unity, espousing a belief in holism and in the innate capabilities, purpose, and worth of human beings. Her pediatric clinical experience has fostered a belief in the resiliency of the human body and spirit. It was from her clinical experience in nursing and a review of the literature that she derived her concepts of person, environment, health, and nursing (Andrews & Roy, 1991a, 1986; Roy, 1991a, 1987a; Roy & Andrews, 1999).

Roy began her work on the adaptation model in the 1960s, when she was a graduate student at the University of California, Los Angeles. Drawing upon the works of experts in the areas of systems theory (von Bertalanffy, 1968) and adaptation (Dohrenwend, 1961; Helson, 1964; Lazarus, 1966; Mechanic, 1970; Selye, 1978), she formulated a beginning conceptualization and has continued developing the model. During the last 30 years, the model has been developed as a framework for nursing education, research, and practice using a variety of strategies, including model construction, theory development, philosophical explication, and research. During this time nurses in the United States and around the world have helped to clarify, refine, and extend the model. Use of the model in practice and research has provided data to help validate the model (Andrews & Roy, 1991a; Roy, 1991a; Roy & Andrews, 1991, 1999; Roy & McLeod, 1981).

BASIC CONSIDERATIONS IN THE MODEL
Definitions of Person, Nursing, Health, and Environment

Person. Within the model, person (human) is described as a holistic adaptive system, which is in constant interaction with the environment (Andrews & Roy, 1991a). More specifically, the person is defined as "an adaptive system, with regulator and cognator acting to maintain adaptation in the four adaptive modes; physiologic function, self-concept, role function, and interdependence" (Roy, 1984, p. 12).

The definition of person has evolved as the model has been developed. Although Roy has always described the person in terms of systems and adaptation, initial definitions and descriptions focused on the person as a biopsychosocial being in constant interaction with a changing environment (Roy, 1976a). Although Roy no longer specifically defines person as a biopsychosocial being, the biopsychosocial nature of the person as an adaptive system is reflected in the four adaptive modes: *physiological* (biologic), *self-concept* (psychological), *role function* (social), and *interdependence* (social).

Nursing. Roy has described nursing as a scientific discipline with a practice orientation. The science of nursing is interested in understanding life processes, which promote adaptation and health, how persons cope with health and illness, and nursing interventions to promote or enhance adaptive coping and health. As a practice discipline nursing uses this scientific knowledge to provide a service to people. More specifically, Roy has defined nursing as the science and practice of promoting adaptation for the purpose of affecting health positively. Thus, the adaptation model provides guidelines for the development of nursing knowledge (science) and the practice of nursing based on that knowledge. The theoretical and scientific domains of nursing and the nursing process distinguish it from other health disciplines (Andrews & Roy, 1991b; Roy, 1984, 1986, 1988, 1991a, 1991b; Roy & Andrews, 1999).

Within the model nursing consists of both the goal of nursing and nursing activities. Roy (Roy & Andrews, 1999) has defined the goal of nursing as "the promotion of adaptation in each of the four modes, thereby contributing to the person's health, quality of life, and dying with dignity" (p. 55). The nurse's role is to promote health by promoting adaptation and enhancing interaction of the human system with the environment through acceptance, protection, and fostering of interdependence, thereby promoting personal and environmental transformations. Nursing activities specified by the model are referred to as the nursing process (Andrews & Roy, 1991b; Roy & Andrews, 1999).

Although Roy has continued to refine her definition and description of nursing, there have been no major changes in this area of the model. The goals of nursing and nursing activities have been consistently identified as aspects of the concept of nursing and the fundamental description of these aspects of nursing has remained the same. Her more recent writings have put increased emphasis on describing the science of nursing and its relationship to nursing practice and have more clearly delineated how the adaptation model guides the development of the science of nursing. More recent writings also reflect the new assumptions for the 21st century (Andrews & Roy 1991a, 1991b; Roy, 1991a, 1991b, 1997; Roy & Andrews, 1999).

Health. An understanding of the concepts of the human adaptive system and environment and an appreciation of the scientific and philosophic assumptions of the model are essential to an understanding of health as explicated within the model (Roy & Andrews, 1999). According to Roy (Roy & Andrews, 1999), health is defined as "a state and a process of being and becoming an integrated and whole person" (p. 54). Health can be viewed as a reflection of the interaction or adaptation of human adaptive systems within a changing environment. Being integrated is a state that reflects the adaptation process and can be described at any given point in time as it is manifested in the wholeness and integration of the four adaptive modes. Becoming integrated is a continuous process consisting of a systematic series of actions directed toward the human goals or survival, growth, reproduction, mastery, and person and environment transformations and the purposefulness of human existence (Andrews & Roy, 1991a; Roy, 1990; Roy & Andrews, 1999).

Being integrated implies a soundness or unimpaired condition leading to wholeness. Integration and wholeness can lead to completeness or unity and the highest possible fulfillment of human potential. Thus, integration is health, whereas the absence of integration is a lack of health. Health is defined without reference to illness and includes emphasis on states of wellbeing (Andrews & Roy, 1991a; Roy, 1984,1990; Roy & Andrews, 1999).

Environment. Environment is defined as "all conditions, circumstances, and influences that surround and affect the development and behavior of human adaptive systems with particular consideration of person and earth resources" (Roy & Andrews, 1999, p. 52). As the world around and within human adaptive systems, the environment is viewed as input for the human adaptive system and may be described as internal and external stimuli. These stimuli may be further classified as focal, contextual, and residual (Andrews & Roy, 1991a, Roy & Andrews, 1999).

Additional Understanding of Nursing

Nursing science. Roy's (1988) perspective of the discipline of nursing is "that of an integrated metaparadigm that has the dynamics of life processes at its heart and the functional life patterns emanating from that center and being manifested in human responses to actual or potential health problems" (p. 28). This perspective includes both the basic and the clinical science of nursing.

The basic science of nursing focuses on human life processes and patterns that promote health; that is, understanding persons as adaptive systems. Life processes include regulating, thinking, becoming, valuing, relating, feeling, and acting. Functional life patterns emerge from the development and use of these life processes, and the person's response to health problems arises from these patterns (Roy, 1988, 1990, 1991a, 1991b; Roy & Andrews, 1999).

The clinical science of nursing focuses on the diagnosis of effective and ineffective adaptation and on intervention strategies to enhance adaptation in situations of health and illness (Roy, 1988, 1990, 1991a, 1991b; Roy & Andrews, 1999). Roy (1988) has described the clinical science of nursing as the "diagnosis and treatment of the patterning of life processes" (p. 28), or the "diagnosis and treatment of human responses within the functional health patterns" (p. 29).

Nursing activities. The recipient of nursing is a holistic, adaptive system, which may be an individual, family, group, community, or society (Andrews & Roy, 1991a; Roy & Andrews, 1999). Although the discussion in most of Roy's writings has focused on the individual, the principles can be applied to families, groups, communities, and society. The focus on collectives has become more evident as the model has been developed (Roy, 1983; Roy & Andrews, 1999; Roy & Anway, 1989).

Nursing is concerned with the human-environment interaction, where input and internal and external stimuli from the environment activate coping processes that act to maintain adaptation. Situations of particular concern to nursing are those in which the environmental changes strain the person's coping mechanisms; that is, situations in which unusual stressors (focal stimuli) or weakened coping mechanisms make a person's usual attempts to cope ineffective. This should not be interpreted to mean that nursing activities are needed or occur only when the person is ill or not coping effectively. According to Roy, nursing's holistic approach looks at processes for maintaining well-being and high-level functioning. This focus on positive adaptation is particularly evidenced by the recent development of typologies of indicators of positive adaptation (Andrews & Roy, 1991a, 1991b; Roy & Andrews, 1999; Roy & Roberts, 1981).

The goal of nursing—promoting adaptation by enhancing the interaction of human systems with the environment—is fostered by nursing activities; that is, the use of the nursing process: assessment, nursing diagnosis, goal-setting, intervention, and evaluation. The adaptation model provides specific guidelines for use of the nursing process (Andrews & Roy, 1991a, 1991b; Roy & Andrews, 1999).

Roy has consistently described a six-step nursing process. Although each step is described separately, Roy (Andrews & Roy, 1991b; Roy & Andrews, 1999) emphasizes that the process is ongoing and simultaneous.

The units of analysis for the two-level assessment (steps 1 and 2) are the person in interaction with his or her environment. The first level of assessment is the *collection of data about the person's behavior (observable and nonobservable) in each of the four adaptive modes.* The primary concern is with behaviors that are ineffective; however, identification of adaptive behaviors is also important. The second level of assessment is the *collection of data regarding the focal, contextual, and residual stimuli.* It is particularly important to determine factors that influence the behavior of concern (ineffective behavior), although it is also important to identify factors influencing adaptive behaviors (Andrews & Roy, 1991b; Roy & Andrews, 1999).

The third step of the nursing process, nursing diagnosis, involves *interpretation of* the *assessment* data. This step involves "a judgment process resulting in statements conveying the adaptation status of the human adaptive system" (Roy & Andrews, 1999, p. 77). *Goal-setting,* step 4 of the nursing process, involves establishing a clear statement of the behavioral outcomes for the person as a result of nursing care. This goal statement has three parts: behavior, expected change, and time frame (Andrews & Roy, 1991b; Roy & Andrews, 1999).

Nursing intervention, step 5, focuses on stimuli influencing behavior and the ability to cope (i.e., the coping processes). Management of stimuli (internal and external) involves removing, increasing, decreasing, maintaining, or altering stimuli. Focal or contextual stimuli may be the focus of nursing intervention; however, when possible the focus should be the focal stimulus. Managing stimuli promotes adaptive behavior by bringing the stimuli within the ability of the coping processes of the human system. Interventions also may be designed specific to the coping processes of regulator-stabilizer and cognator-innovator systems (e.g., providing knowledge to alter perception, thus influencing the cognator). In step 6, *behavioral outcomes are evaluated* and *approaches modified as needed* (Andrews & Roy, 1991b; Roy & Andrews, 1999).

Within the model the person is viewed as an active participant in personal care. There is emphasis on the importance of collaboration with the person throughout the steps of the nursing process and manipulation of stimuli is not seen as manipulation of the person (Andrews & Roy, 1991b; Roy & Andrews, 1999; Roy & Roberts, 1981).

Understanding of Person

To gain a clearer understanding of humans (person), as conceptualized within the model, it is necessary to examine in more detail the description of humans as holistic adaptive systems The term *holistic* comes from the philosophic assumptions of the model and conveys the idea that human systems function as wholes in one unified expression of meaningful behavior. As a *system,* humans can be described as a set of interrelated parts with inputs, control and feedback processes, and outputs functioning as a whole for some purpose. As *adaptive* systems, humans not only have the capacity to adjust effectively to environmental changes, but also can affect the environment (Andrews & Roy, 1986, 1991a; Roy & Andrews, 1999).

Input for the system is stimuli, which are received externally from the environment (external stimuli) and from the internal environment (internal stimuli). A specific input to the system is the human's adaptation level, which results from the pooling of certain relevant stimuli—focal, contextual, and residual. It represents the condition of life processes and may be described in three levels: integrated, compensatory, and compromised. This constantly changing adaptation level affects the ability of the human system to respond positively (Andrews & Roy, 1991a, 1991b; Roy, 1984; Roy & Andrews, 1999).

The control processes of the system are two coping mechanisms for adapting or coping with a changing environment. These control processes are the *regulator* and *cognator subsystems for individuals* and the *stabilizer* and *innovator subsystems for groups*. In the individual these mechanisms are viewed as biological, psychological, and social in origin and are both innate and acquired. The regulator is viewed as responding automatically through neural, chemical, and endocrine channels. The cognator is viewed as responding through cognitive-emotive channels that include perceptual-information processing, learning, judgment, and emotion. The stabilizer and innovator subsystems of groups parallel those of the regulator and cognator subsystems of the individual and are related to goals of stability and change. The responses of the regulator-cognator and stabilizer-innovator are manifested or carried out through four adaptive or effector modes (Andrews & Roy, 1991a; Roy, 1976a; Roy & Andrews, 1999).

Four adaptive modes were initially developed for individual human systems based on the analysis and categorization of samples of patient behavior and have been expanded to include groups. These four modes—*physiological-physical, self-concept-group identity, role function,* and *interdependence*—are seen as providing the particular form or manifestation of regulator-cognator or stabilizer-innovator activity. Beneath each of the adaptive modes is a basic need for integrity that includes physiological, psychic, and social integrity (Andrews & Roy, 1991a; Roy & Andrews, 1999).

Relationships among the regulator and cognator and the four adaptive modes are complex. Processes of the regulator and cognator, defined in a series of propositions, link together the regulator and cognator with the four adaptive modes. The regulator is viewed as related predominantly to the physiological mode. The propositions of the regulator are applied to each of the physiological functions and are related to adaptive and ineffective responses. The cognator is viewed as related to each adaptive mode in at least three ways: (a) each mode provides specific, relevant input for the cognator; (b) the adaptive mode under consideration will specify the relevant pathways and apparatus; and (c) within each mode it is possible to view specific cognator processes (Roy & McLeod, 1981; Roy & Roberts, 1981).

The process of perception is found in both the regulator and cognator and is viewed as the process linking these two subsystems. "Inputs to the regulator are transformed into perception. Perception is a process of the cognator. The responses following perception are feedback into both the cognator and the regulator" (Roy & McLeod, 1981, p. 67). Thus, the relationship between the regulator and cognator is a hierarchical relationship (Roy & McLeod, 1981).

Three relationships can be observed among the four modes. These relationships are that (a) internal and external stimuli may affect more than one adaptive mode simultaneously, (b) one behavior may be a manifestation of disruption in more than one mode, and (c) each adaptive mode may act as a focal, contextual, or residual stimulus for each of the other modes. The complex relationships among the adaptive modes and the regulator and cognator subsystems reflect the integrated, holistic nature of the person. Examples of the various relationships may be found in the writings of Roy and others (Andrews & Roy, 1991a; Roy & McLeod, 1981; Roy & Roberts, 1981; Tiedeman, 1989). The same complexity exists between the stabilizer and innovator and the four adaptive modes of a group (Roy & Andrews, 1999).

Outputs of the system are responses called *behavior*. Behavior is viewed as "internal and external actions and reactions under specified circumstances" (Roy & Andrews, 1999, p. 43). Behaviors result from the control processes; are manifested in the four adaptive modes; and can be observed, measured, or subjectively reported. In collaboration with the person, behaviors can be judged as adaptive or ineffective. Adaptive responses maintain or promote integrity, whereas ineffective responses disrupt integrity. Through feedback processes behaviors (responses) provide further input for the person as a system (Andrews & Roy, 1991a; Roy & Andrews, 1999). A schematic representation of the person as an adaptive system is shown in Figure 8–1 of the model.

Understanding of Environment

In defining environment, three classes of stimuli are described: focal, contextual, and residual. These stimuli may be either internal or external. The stimulus most immediately confronting the person is called the *focal stimulus*. The focal stimulus is the focus of the person's attention, and the person expends energy to deal with it. All other stimuli present in the situation that are contributing to the effect of the focal stimulus are called *contextual stimuli*. Although not the center of the person's attention and energy, contextual stimuli influence how the person is able to deal with the focal stimulus. Stimuli whose effects on the given situation are unclear are called *residual stimuli*. This category is useful for considering possible influencing stimuli based on general knowledge and/or intuitive impressions (Andrews & Roy, 1991a).

As the environment changes, the significance of any one stimulus changes. In a rapidly changing environment stimuli may readily switch from one category of stimuli to another. The identification and classification of relevant stimuli is important for providing nursing care within the framework of the model (Andrews & Roy, 1991a).

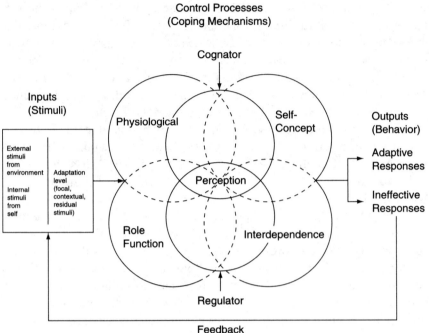

FIGURE 8–1 The person as an adaptive system.

Adaptation

The definition of adaptation, the core concept of the adaptation model, has been expanded recently to reflect the mission of nursing in a new epoch and the scientific and philosophic assumptions of the 21st century (Roy, 1997). Adaptation is defined as "the process and outcome whereby thinking and feeling persons, as individuals or in groups, use conscious awareness and choice to create human and environmental integration" (Roy & Andrews, 1999, p. 30). The concept of adaptation is closely linked to the concept of health. The person, as an adaptive system, is in constant interaction with a changing environment. Health is a reflection of this interaction. Adaptive responses promote integrity relative to the goals of the human system—survival, growth, reproduction, mastery, and person environment transformations—thereby promoting health. Ineffective responses do not promote integrity or contribute to the goals of adaptation. In addition, adaptive responses free energy from ineffective coping and allow the person to respond to other stimuli. This freeing of energy can promote healing and enhance health. It is the freeing of energy that links the concepts of adaptation and health (Andrews & Roy, 1991a; Roy, 1984, 1990; Roy & Andrews, 1999).

Within the model adaptation is viewed as both a *process* and an *outcome*. As a process, it involves a systematic series of actions directed toward the goals of adaptation, thus promoting integrity and affecting health positively. The process of adaptation includes all of the person's interactions with the environment. It is a two-part process, which is a function of the focal stimulus and the person's adaptation level. The first part of the process is initiated by changes in the internal or external environment (focal stimuli) that demand a response. The impact of these focal stimuli is mediated by contextual and residual factors. The second part of the process is coping mechanisms that are triggered to produce adaptive or ineffective responses. Although this process is described in terms of responding to stimuli, Roy indicates that it is not a passive process, but is always positive, active, and creative. The emphasis is on purposefulness of human existence in a universe that is creative and views persons as coextensive with their physical and social environments (Andrews & Roy, 1991a; Roy, 1990; Roy & Andrews, 1999; Roy & McLeod, 1981).

Adaptation also is considered an outcome in that the condition of the person with respect to the environment may be viewed at any given point in time. It is a state of dynamic equilibrium, which is the result of the cumulative effect of the ongoing process of adaptation and can be described in terms of conditions, which promotes the goals of the human system and the individualized goals of the person. Each new adaptive state affects the adaptation level of the person, resulting in the dynamic equilibrium of the person being at an even higher level and allowing greater ranges of stimuli to be dealt with successfully by the person as an adaptive system. Thus, promoting adaptation leads to higher level of well-being or health (Andrews & Roy, 1991a; Roy, 1990; Roy & McLeod, 1981; Roy & Roberts, 1981).

Interrelationships Among the Concepts

Adaptation is the central and unifying concept within the model. The recipient of nursing care is the person (or group) as an adaptive system in constant interaction with a changing environment. Stimuli from the external and internal environment activate the coping processes of regulator-cognator (or stabilizer-innovator), which produce behavior observed in the four adaptive modes. This behavior is a function of input (stimuli) and the individual or group adaptation level. When adaptive responses occur, energy is freed for response to other stimuli, thus promoting integrity or health. Nursing enhances adaptation through the use of the nursing process, thereby promoting health through the management of stimuli (environment) or the strengthening of coping processes (Andrews & Roy,

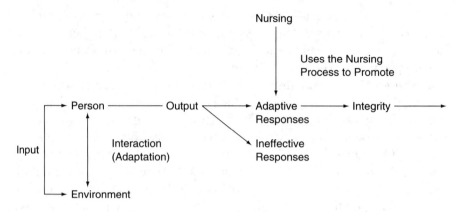

FIGURE 8–2   Relationships among the basic components of the adaptation model of nursing.

1991a, 1991b; Roy, 1984, 1990; Roy & Andrews, 1999). The relationships among the basic concepts of the model are shown in Figure 8–2.

INTERNAL ANALYSIS AND EVALUATION

Underlying Assumptions

The assumptions of the adaptation model include both scientific and philosophical assumptions. The scientific assumptions are associated with systems theory and adaptation-level theory; the philosophical assumptions are associated with humanism and veritivity (Andrews & Roy, 1991a; Roy, 1986; Roy & Andrews, 1999).

Underlying assumptions associated with systems theory include holism, interdependence, control processes, information feedback, and complexity of living systems. Underlying assumptions associated with adaptation-level theory include behavior as adaptive; adaptation as a function of stimuli and adaptation level; individual, dynamic adaptation levels; and positive and active processes of responding. These notions have been expanded to include views of the universe progressing in structure, organization, and complexity, and the purposefulness of human existence (Roy, 1997; Roy & Andrews, 1999). Scientific assumptions for the 21st century are more explicitly identified in Table 8–1.

Underlying assumptions associated with humanism include creativity, purposefulness, holism, and interpersonal process, whereas those associated with veritivity include purposefulness of human existence; unity of purpose; activity and creativity; and value and meaning of life. Philosophic concepts also have been expanded. Philosophic assumptions for the

TABLE 8-1   Scientific Assumptions of the Roy Adaptation Model for the 21st Century

1. Systems of matter and energy progress to higher levels of complex self-organization.
2. Consciousness and meaning are constitutive of person and environment integration.
3. Awareness of self and environment is rooted in thinking and feeling.
4. Human decisions are accountable for the integration of human processes.
5. Thinking and feeling mediate human action.
6. System relationships include acceptance, protection, and fostering of interdependence.
7. Persons and earth have common patterns and integral relations.
8. Person and environment transformations are created in human consciousness.
9. Identification of human and environment meanings results in adaptation.

Roy (1997, p. 44); Roy & Andrews (1999, p. 35).

TABLE 8-2   Philosophic Assumptions of the Roy Adaptation Model for the 21st Century

1. Persons have mutual relationships with the world and with a God—figure.
2. Human meaning is rooted in an omega point convergence of the universe.
3. God is intimately revealed in the diversity of creation and in the common destiny of creation.
4. Persons use human creative abilities of awareness, enlightenment, and faith.
5. Persons are accountable for the processes of deriving, sustaining, and transforming the universe.

Roy (1997, p. 45); Roy & Andrews (1999, p. 35).

21st century are more explicitly identified in Table 8–2 (Andrews & Roy, 1991a; Roy, 1986, 1988).

According to Barnum (1998), identification of the underlying assumptions is necessary to both the internal and external evaluation of the theory. Internal criticism deals with logic and consistency of the theory given the underlying assumptions. External criticism involves the congruence of the assumptions with the "real world." Internal and external criticisms will be addressed later.

The philosophical orientation most compatible with the adaptation model appears to be that of logical positivism. Within this philosophical orientation concepts are used in describing phenomena, statements or propositions are developed to propose how concepts are related, and propositions are related to each other in a systematic way (Barnum, 1998; Jacox, 1974). A clearer understanding of the philosophical orientation of the model can be obtained by examining it in terms of principle, interpretation, and method (Barnum, 1998). The key principle in the adaptation model is adaptation. Adaptation is the process and outcome of coping with a changing environment and, thus, it is located in the person-environment interaction. The outcome of adaptation is viewed as a state of dynamic equilibrium. Therefore, the nature of the principle of adaptation as explicated within the model is reflexive; that is, the principle is located in the interaction of the person and circumstances (changing environment). The principle of adaptation also may be classified as a simple principle—one that explains the principle in terms of component parts; for example, the inputs (stimuli), control and feedback processes (coping mechanisms), and outputs (responses) characterizing the process of adaptation (Andrews & Roy, 1991a; Barnum, 1998; Roy, 1990; Roy & Andrews, 1999).

In examining the interpretation of the model, one needs to consider how the author views the reality of the phenomenon under consideration. The phenomena of Roy's model fall within the human experience (as distinct from phenomena beyond it) and would be termed *phenomenal*. When the essence of the subject matter is phenomenal, the model may be interpreted as existential or essential. An *essential* interpretation is one in which the phenomenon is explained by reference to the circumstances in which it occurs (Barnum, 1998). Within the adaptation model, the person's adaptation occurs in response to a changing environment or by affecting the environment (Andrews & Roy, 1991a; Roy & Andrews, 1999). Therefore, the adaptation model is an essential model.

The method of the adaptation model is less easily identified. The logistic method is evident in the earlier scientific assumptions of the model, particularly the assumptions related to systems theory. The logistics method is one in which parts are used to organize the whole so that "a system, event, or entity is organized by reference to its parts and their interrelationships" (Barnum, 1998, p. 133). This method is less clear in the scientific assumptions for the 21st century, which appear to be moving toward the dialectic method by describing person and earth as having common patterns and integral relationships. The philosophical assumptions are more in keeping with the dialectic method. Within the dialectic method all components are parts of a larger whole, "a whole that is different from and greater than a mere summation of those parts" (Barnum, 1998, p. 132).

Relative Importance of the Basic Components

The components of the adaptation model that receive the most emphasis are the concepts of person as an adaptive system and adaptation. Roy has discussed these concepts in detail and depth and they have received much attention as she has clarified and refined the model. Adaptation is viewed as the central and unifying concept of the model. It is the concept of adaptation that links the concepts of person, environment, health, and nursing.

The nursing process has been delineated clearly within the model and has undergone little change as the model has been clarified and refined. In her more recent writings, Roy has placed more emphasis on the science of nursing, describing both the basic and clinical science of nursing.

The concepts of health and environment have received more attention as the model has developed. Although environment is defined in terms of stimuli, there is more emphasis on the discussion of stimuli as related to the person as an adaptive system rather than as related to the environment. The concept of health, as explicated within the model, is viewed by Roy as being in the developing stages, and according to Roy, an understanding of the concept of health is contingent upon an understanding of the concepts of person and environment. The concept of health is closely related to the concept of adaptation and has been explicitly defined within the model since 1983 (Andrews & Roy, 1991a; Roy, 1983; Roy & Andrews, 1999).

Analysis of Consistency

It is important to examine the clarity and consistency (congruence) of a model (Barnum, 1998; Meleis, 1991). To assess clarity and consistency, one needs to determine if the concepts are clearly and consistently defined, if the relationships between the concepts are clear and consistent, and if the assumptions are consistent with the concepts and the relationships between the concepts.

The concepts of person, adaptation, health, environment, and nursing are clearly defined and can be readily understood; however, there are some inconsistencies. Within the adaptation model, person is described as an adaptive system, a whole made up of parts that adapts to changes in the environment and also affects the environment (Andrews & Roy, 1991a; Roy & Andrews, 1999). A mechanistic view of person is inconsistent with the holistic view espoused by Roy. However, Roy has stated that the focus on parts is only for descriptive purposes and that the model is based on a holistic view of person. The philosophic assumptions of the model support the holistic view espoused by Roy that behavior is purposeful and not a chain of cause and effect. Thus, to explicate relationships, the person's behavior is described as both purposeful and as cause and effect or response to stimulus. Although Roy has stated that the person affects the environment, she has placed much greater emphasis on the person's response to the environment (Andrews & Roy, 1991a; Roy, 1986, 1988; Roy & Andrews, 1999). Roy (1988) provided further support for the holistic view of person by stating that "the complexities and subtleties of the process whereby the person takes in and responds to the environment precludes . . . a behavioristic interpretation" (p. 32).

In the model, environment is defined as internal and external stimuli, and the person is described as receiving inputs from the external and internal environments (Andrews & Roy, 1991a; Roy & Andrews, 1999). In her earlier writings, Roy (Roy & Roberts, 1981) stated that further work was needed to clarify environment as distinct from internal stimuli. It would seem that internal stimuli are now viewed as part of the environment. This raises the following question: If internal stimuli are part of the environment, how is this internal environment differentiated from the person as an adaptive system; that is, how does one determine what is part of the internal environment and what is part of the person? This is a particularly important question because within the model, nursing intervention is viewed as the management of stimuli, and Roy (Roy & Roberts, 1981) has clearly indicated that the manipulation of stimuli is not manipulation of the person. It also is not clear how environment is distinguished from the person's adaptation level, given that both are defined and described in terms of focal, contextual, and residual stimuli (Andrews & Roy, 1991a; Roy & Andrews, 1999).

The relationships among the concepts vary in clarity but there are no discrepancies or contradictions within the relationships. The relationships among person, adaptation, and nursing are clear. The person adapts and nursing promotes this adaptation. The relationship between adaptation and health also is fairly clear. Adaptation promotes integrity and integrity is health. Thus, adaptation leads to health. Because nursing promotes adaptation, the relationship between nursing and health also is clear; that is, nursing promotes health (Andrews & Roy, 1991a; Roy & Andrews, 1999). The relationship between person and health is less clear but appears to be an indirect relationship linked by the concept of adaptation.

There is a question with regard to the concept of adaptation, especially as it is related to the other concepts in the model. Adaptation refers to the person-environment interaction. In this interaction the person may respond adaptively or ineffectively; however, Roy (Andrews & Roy, 1991a; Roy & Andrews, 1999) has indicated that the person adapts and that nursing promotes this adaptation for the purpose of enhancing health. It seems that nursing is actually promoting successful adaptation or adaptive responses rather than adaptation per se.

The relationships between the regulator and cognator and the four adaptive modes are not always specified. This is particularly true of the relationship between the regulator and the physiological mode. The propositions of the regulator and the physiological mode need additional distinction (Limandri, 1986).

The definitions of the concepts within the model and the relationships among them are consistent with the model's scientific assumptions. The definitions of the concepts and the relationships among them are not always clearly consistent with the philosophical assumptions that emphasize holism. Integration of these assumptions within the model would help clarify the congruence of the more part-focused systems theory and adaptation-level theory with the more whole-focused philosophical assumptions (Whall, 1992). With the new definition of adaptation and the scientific assumptions for the 21st century, the model is moving in that direction.

Analysis of Adequacy

According to Barnum (1998), "a theory is adequate if it accounts for the subject matter with which it purports to deal" (p. 174) and "if its prescriptions are extensive enough to cover the scope claimed by its author" (p. 174). Using this definition, the adaptation model meets the criterion of adequacy. The model views nursing as promoting adaptation in situations related to health, and it deals with the concept of adaptation in a careful and detailed manner. The model is viewed as broad in scope and the identification of interventions as the management of stimuli or the strengthening of coping processes would support the broad scope inferred by the author of the model (Andrews & Roy, 1991a; Roy, 1984; Roy & Andrews, 1999).

Hardy (1974) described two criteria for assessing the adequacy of a model—meaning and logical adequacy, and operational-empirical adequacy. In assessing meaning and logical adequacy, one needs to examine the validity of the assumptions and the validity of the meaning attributed to the concepts; that is, are the concepts defined in a manner similar to that used by other scientists in the area? In addition, one needs to examine the logic of the theoretical system.

Person, adaptation, health, and nursing are clearly defined and explained in detail within the model. Although each of the concepts has aspects unique to the model, each has aspects similar to those used by other scientists in the area.

The cognator and regulator as coping mechanisms are unique to the model, although there is support for the concept of coping mechanisms in the conceptions of person as specified by other scientists. The idea of persons having four adaptive modes also is unique to the model. Some have stated that they found it difficult to separate the self-concept, role function, and interdependence modes (Gerrish, 1989; Limandri, 1986; Nyqvist & Sjoden, 1993; Wagner, 1976). These modes were identified based on the analysis and categorization of patient behaviors (Roy, 1991a). Therefore, there is a question that if a person's behavior cannot be absolutely categorized, are these modes mutually exclusive?

Two aspects of nursing are unique to the model: the two-level assessment in the nursing process and intervention as management of stimuli. The two-level assessment provides for evaluation of patient behavior (responses) and the stimuli to which the person is responding. This is appropriate to a model that focuses on persons responding to stimuli. The specification within the model of nursing intervention as management of focal and contextual stimuli, both internal and external, raises a question. Can internal stimuli be manipulated without manipulating the person? It is clearly stated that the manipulation of stimuli is different from the manipulation of people (Roy & Roberts, 1981). An example would serve to clarify this point. This question still remains, although internal stimuli have now been conceptualized as part of the environment (Andrews & Roy, 1991a; Roy & Andrews, 1999).

The concept of adaptation as process and outcome draws upon the definitions of other theorists, such as Dohrenwend (1961). Lazarus (1966), Mechanic (1970), and Selye (1978), who defined adaptation as a process, and Helson (1964), who defined it as a product (outcome). The model combines the various aspects of the definitions in a logical manner and has developed the concept further in a manner that is consistent with the definitions of these theorists.

The logical adequacy of the model also can be assessed by examining the relationships among the concepts. Roy has described most of the relationships clearly. There are no apparent discrepancies or contradictions.

In assessing operational and empirical adequacy, one asks the following questions. Can the concepts be measured? Do operational definitions reflect theoretical concepts? Does the evidence support the model or the theories derived from it; that is, do the empirical data conform to hypothesized expectations (Calvillo & Flaskerud, 1993; Hardy, 1974)? Because this is a broad model for nursing, the adaptation model does not define the major concepts operationally. However, general propositions have been developed in the model and from these propositions it is possible to deduce testable hypotheses. Thus, concepts contained in these hypotheses could be defined in a manner that would be theoretically consistent with the concepts and would be measurable. Testable hypotheses have been derived from the model and have provided evidence (empirical data) that supports portions of the model (Fawcett & Tulman, 1990; Frederickson, Jackson, Strauman, & Strauman, 1991; Hill & Roberts, 1981; Smith, 1988; Thornbury & King, 1992).

Another aspect of adequacy is pragmatic adequacy; that is, the usefulness of the model, including its usefulness in generating innovative actions from the research, which could be used in practice (Calvillo & Flaskerud, 1993). A number of studies have used the model to derive interventions and then tested these interventions in practice. These studies supported the usefulness of interventions derived from the model (Smith, 1988; Thornbury & King, 1992).

EXTERNAL ANALYSIS

Relationship to Nursing Research

The usefulness of a model for research depends on its ability to guide all phases of a study. It should provide a perspective for research by suggesting the subject matter or phenomena to be studied, identifying the nature of the problems to be studied or the research questions to be asked, and identifying appropriate methods of inquiry (Barnum, 1998; Fawcett & Tulman, 1990; Roy, 1991a). The elements and assumptions of the adaptation model provide such a perspective for research in both the basic and clinical science of nursing. The phenomena of study, as identified by the model, are persons (both individuals and groups). The distinctive nature of the problems to be studied or the research questions to be asked are related to basic life processes and patterns, coping with health and illness, and enhancing adaptive coping (positive life processes and patterns) (Roy, 1987b, 1988, 1990, 1991a). According to Roy (1991a), multiple methods are appropriate and desirable when conducting research based on the model. The concepts Roy (1970) articulated provide a model for the long-term process of observation and clarification of facts leading to postulates regarding (a) the occurrence of adaptation problems; (b) coping mechanisms; and (c) interventions based on laws derived from factors composing the response potential; that is, focal, contextual, and residual stimuli. Using this framework, typologies of adaptation problems or nursing diagnoses have been developed as well as typologies of indicators of positive adaptation (Andrews & Roy, 1991b; Roy & Andrews, 1991). In 1981, Roy and Roberts noted the need to develop an organization of categories of interventions that would fit within the model. Some research has been done in this area. Data on cognitive deficits have been used to design intervention protocols for cognitive recovery from head injury (Roy, 1991a). Others have used the framework to develop and test interventions to help promote adaptation based on managing stimuli (Fawcett, 1990; Kuhns, 1997; Samarel et al., 1998; Smith, 1988; Thornbury & King, 1992).

Within the tradition of logical empiricism, to be useful for research, a model must be able to generate testable hypotheses (Silva & Rothbart, 1984). This is consistent with the verificationist perspective of logical positivism, in which the meanings of propositions depend on their method of verification. A number of general propositions have been developed from the adaptation model (Roy & McLeod, 1981; Roy & Roberts, 1981). From these general propositions, specific propositions or testable hypotheses can be developed. Roy (Roy & Roberts, 1981) has cited examples of such testable hypotheses, which she has stated are relevant for specifying prescriptions for practice. Others also have demonstrated the development of testable hypotheses from the model. Testing of these hypotheses has provided data to validate or support the model (Frederickson et al., 1991; Hill & Roberts, 1981; Smith, 1988; Thornbury & King, 1992; Zhan, 2000).

The model has been used as a framework for research by Roy and others. During the last 30 years it has been used in more than 200 quantitative research studies (Frederickson, 2000; Roy & Andrews, 1999). (See Table 8–3 for a partial list of studies using the model.) Roy (1991a) has provided

TABLE 8–3 Use of the Adaptation Model in Research

Focus of research	Researcher
Cross-cultural pain	Cavillo & Flaskerud (1993)
Caesarean birth	Fawcett (1990)
Child-bearing women	Fawcett & Tulman (1990), Tulman et al. (1998)
Cancer patients	Frederickson et al. (1991), Samarel et al. (1998)
Spinal cord injury patients	Harding-Okimoto (1997)
Abused women	Limandri (1986)
Well adolescents	Modrcin et al. (1998)
Breast-feeding women	Nyqvist & Sjoden (1993)
Spouses of surgical patients	Silva (1987)
Elderly persons	Smith (1988), Zhan (2000)
Person with Alzheimer's disease	Thornbury & King (1992)

research examples from both basic and clinical nursing science. In basic nursing science the model has been used as a framework for exploring how the cognator coping mechanism acts to promote adaptation and its relationship to the four adaptive modes, and for examining the relationship of adaptation to health. In clinical nursing science the model has been used in a program of research related to cognitive recovery of patients with head injury. Specifically, this research focused on gaining an understanding of basic human cognitive processes and how nurses can assist persons to positively affect their health by use of these processes.

Scholars who have used the adaptation model as the conceptual basis for their research have found it to be useful in identifying the concepts and variables to study and in selecting instruments to measure or operationalize these variables (Calvillo & Flaskerud, 1993; Fawcett, 1990; Fawcett & Tulman, 1990; Harding-Okimoto, 1997; Limandri, 1986; Modrcin-Talbott, Pullen, Ehrenberger, Zandstra, & Muenchen, 1998; Tulman, Morin, & Fawcett, 1998; Vicenzi & Thiel, 1992). In addition, it has been found to be useful in suggesting the design or methodology for research studies (Fawcett & Tulman, 1990; Roy, personal communication, March 6, 1986) and in structuring and organizing data into themes and categories (Nyqvist & Sjoden, 1993; Silva, 1987). The model also is useful for deriving testable hypotheses and propositions. The model clearly has demonstrated its usefulness in research to date. As the model continues to develop it will serve as a framework for both quantitative and qualitative research.

Relationship to Nursing Education

The adaptation model has demonstrated its usefulness in education. As a theoretical framework for nursing education, it is one the most widely used models in the United States and is being used increasingly in other countries (Roy, 1982; Roy & Andrews, 1991). A combination of nursing process and adaptation problems provide the framework for nursing curricula based on the model, and form the units and strands of knowledge and practice that are developed throughout the educational program (Roy, 1973).

The model is currently the basis for the nursing curricula at Mount Saint Mary's College, Los Angeles, and the Royal Alexandra Hospitals School of Nursing, Edmonton, Alberta, Canada (Roy & Andrews, 1991). The model also has been used in a geriatric nurse-practitioner program (Brower & Baker, 1976), and in the first-year nursing course of a generic baccalaureate program at the University of Ottawa School of Nursing, Ottawa, Ontario, Canada (Morales-Mann & Logan, 1990).

According to Roy (1973, 1976b, 1979), the curriculum at Mount Saint Mary's has clearly demonstrated the relationship of nursing theory to nursing education. The model allows for increasing knowledge in the areas of both theory and practice, and it helps students test theory and develop new theoretical insights. In addition, the model distinguishes between nursing science and medical science. Brower and Baker (1976) stated that the adaptation model for nursing integrated nursing theory, thereby decreasing students' anxiety. They also stated that the model provided some distinction between nursing and medicine, although there was some overlap.

Although the model has demonstrated its usefulness in education, challenges faced by educators when implementing the model have been identified. These challenges include (a) developing or adapting courses to be congruent with the model; (b) developing teaching tools that are consistent with the model and suitable for student learning; (c) sequencing content to facilitate student learning about the model, course content, and the relationship between them; and (d) obtaining competent role models in the application of the model (Morales-Mann & Logan, 1990).

Relationship to Professional Nursing Practice

The clinical application of an explicit model improves nursing practice by integrating theory into everyday processes of patient care and nursing administration, providing a distinctive focus for nursing practice, helping to define nursing roles and goals, facilitating communication among nurses, and fostering development of common goals for patient care. A model provides structure to guide practice by providing direction for the nursing process (Connerly, Ristau, Lindberg, & McFarland, 1999; Keen et al., 1998). The adaptation model provides this direction based on its well-developed guidelines for the use of the nursing process. The two-level assessment process focuses on the assessment of behaviors and stimuli and leads to the identification of nursing diagnoses (behaviors related to stimuli) and the establishment of goals (behavioral outcomes). The model provides the framework for intervention, which is focused on the management

TABLE 8–4 Use of the Roy Adaptation Model in Practice

Focus of research	Researcher
Cancer patients	Cook (1999), Gerrish (1989)
Patients undergoing amputation	Dawson (1998)
Occupational health, work environment	Doyle & Rejacich (1991)
Patients with anxiety	Frederickson (1993)
Hospitalized children	Galligan (1979), Starn & Niederhauser (1990)
Coronary care unit	Hamner (1989)
Adolescents with asthma	Hennessy-Harstad (1999)
Adult hemodialysis patients	Keen et al. (1998)
Home care	Lankester & Sheldon (1999), Schmitz (1980)
Abused women	Limandri (1986)
Patients with Kawasaki disease	Nash (1987)
Adolescents with bulimia nervosa	Pilote (1998a, 1998b)
Elderly in apartment complexes	Smith (1988)
Patients with Alzheimer's disease	Thornbury & King (1992)

of stimuli or strengthening the adaptive processes. Evaluation assesses the effectiveness of the intervention by examining behavior relative to the goals. As the model has been developed, there has been a refinement of the approaches to nursing diagnosis, an identification of major stimuli for each mode, and development of intervention protocols based on the model (Andrews & Roy, 1991b; Gray, 1991; Roy & Andrews, 1991, 1999).

The usefulness of the adaptation model in practice has been demonstrated in a variety of clinical settings with various populations (see Table 8–4). In addition, the model has been adopted by a number of healthcare agencies in the United States and abroad, where it serves as a basis for practice (Connerly et al., 1999; Frederickson, 1991; Frederickson & Williams, 1997; Nyqvist & Sjoden, 1993; Roy, 1986; Weiss, Hastings, Holly, & Craig, 1994).

Use of this comprehensive, holistic model in practice has advantages and disadvantages. The model has been found to facilitate thorough and holistic assessments by providing a comprehensive framework, which includes psychosocial aspects as well as physiological aspects (Dawson, 1998; Doyle & Rajacich, 1991; Galligan, 1979; Gerrish, 1989; Hamner, 1989; Smith, 1988; Thornbury & King, 1992). This holistic approach may foster earlier identification of problems (Frederickson, 1993). In addition, as the model has developed, coping processes and adaptive modes have been defined for groups that parallel those of the individual human adaptive system. This expansion of the model offers a framework for systematic healthcare delivery to aggregates, making it more amenable to community health nursing applications (Dixon, 1999).

The adaptation model has been used in practice to design nursing interventions based on the management or manipulation of stimuli or the strengthening of adaptive processes that were identified during assessment and formulation of nursing diagnoses. This approach to intervention, which is specific to the individual and the diagnosis, helps individualize care and may be more effective than more general, standardized approaches to care (Cook, 1999; Frederickson, 1993; Hennessy-Harstad, 1999; Lankester & Sheldon, 1999; Smith, 1988; Starn & Niederhauser, 1990; Thornberry & King, 1992).

A number of additional advantages have been identified by nurses who have used the model in practice. The holistic approach of the model helps prevent putting too much emphasis on aspects of illness and allows for the inclusion of health promotion. In addition, it is easy to apply as a family-centered model (Lankester & Sheldon, 1999). Other advantages are a perceived improvement in efficiency and effectiveness of the nursing process and quality of patient outcomes, and improved patient and/or family satisfaction (Frederickson & Williams, 1997; Weiss et al., 1994).

Despite its usefulness in facilitating thorough and holistic assessments, application of the nursing process based on the model can be lengthy, repetitious, and time consuming, especially during the assessment phase. In addition, the process may include elements not considered necessary or relevant to the actual care of the patient. These concerns have been found to be most problematic in intensive care units, where there are rapid changes in patient's conditions, and least problematic in outpatient and long-term care settings (Gerrish, 1989; McIver, 1987; Wagner, 1976; Weiss et al., 1994).

Some difficulty in using the model in practice arises from some apparent overlap in modes, which can make it difficult to structure the assessment to cover one mode at a time and/or to decide which mode is appropriate for a given behavior (Gerrish, 1989; Limandri, 1986; Nyqvist & Sjoden, 1993; Wagner, 1976). Because of the possible overlap in modes, Nyqvist and Sjoden (1993) expressed doubt about the appropriateness of the model for daily patient assessment. Others expressed difficulty in using the model for identification and classification of stimuli as focal, contextual, or residual (Gerrish, 1989; Lankester & Sheldon, 1999). Despite some difficulties in using the model in practice, the advantages in using the model clearly outweigh the disadvantages.

Nursing Classification Systems and the Model

Nursing practice is conducted through the nursing process (Roy & Andrews, 1999). Three American Nurses Association (ANA)-approved classification systems focus on components of the nursing process. These classification systems include the North American Nursing Diagnosis Association (NANDA) classification of nursing diagnoses, the Nursing Outcomes Classification (NOC), and the Nursing Interventions Classification (NIC). These classification systems have been linked to one another given that they all suggest specific interventions and outcomes for specific diagnoses (Wilkinson, 2000).

Roy (Roy & Andrews, 1999) defines nursing diagnosis as "a judgment process resulting in a statement conveying the person's adaptation status" (p. 77). Although this definition reflects both process and outcome, the emphasis is on the outcome or product. This outcome has been described as a summary statement or conclusion about the person based on the interpretation of assessment data. The concept of nursing diagnoses is also applicable to groups.

The framework provided by the adaptation model for establishing nursing diagnoses is that of behavior related to stimuli. It is the "related to" portion of the diagnosis that serves as the focus for nursing intervention within the model. Within this framework three alternatives for establishing nursing diagnoses are described. One method of establishing a nursing diagnoses is a statement of a specific observed behavior with the relevant influencing stimuli for that behavior; for example, "pulse 120 due to hemorrhage from injury." This method allows for the lack of completeness of the typologies of nursing diagnoses and provides specific indications for nursing intervention. Another method of establishing a nursing diagnosis is to cluster assessment data to provide a summary label for behaviors rather than a statement of individual behaviors. This summary label reflects the typology of commonly recurring adaptive problems within each of the four modes. "Hypoxia related to hemorrhage from injury" would be an example of this method. This method is useful in complex situations for which the label represents a multifaceted clinical situation. Established sets of cues, signs, and symptoms, possible causes or etiologies, and scientific nursing knowledge useful in planning interventions are associated with these summary labels (Andrews & Roy, 1991b; Carpenito, 1997; Roy & Andrews, 1999).

The definition and description of nursing diagnoses within the adaptation model is consistent with NANDA's definition of nursing diagnosis. According to NANDA, "nursing diagnosis is a clinical judgment about individual, family, or community responses to actual or potential health problems/life processes. A nursing diagnosis provides the basis for selection of nursing interventions to achieve outcomes for which the nurse is accountable" (NANDA, 2001, p. 245).

Based on the model, Roy (Andrews & Roy, 1991b; Roy & Andrews, 1991, 1999) has developed a typology of commonly recurring adaptation problems as well as a typology of indicators of positive adaptation. As a whole, NANDA diagnoses are congruent with the adaptation model, given that these diagnostic labels are reflective of the person's responses or behaviors. Roy herself (Roy & Andrews, 1999) relates the NANDA diagnoses to the typology of commonly recurring adaptation problems. Not all diagnoses included in the typology developed within the adaptation model are NANDA-approved diagnoses, and not all NANDA-approved diagnoses are included in the typology based on the model. Diagnoses appearing in both classification systems include "activity intolerance," "body image disturbance," and "anxiety." A diagnosis of "shock" is included in Roy's typology but is not an approved NANDA diagnosis, whereas "impaired parenting" is an approved NANDA diagnosis that is not included in Roy's typology.

There are some differences in how the "related to" portion of the nursing diagnosis is viewed in Roy's typology compared with approved NANDA diagnoses. In the adaptation model, the "related to" portion of the statement is the stimuli most directly affecting behavior and is the focus of intervention. This connection is less direct with approved NANDA diagnoses. The "related to" portion of the statement indicates what should change for the person to return to optimal health and helps the nurse select effective nursing interventions. It is not clear that the "related to" portion of the statement is the specific focus of nursing intervention (Andrews & Roy, 1991b; NANDA, 2001; Roy & Andrews, 1999; Wilkinson, 2000).

Roy (Roy & Andrews, 1999) defines goal setting as the "establishment of clear statements of behavioral outcomes of nursing care" (p. 81). The focus is on behavior of the human adaptive system—either changing ineffective behavior to adaptive behavior or maintaining and enhancing adaptive behavior. Each goal statement contains three parts: the behavior to be observed, that manner in which it will change, and the time frame. Change may be observed, measured, or subjectively reported (Roy & Andrews, 1999). NOC describes nursing-sensitive outcomes rather than goals. A nursing-sensitive patient outcome describes a measurable patient or family state, behavior, or perception labeled as concepts that can be measured along a continuum; for example, "activity tolerance." Nursing-sensitive outcome indicators are specific variables referent to a nursing-sensitive patient outcome and characterize a patient's state at a concrete level; for example, "heart rate in expected range in response to activity." Nursing-sensitive outcome measures are operations or activities that describe precisely what outcome indicator is to be measured and how; for example, extremely compromised (1) to not compromised (5) (Johnson, Maas, & Moorhead, 2000). Outcomes, outcome indicators, and outcome measures are all needed to establish patient outcomes or goals.

There are similarities between goals as defined by the adaptation model and outcomes as defined by NOC. Both address individuals and family (groups) and both are holistic with physiological and psychosocial goals and outcomes. Other commonalities are that both state goals or outcomes in terms of behavior and both measure change in behavior in response to nursing care.

Although not specifically stated, the goals in the adaptation model would appear to represent a resolution of a nursing diagnosis. Within NOC the majority of outcomes represent the resolution of nursing diagnosis, whereas others are more generic and not necessarily related to nursing diagnoses (Johnson et al., 2000). Although the adaptation model states that a time frame is an essential part of the goal statement, establishing an appropriate time frame for measuring outcomes is still being studied by NOC.

In the adaptation model the focus of intervention is on stimuli, which are influencing behavior and the coping processes of regulator and cognator. More specifically, Roy (Roy & Andrews, 1999) describes intervention as "the selection of nursing approaches to promote adaptation by changing stimuli or strengthening adaptive processes" (p. 86). NIC defines nursing intervention as "any treatment, based upon clinical judgment and knowledge, that the nurse performs to enhance patient/client outcomes" (McCloskey & Bulechek, 2000, p. 3).

There are some similarities between interventions as defined in the adaptation model and NIC interventions. Both include a holistic approach with interventions aimed at physiological problems and psychosocial problems, and both address interventions with groups as well as individuals. Another commonality is the purpose of the intervention, which is enhancing client outcomes, although the adaptation model specifies this outcome in terms of promoting adaptation. The most obvious difference between the two approaches is the focus of the intervention. Within the adaptation model the focus in on the stimuli or coping processes, whereas NIC interventions are linked to specific diagnostic labels rather than related to the portion of the diagnosis.

Relationship to Theory-driven, Evidence-based Practice

The topic of evidence-based practice is generating much discussion in the nursing literature today. The current emphasis is on an atheoretical, empirical model of evidence, which focuses on the randomized clinical trials as the most legitimate form of evidence. This narrow view of evidence-based practice fails to address the scope of knowledge (evidence) needed for holistic nursing practice. Furthermore, the lack of a theoretical perspective widens the theory-practice gap when a theory-based approach to nursing is needed. Nursing models can be used to create a theory-guided, evidence-based practice (Dixon, 1999; Fawcett, Watson, Neuman, Walker, & Fitzpatrick, 2001; Hennessy-Harstad, 1999; Ingersoll, 2000; Walker & Redman, 1999; Upton, 1999)

Carper (1978) identified four patterns of knowing, all of which are important for knowing in nursing (Chinn & Kramer, 1999; Fawcett et al.,

2001; Stein, Corte, Colling, & Whall, 1998). Models of nursing can be examined to determine their contribution to evidence in the four patterns of knowing. The Roy adaptation model is clearly able to guide research, which produces scientific data as evidence for empirical knowing or theories. The model has been used to guide numerous research studies, which have generated publicly verifiable, factual descriptions, explanations, or predictions. Furthermore, the model provides a framework for developing and answering questions that are important to both theorists and practicing nurses (see Relationship to Nursing Research, p. 162). Ethical knowledge is evident in the adaptation model in the philosophic assumptions. These assumptions are clearly articulated values, which can serve as a foundation for future dialogue about values and beliefs, thus generating additional ethical knowledge or theories (Fawcett et al., 2001; Stein et al., 1998; Roy, 1997; Roy & Andrews, 1999; Upton, 1999).

The relationship of the adaptation model to personal knowing or theories is less clear; however, the focus of the interdependence mode is on relationships, which would include the interpersonal relationships of nursing. In addition, the philosophic assumptions clearly communicate the valuing of persons, suggesting the value of listening to responses from others and reflecting on those thoughts and responses. Aesthetic knowledge or theories encompass the art or act of nursing that is the knowledge underlying the performance of nursing practice or "knowing how." Emphasis is on the nurse's perceptions of what is significant in the behavior of an individual patient. The adaptation model provides a framework for the nurse to rehearse the art of nursing via the nursing process explicated in the model (Fawcett et al., 2001; Stein et al., 1998; Roy & Andrews, 1999).

SUMMARY

There is disagreement whether a nursing theory should have a broad or limited scope (Barnum, 1998). Jacox (1974) originally supported a limited scope, whereas Ellis (1968) supported a broad scope and considered both scope and complexity as characteristic of significant theory. The adaptation model would be viewed as broad in scope, given that it can be applied to any situations related to adaptation and health in any setting.

There also is lack of agreement within nursing regarding whether the complexity of theory should be distinct from parsimony. An appropriate balance should be determined based on the complexity of the subject matter (Barnum, 1998). The model is complex, dealing with multiple complex concepts and relationships. This complexity is in keeping with the nature of the subject matter and does not deter the essence of the theory from being explained in parsimonious terms.

   It has been shown that the adaptation model for nursing is a complex model that deals with multiple concepts and relationships. The individual concepts also are complex. Within this complexity are few inconsistencies in the definitions with little vagueness in the description of the relationships between the concepts. However, the model is broad in scope and can be applied in many situations. In practice, it has been found very useful in inpatient and outpatient settings as well as in work settings and in the community. The model also has been used extensively to guide research, which has provided some confirmation for the model and demonstrated its ability to generate new information. The Roy Adaptation Model thus makes a significant contribution to nursing's body of knowledge.

REFERENCES

Andrews, H. A., & Roy, C. (1986). *Essentials of the Roy Adaptation Model.* East Norwalk, CT: Appleton-Century-Crofts.

Andrews, H. A., & Roy, C. (1991a). Essentials of the Roy Adaptation Model. In C. Roy & H. A. Andrews (Eds.), *The Roy Adaptation Model: The definitive statement.* Norwalk, CT: Appleton & Lange.

Andrews, H. A., & Roy, C. (1991b). The nursing process according to the Roy Adaptation Model. In C. Roy & H. A. Andrews (Eds.), *The Roy Adaptation Model: The definitive statement.* Norwalk, CT: Appleton & Lange.

Barnum, B. S. (1998). *Nursing theory: Analysis, application, evaluation* (5th ed.). Philadelphia: J. B. Lippincott.

Brower, H. T. F., & Baker, B. J. (1976). The Roy Adaptation Model: Using the adaptation model in a practitioner curriculum. *Nursing Outlook, 24,* 686–689.

Calvillo, E. R., & Flaskerud, J. H. (1993). The adequacy and scope of Roy's adaptation model to guide cross-cultural pain research. *Nursing Science Quarterly, 6,* 118–129.

Carpenito, L. H. (1997). *Nursing diagnosis: Application to clinical practice* (7th ed.). Philadelphia: J. B. Lippincott.

Carper, B. A. (1978). Fundamental patterns of knowing in nursing. *Advances in Nursing Science, 1,* 13–23.

Chinn, P. L., & Kramer, M. K. (1999). *Theory and nursing: Integrated knowledge development* (5th ed.). St. Louis, MO: Mosby.

Connerley, K., Ristau, S., Lindberg, C., & McFarland, H. (1999). The Roy model in practice. In C. Roy & H. A. Andrews. *The Roy Adaptation Model* (2nd ed., pp. 515–534). Stanford, CT: Appleton-Lange.

Cook, N. F. (1999). Self-concept and cancer: Understanding the nursing role. *British Journal of Nursing, 8,* 318–324.

Dawson, S. (1998). Pre-amputation assessment using Roy's Adaptation Model. *British Journal of Nursing, 7,* 536, 538–542.

Dixon, E. L. (1999). Community health nursing practice and the Roy Adaptation Model. *Public Health Nursing, 16,* 290–300.

Dohrenwend, B. P. (1961). The social psychological nature of stress: A framework for causal inquiry. *Journal of Abnormal and Social Psychology, 62,* 294–302.

Doyle, R., & Rajacich, D. (1991). The Roy Adaptation Model: Health teaching about osteoporosis. *AAOHN Journal, 39,* 508–512.

Ellis, R. (1968). Characteristics of significant theories. *Nursing Research, 17,* 217–222.

Fawcett, J. (1990). Preparation for Caesarean childbirth: Derivation of a nursing intervention from the Roy Adaptation Model. *Journal of Advanced Nursing, 15,* 1418–1425.

Fawcett, J., & Tulman, L. (1990). Building a programme of research from the Roy Adaptation Model of nursing. *Journal of Advanced Nursing, 15,* 720–725.

Fawcett, J., Watson, J., Neuman, B., Walker, P. H., & Fitzpatrick, J. J. (2001). On nursing theories and evidence. *Journal of Nursing Scholarship, 33,* 115–119.

Frederickson, K. (1991). Nursing theories-a basis for differentiated practice: Application of the Roy Adaptation Model in nursing practice. In I. E. Goertzen (Ed.), *Differentiating nursing practice into the twenty-first century.* Kansas City, MO: American Academy of Nursing.

Frederickson, K. (1993). Using a nursing model to manage symptoms: Anxiety and the Roy Adaptation Model. *Holistic Nurse Practitioner, 7*(2), 36–43.

Fredrickson, K. (2000). Nursing knowledge development through research: Using the Roy Adaptation Model. *Nursing Science Quarterly, 13,* 12–17.

Frederickson, K., Jackson, B. S., Strauman, T., & Strauman, J. (1991). Testing hypotheses derived from the Roy Adaptation Model. *Nursing Science Quarterly, 4,* 168–174.

Frederickson, K., & Williams, J. K. (1997). Nursing-theory guided practice: The Roy Adaptation Model and patient/family experiences. *Nursing Science Quarterly, 10,* 53–54.

Galligan, A. C. (1979). Using Roy's concept of adaptation to care for young children. *MCN: The American Journal of Maternal-Child Nursing, 4,* 24–28.

Gerrish, C. (1989). From theory to practice. *Nursing Times, 85*(30), 42–45.

Gray, J. (1991). The Roy Adaptation Model in nursing practice. In C. Roy & H. A. Andrews (Eds.), *The Roy Adaptation Model: The Definitive Statement.* Norwalk, CT: Appleton & Lange.

Hamner, J.B. (1989). Applying the Roy Adaptation Model to the CCU. *Critical Care Nurse, 9,* 51–52, 54–61.

Harding-Okimoto, M. B. (1997). Pressure ulcers, self-concept and body image in spinal cord injury patients. *SCI Nursing, 14,* 111–117.

Hardy, M. E. (1974). Theories: Components, development, evaluation. *Nursing Research, 23,* 100–107.

Helson, H. (1964). *Adaptation-level theory: An experimental and systematic approach to behavior.* New York: Harper & Row.

Hennessy-Harstad, E. B. (1999). Empowering adolescents with asthma to take control through adaptation. *Journal of Pediatric Health Care, 13,* 273–277.

Hill, B. J., & Roberts, C. S. (1981). Formal theory construction: An example in process. In C. Roy & S. L. Roberts (Eds.), *Theory construction in nursing: An adaptation model.* Englewood Cliffs, NJ: Prentice-Hall.

Ingersoll, G. L. (2000). Evidence-based nursing. What it is and what it isn't. *Nursing Outlook, 48,* 151–152.

Jacox, A. (1974). Theory construction in nursing: An overview. *Nursing Research, 23,* 4–13.

Johnson, M., Maas, M., & Moorhead, S. (Eds.). (2000). *Nursing Outcomes Classification (NOC)* (2nd ed.). St. Louis, MO: Mosby.

Keen, M., Breckenridge, D., Frauman, A. C., Hartigan, M. F., Smith, L., Butera, E., et al. (1998). Nursing assessment and intervention for adult hemodialysis patients: Application of Roy's Adaptation Model. *ANNA Journal, 25,* 311–319.

Kuhns, M. L. (1997). Treatment outcomes with adult children of alcoholics: Depression. *Advanced Practice Nursing Quarterly, 3,* 64–69.

Lankester, K., & Sheldon, L. M. (1999). Health visiting with Roy's model: A case study. *Journal of Child Health Care, 3,* 28–34.

Lazarus, R. S. (1966). *Psychological stress and the coping process.* New York: McGraw-Hill.

Limandri, B. J. (1986). Research and practice with abused women: Use of the Roy Adaptation Model as an explanatory framework. *Advances in Nursing Science, 8*(4), 52–61.

McCloskey, J. C., & Bulechek, G. M. (Eds.). (2000). *Nursing Interventions Classification (NOC)* (3rd ed.). St. Louis, MO: Mosby.

McIver, M. (1987). Putting theory into practice. *Canadian Nurse, 83*(10), 36–38.

Mechanic, D. (1970). Some problems in developing a social psychology of adaptation to stress. In J. McGrath (Ed.), *Social and psychological factors in stress.* New York: Holt, Rinehart & Winston.

Meleis, A. I. (1991). *Theoretical nursing: Development and progress* (2nd ed.). Philadelphia: J. B. Lippincott.

Modrcin-Talbott, M. A., Pullen, L, Ehrenberger, H., Zandstra, K., & Muenchen, B. (1998). Self-esteem in adolescents treated in an outpatient mental health setting. *Issues in Comprehensive Pediatric Nursing, 21,* 159–171.

Morales-Mann, E. T., & Logan, M. (1990). Implementing the Roy model: Challenges for nurse educators. *Journal of Advanced Nursing, 15,* 142–147.

Nash, D. J. (1987). Kawasaki disease: Application of the Roy Adaptation Model to determine interventions. *Journal of Pediatric Nursing, 2,* 308–315.

North American Nursing Diagnosis Association (NANDA). (2001). *NANDA nursing diagnoses: Definitions & classification 2001–2002.* Philadelphia: Author.

Nyqvist, K. H., & Sjoden, P. (1993). Advice concerning breastfeeding from mothers of infants admitted to a neonatal intensive care unit: The Roy Adaptation Model as a conceptual structure. *Journal of Advanced Nursing, 18,* 54–63.

Pilote, R. A. (1998a). Adolescent bulimia nervosa—Part 1: A comprehensive review of the literature. *Journal of Addictions Nursing, 10,* 180–189.

Pilote, R. A. (1998b). Adolescent bulimia nervosa—Part 2: A proposed group nursing intervention. *Journal of Addictions Nursing, 10,* 190–196.

Roy, C. (1970). Adaptation: A conceptual framework for nursing. *Nursing Outlook, 18,* 42–45.

Roy, C. (1973). Adaptation: Implications for curriculum change. *Nursing Outlook, 21,* 163–168.

Roy, C. (1976a). *Introduction of nursing: An adaptation model.* Englewood Cliffs, NJ: Prentice-Hall.

Roy, C. (1976b). The Roy Adaptation Model: Comment. *Nursing Outlook, 24,* 690–691.

Roy, C. (1979). Relating nursing theory to nursing education: A new era. *Nurse Educator, IV*(2), 16–21.

Roy, C. (1982). Foreword. In B. Randall, M. P. Tedrow, & J. Landingham (Eds.), *Adaptation nursing: The Roy conceptual model applied.* St. Louis, MO: Mosby.

Roy, C. (1983). Roy Adaptation Model. In I. M. Clements & B. R. Roberts (Eds.), *Family health: A theoretical approach to nursing.* Englewood Cliffs, NJ: Prentice-Hall.

Roy, C. (1984). *An introduction to nursing: An adaptation model* (2nd ed.). Englewood Cliffs, NJ: Prentice-Hall.

Roy, C. (1986, August). *Overview of the Roy Adaptation Model and its contributions to nursing as a practice discipline.* Paper presented at meeting of Nursing Theory Conference. Toronto, Ontario, Canada.

Roy, C. (1987a). Response to "needs of spouses of surgical patients: A conceptualization within the Roy Adaptation Model." *Scholarly Inquiry for Nursing Practice: An International Journal, 1,* 45–50.

Roy, C. (1987b). Roy's Adaptation Model. In R. R. Parse (Ed.), *Nursing science: Major paradigms, theories, and critiques.* Philadelphia: W. B. Saunders.

Roy, C. (1988). An explication of the philosophical assumptions of the Roy Adaptation Model. *Nursing Science Quarterly, 1,* 26–34.

Roy, C. (1990). Strengthening the Roy Adaptation Model through conceptual clarification-response: Conceptual clarification. *Nursing Science Quarterly, 3,* 64–66.

Roy, C. (1991a). The Roy Adaptation Model in nursing research. In C. Roy & H. A. Andrews (Eds.), *The Roy Adaptation Model. The definitive statement.* Norwalk, CT: Appleton & Lange.

Roy, C. (1991b). Structure of knowledge: Paradigm, model, and research specifications. In I. E. Goertzen (Ed.), *Differentiating nursing practice into the twenty-first century.* Kansas City, MO: American Academy of Nursing.

Roy, C. (1997). Future of the Roy model: Challenge to redefine adaptation. *Nursing Science Quarterly, 10,* 42–48.

Roy, C., & Andrews, H. A. (1991). *The Roy Adaptation Model: The definitive statement.* Norwalk: CT: Appleton & Lange.

Roy, C., & Andrews, H. A. (1999). *The Roy Adaptation Model* (2nd ed.). Stanford, CT: Appleton & Lange.

Roy, C., & Anway, J. (1989). Roy's Adaptation Model: Theories for nursing administration. In B. Henry, C. Arndt, M. DiVincenti, & A. Marriner-Tomey (Eds.), *Dimensions of nursing administration: Theory, research, education, practice.* Boston: Blackwell Scientific.

Roy, C., & McLeod, D. (1981). Theory of person as an adaptive system. In C. Roy & S. L. Roberts (Eds.), *Theory construction in nursing: An adaptation model.* Englewood Cliffs, NJ: Prentice-Hall.

Roy, C., & Roberts, S. L. (1981). *Theory construction in nursing: An adaptation model.* Englewood Cliffs, NJ: Prentice-Hall.

Samarel, N., Fawcett, J., Kreppendorf, K., Piacentino, J. C., Eliasof, B., Hughes, P., et al. (1998). Women's perceptions of group support and adaptation to breast cancer. *Journal of Advanced Nursing, 28,* 1259–1268.

Schmitz, M. (1980). The Roy Adaptation Model: Application to a community setting. In J. P. Riehl & C. Roy (Eds.), *Conceptual models for nursing practice* (2nd ed.). New York: Appleton-Century-Crofts.

Selye, H. (1978). *The stress of life.* New York: McGraw-Hill.

Silva, M. C. (1987). Needs of spouses of surgical patients. A conceptualization within the Roy Adaptation Model. *Scholarly Inquiry for Nursing Practice: An International Journal, 1,* 29–43.

Silva, M. C., & Rothbart, D. (1984). An analysis of changing trends in philosophies of science on nursing theory development and testing. *Advances in Nursing Science, 6*(2), 1–13.

Smith, M. C. (1988). Roy's Adaptation Model in practice. *Nursing Science Quarterly, 1,* 97–98.

Starn, J., & Niederhauser, V. (1990). An MCN model for nursing diagnosis to focus intervention. *MCN: The American Journal of Maternal-Child Nursing, 13,* 180–183.

Stein, K. F., Corte, C., Colling, K. B., & Whall, A. (1998). A theoretical analysis of Carper's ways of knowing using a model of social cognition. *Scholarly Inquiry for Nursing Practice: An International Journal, 12,* 43–60.

Thornbury, J. M., & King, L. D. (1992). The Roy Adaptation Model and care of persons with Alzeheimers disease. *Nursing Science Quarterly, 5,* 129–133.

Tiedeman, M. E. (1989). The Roy Adaptation Model. In J. J. Fitzpatrick & A. L. Whall (Eds.), *Conceptual models of nursing: Analysis and application* (2nd ed.). Norwalk, CT: Appleton & Lange.

Tulman, L., Morin, K. H., & Fawcett, J. (1998). Prepregnant weight and weight gain during pregnancy: Relationship to functional health status, symptoms, and energy. *JOGNN: Journal of Obstetric, Gynecologic, and Neonatal Nursing, 27,* 629–634.

Upton, D. J. (1999). How can we achieve evidence-based practice if we have a theory-practice gap in nursing today? *Journal of Advanced Nursing, 29,* 549–555.

Vicenzi, A. E., & Thiel, R. (1992). AIDS education on the college campus. Roy's Adaptation Model directs inquiry. *Public Health Nursing, 9,* 270–276.

von Bertalanffy, L. (1968). *General Systems Theory.* New York: Braziller.

Wagner, P. (1976). The Roy Adaptation Model: Testing the application of the model in practice. *Nursing Outlook, 24,* 661–685.

Walker, P. H., & Redman, R. (1999). Theory-guided, evidence-based reflective practice. *Nursing Science Quarterly, 12,* 298–303.

Weiss, M. E., Hastings, W. J., Holly, D. C., & Craig, D. I. (1994). Roy's Adaptation Model in practice: Nurses' perspectives. *Nursing Science Quarterly, 7,* 80–86.

Whall, A. L. (1992). Book review: *The Roy Adaptation Model: The definitive statement.* Norwalk, CT: Appleton & Lange. *Nursing Science Quarterly, 5,* 190–191.

Wilkinson, J. M. (2000). *Nursing diagnosis handbook with NIC interventions and NOC outcomes* (3rd ed.). St. Louis, MO: Mosby.

Zhan, L. (2000). Cognitive adaptation and self-consistency in hearing-impaired older persons: Testing Roy's Adaptation Model. *Nursing Science Quarterly, 13,* 158–165.

ADDITIONAL REFERENCES

Roy, C. (1971). Adaptation: A basis for nursing practice. *Nursing Outlook, 19,* 254–257.

Roy, C. (1975a). A diagnostic classification system for nursing. *Nursing Outlook, 23,* 90–94.

Roy, C. (1975b). The impact of nursing diagnosis. *AORN Journal, 21,* 1023–1030.

Roy, C. (1976a). The impact of nursing diagnosis. *Nursing Digest, 4,* 67–79

Roy, C. (1976b). *The Roy Adaptation Model: Past, present, and future.* Taped at Wayne State University, Detroit, MI.

Roy, C. (1980). The Roy Adaptation Model. In J. P Riehl & C. Roy (Eds.), *Conceptual models for nursing practice* (2nd ed.). New York: Appleton-Century-Crofts.

9

Leininger's Transcultural Nursing

Cynthia Cameron and Linda Luna

Leininger's theory of transcultural care diversity and universality is the creative outcome of some four decades of evolutionary development and refinement. Historically, the roots of the theory can be traced back to Leininger's experience as a staff nurse on a medical-surgical unit in a large general hospital in the mid-1940s. Through direct observation and experiences with patients with a variety of health problems, Leininger realized that human care was an important aspect of nursing that helped people to maintain health and recover from illness (Leininger, 1991, p. 7). Later, Leininger worked as a clinical specialist in child mental health in a child guidance center in the mid-1950s. Through working with emotionally disturbed children of diverse cultural backgrounds, Leininger noted definite behavioral differences that began to raise questions about cultural aspects of care (Leininger, 1978, p. 21). According to the theorist, psychoanalytic and mental health theories popular in nursing at the time failed to explain the observed differences in the behavior of the children. As a mental health nurse specialist, Leininger continued to question the influence of culture and care in explaining human behavior. Through linking the concepts of human care and culture, the theory of culture care was born.

Realizing that nursing could greatly benefit from anthropological, theoretical, and research findings, Leininger sought higher education in this discipline. Upon completion of a doctoral program at the University of

This chapter is reprinted from *Conceptual Models of Nursing: Analysis and Application,* 3rd ed.

Washington, Leininger pioneered in establishing and developing the new field of transcultural nursing. Through synthesis and creative formulation of selected concepts, themes, and paradigms from anthropology and nursing, she developed this new and different area of study and research in nursing. At the same time, she initiated the idea of linking care to culture to generate substantive knowledge for the discipline of nursing (1991, p. 15).

Leininger's theory of *transcultural care diversity* and *universality* provides a unique and important and conceptual, theoretical, and research approach to study nursing phenomena (Leininger, 1985a, p. 44). Emphasis is given to the historical, social, and cultural context of human beings to explain and predict the broad dimensions of human care behaviors. A major goal of the theory is to improve and advance the quality of care to people through the deliberate and creative use of transcultural nursing knowledge that reflects culturally congruent care based on the values, beliefs, and lifestyles of people from diverse cultures (1991, p. 37). According to the theory, culturally derived nursing care based on transcultural human care knowledge is predicted to maintain client health and well-being or to help clients face death in culturally appropriate ways (1991, p. 39).

BASIC CONSIDERATIONS INCLUDED IN THE MODEL

During the last few decades, nurses have devoted much attention to developing a scientific knowledge base that reflects the distinctiveness of nursing as a discipline (Algase & Whall, 1993). Certain nurse-scholars have embraced the concepts of person, environment, health, and nursing as constituting a metaparadigm of nursing (Fawcett, 1989; Fitzpatrick & Whall, 1989). Leininger, however, has firmly held, over an extended period of time, to the position that human care is the critical and essential element of nursing and is a central concept of a metaparadigm of the discipline. Moreover, she rejects the idea that nursing can be a concept of the metaparadigm because this is the phenomenon to be explained and predicted and thus violates the discovery process (1991, p. 39). For Leininger, care is the essence of nursing, and culturally based care can be predicted to enable health and well-being for humans of diverse cultures. Furthermore, care has the greatest potential for explaining nursing phenomena and for predicting health outcomes of individuals, families, groups, and communities.

Definition of Nursing

As previously mentioned, Leininger holds that nursing is the phenomenon to be explained by concepts of the metaparadigm. Nursing is defined as "a learned humanistic and scientific profession and discipline which is focused on human care phenomena and activities in order to assist, support, facilitate, or enable individuals or groups to maintain or regain their well being (or health) in culturally meaningful and beneficial ways, or to help people face handicaps or death" (1991, p. 47). The idea that nursing's focus is *human care* is central to the definition. Leininger believes that nursing is essentially a transcultural care phenomenon and lived experience, the uniqueness of which centers on providing human care to people in a way that is meaningful, congruent, and respectful of cultural values and lifestyles.

Description of Nursing Activity

Health and care behaviors tend to vary transculturally and take on different meanings in different contexts. Therefore, culturally congruent nursing care cannot be determined through superficial knowledge and limited contact with a cultural group (Leininger, 1992a). Nursing care must be based on transcultural knowledge discovered by examining social structure, worldview, cultural values, language, and environmental contexts, as depicted in the sunrise model (1991, p. 49). According to Leininger, nursing care actions and decisions that recognize and respect cultural care values of people will result in congruency and will prevent cultural imposition, cultural care negligence, and cultural care conflicts (1991, p. 41).

Leininger identifies three major modes to guide nursing judgments, decisions, or actions to provide culturally congruent care to clients (1991, p. 41):

1. *Cultural care preservation (or maintenance)* refers to those assistive, supporting, facilitative, or enabling professional notions and decisions that help people of a particular culture to retain and/or preserve relevant care values so that they can maintain their well-being, recover from illness, or face handicaps and/or death.

2. *Cultural care accommodation (or negotiation)* refers to those assistive, supporting, facilitative, or enabling creative professional actions and decisions that help people of a designated culture to adapt to, or to negotiate with others for a beneficial or satisfying health outcome with professional care providers.

3. *Cultural care repatterning (or restructuring)* refers to those assistive, supporting, facilitative, or enabling professional actions and decisions that help a client(s) reorder, change, or greatly modify their lifeways for new, different, and beneficial health care patterns while respecting the client(s) cultural values and beliefs and still providing a more beneficial or healthier lifeway than before the changes were coestablished with the client(s).

The *care modalities* require that the nurse and client work together to identify, plan, and implement care that is congruent with and fits the client's lifeways. Leininger does not use the term *nursing intervention* because she feels it to be culture bound to Western professional nursing orientations and tends to communicate ideas of cultural interferences and imposition practices (1991, p. 55).

Definition and Description of Person

Leininger's theory of transcultural care diversity and universality addresses clients as *humans* who are "cultural beings who have survived through time and place because of their ability to care for infants, young and older adults in a variety of environments and ways" (Leininger, 1985b, p. 210). Viewing humans as cultural beings supports the idea that humans cannot be separated and viewed apart from this cultural background. Humans need to be viewed and understood in their total context, and culture is the broadest and most holistic perspective that allows this.

Leininger believes that the use of the term *person* in the transcultural sense is problematic because "many non-Western cultures do not focus on or believe in the concept person, and often there is no linguistic term for person" in some cultures (1991, p. 39). From Leininger's perspective, human beings include individuals, families, groups, communities, and total cultures and institutions, a dimension that gives considerable scope to the theory. Culture and human care are seen as a holistic and unifying perspective to reflect individuals' or groups' total caring lifeways. Because humans vary with regard to cultural values, beliefs, and lifestyles, professional care must first be conceptualized, defined, and studied from a cultural perspective. From this body of knowledge, specific nursing care is planned and implemented in a way that recognizes and respects cultural differences and similarities. The term *cultural care universality* refers to those attributes found to be more common or potentially universal with respect to care meanings and patterns, whereas *cultural care diversity* refers to the variabilities and/or differences in care meanings and patterns (1991, p. 47).

Definition and Description of Environment

Environment in Leininger's theory becomes important as it influences health and care patterns of individuals, families, and cultural groups. For Leininger, human behavior is meaningful only within specific environmental and cultural contexts. *Environmental context* is defined as ". . . the totality of an event, situation, or particular experiences that gives meaning to human expressions, interpretations, and social interactions in particular physical, ecological, sociopolitical and/or cultural settings" (1991, p. 48). Human behaviors such as health and care patterns must be appropriately studied in context and by methods that prevent context stripping. Leininger stresses that studying an individual, family, or group without reference to the environmental or cultural context limits a full and accurate understanding of human beings. Nurse-researchers using the theory are challenged to tease out culture care meanings and practices as embedded in environmental context, social structure, and other features of the sunrise model.

Definition and Description of Health

From Leininger's perspective, health is more than just the absence of disease or a point on a continuum. *Health* refers to "a state of well-being that is culturally defined, valued, and practiced, and which reflects the ability of individuals (or groups) to perform their daily role activities in culturally expressed, beneficial, and patterned lifeways" (1991, p. 48). Leininger contends that all human cultures have forms, patterns, expressions, and structures of care that allow for knowing, explaining, and predicting health and well-being. If health professionals are to be effective in delivering culturally congruent care, an understanding of health from the people's perspective is important. Such a strategy is referred to as an *emic* approach to building knowledge from the people's view point. The emic dimension of knowledge refers to the local or indigenous cognitions and perceptions about a particular phenomenon, whereas the *etic* dimension refers to the more universal or outside knowledge related to a phenomenon under study (Leininger, 1985a, p. 38). To design and implement culturally congruent care that leads to health, an awareness of the people's view of health is important. Leininger goes further to postulate that caring modalities are so powerful in health, that curing cannot occur without caring (1991, p. 39). Through Leininger's study of some 54 cultures, approximately 172 care constructs have been identified to date. These constructs provide a focus to nursing and enable the primacy and power of care to guide nursing decisions.

Description of Other Basic Concepts

For Leininger, the four metaparadigm concepts previously discussed are inadequate to identify the substantive structure of the discipline of nursing. Leininger recognizes human care as the essential and critical concept central to nursing. For almost four decades, she has held care to be a universal characteristic of human nature, and has believed that care is culturally defined in every culture. According to Leininger, caring for others in need of assistance has been the long-standing focus of nursing. Although care is conceptualized as the central component of the theory, it interrelates closely with the concepts of culture, health, and environmental context.

According to Leininger, the concept of culture is a significant and relevant area to be discovered and used in nursing. *Culture* is defined as "the learned, shared, and transmitted values, beliefs, norms, and lifeways of a particular group that guides their thinking, decisions and actions in patterned ways" (1991, p. 47). The idea of cultural care is described by Leininger as being the broadest and most holistic means to know, explain, interpret, and predict nursing care phenomena to guide nursing practice.

Other concepts important to the theory of *Cultural Care* are *social structure* and *worldview*. A major premise of the theory is that cultural care values, beliefs, and practices are influenced and embedded in worldview and social structure features. Through discovering these features that are specific to various cultures, nursing practices can be provided in a way that blends cultural values and lifeways, and is therefore more meaningful and satisfying to clients (1991, p. 39). Leininger distinguishes between the concepts of generic care (folk care) and professional nursing care in the following definitions (1991, p. 38):

> *Generic care:* refers to culturally learned and transmitted lay, indigenous (traditional) or folk knowledge and skills used to provide assistive, supportive, enabling, facilitative acts (or phenomena) toward or for another individual, group or institution with evident or anticipated needs to ameliorate or improve a human health condition (or well-being), disability, lifeway, or to face death. *Professional nursing care:* refers to formal and cognitively learned professional care knowledge and practice skills obtained through educational institutions that are used to provide assistive, supportive, enabling or facilitative acts to or for another individual or group in order to improve a human health condition (or well-being), disability, lifeway, or to work with dying clients.

It is only through discovering how these systems are alike or different that culturally congruent care can be provided to individuals, groups, or cultural institutions. Leininger's work (1978, 1991, 1993, 1994) as well as the work of others who have used the theory (Bodner & Leininger, 1992; Cameron, 1990; Kloosterman, 1991; Luna, 1989; Rosenbaum, 1990; Spangler, 1991) with various cultural groups has illustrated the importance of discovering generic or traditional folk knowledge in developing professional nursing practices.

INTERNAL ANALYSIS AND EVALUATION

Underlying Assumptions

When asked about the influence of particular persons or philosophies in the development of her theory of culture care, Leininger denies any specific influences, but she does acknowledge the importance of selective personal and professional ideas in guiding her thinking (Leininger, 1991, p. 23). Humanistic, ethical, and moral caring values learned in childhood and in her basic nursing program were carried into early nursing work as a private duty nurse. She explained, ". . . there was always a normative cultural expectation to be humanistic, compassionate, and ethical in doing 'what was best for the patient' and to be morally committed to helping the patient and his or her family" (Leininger, 1991, p. 9). Her studies in cultural, social, and physical anthropology introduced her to the thinking of some outstanding scholars in the field. Consequently, her ". . . philosophical interests and conceptual orientations for the theory of Culture Care were primarily derived from a holistic nursing and anthropological perspective of human beings living in different places and contexts" (Leininger, 1991, p. 21). She stresses the importance of her own creative thinking processes and ability to philosophize from past professional nursing experience as she developed the relationship between culture and care in her theory.

Since 1966, Leininger has been formulating and refining assumptive, theoretical premises to guide nurses in their discovery of culture care phenomena. Some selective premises include (Leininger, 1991; Reynolds & Leininger, 1993) the following:

1. Care is essential for human growth, well-being, and survival, and to face death or disabilities.
2. Care is the essence of nursing and a distinct, dominant, central, and unifying focus.
3. Culture care is the broadest means to know, explain, account for, and predict nursing care phenomena, and guide nursing care practices.
4. Care (caring) is essential to curing and healing, for there can be no curing without caring.
5. Culture care concepts, meanings, expressions, patterns, processes, and structural forms of care are different (diversity) and similar (toward commonalities or universalities) among all cultures of the world.
6. Cultural care values, beliefs, and practices are influenced by and tend to be embedded in the worldview, language, religion (or

spiritual), kinship (social), politics (or legal), education, economic, technology ethnohistory, and environmental context of a particular culture.

7. Culturally congruent or beneficial nursing care can only occur when the individual, group, family, community, or culture care values, expressions, or patterns are known and used appropriately and in meaningful ways by the nurse with the people.

8. The qualitative paradigm provides new ways of knowing and different ways to discover epistemic and ontological dimensions of human care transculturally.

Leininger avoided "tightly constructed theoretical formulations" because such formulations would be inconsistent with the qualitative paradigm and discovery of phenomena in their naturally occurring contexts.

Central Components

Leininger's nursing theory of culture care diversity and universality contains certain central concepts or components that reflect its specific nature and direction. As described previously, orientational definitions have been provided to guide the study of phenomena within the theory. Unique components central to the theory are care and culture. The inextricable link between care and culture concepts in the theory is evident in the related components in Leininger's nursing model: generic and professional care, cultural care diversity and universality, cultural care preservation, accommodations, and repatterning. Environmental context, health, health systems, and nursing are also addressed in the culture care theory. Leininger stresses the importance of regarding individuals, families, and communities within their cultural, ethnohistorical, and social structure so that holistic, cultural congruent nursing care can be given.

Central Concepts: Relative Importance and Relationships

In the Leininger theory, "care is the essence of nursing and the central, dominant, and unifying focus of nursing" (Leininger, 1991, p. 35). The concepts of care, culture, and health are closely linked. She stresses the valuing aspect of care as well as the cultural influence. The culture of an individual or group, with its related values, beliefs, and practices, is assumed by Leininger to be the greatest predictor of health and care patterns. The nurse must have knowledge of culture and of care values to provide therapeutic care and to prevent nontherapeutic cultural stresses, conflict, and imposition practices.

Leininger's definition of theory differs from the traditional view of theory but it is most congruent with anthropology and transcultural nursing. She defines theory as ". . . sets of interrelated knowledge with meanings and experiences that describe, explain, predict, or account for some phenomenon (or domain of inquiry) through an open, creative, and naturalistic discovery process" (1988, p. 154). She emphasizes that "the theory of cultural care diversity and universality is congruent with methods that support the discovery of 'people truths' in human living contexts rather than methods that follow the researcher's preconceived views" (1988, p. 154). Leininger has derived a number of theoretical statements or assumptive premises (described previously) from her conceptual model for nursing, the sunrise model. In using the sunrise model as a cognitive map, the nurse is guided to examine the different influences that describe and explain care with health and well-being outcomes. In the model, social structure and worldview factors influence care and health in the context of language, environment, and ethnohistory. Hence, a systematic view of the phenomenon of care is presented by specifying the interrelationship between social structure, worldview, language, ethnohistory, environment, and care.

Leininger theorizes that sociocultural factors, meanings, and expressions of health and care influence folk (or generic), professional, and nursing health systems. Hence, social structure factors and worldview are meaningfully related to folk and professional care practices.

Ultimately, Leininger's model provides theoretical formulations for nursing care decisions and actions that are consistent with cultural values (1985b, p. 210). Accordingly, she theorizes that there are three modes of actions or decisions to guide nurses in providing culturally congruent care: culture care preservation, accommodation, and repatterning (Leininger, 1993).

By linking concepts and deriving a set of orientational definitions and assumptive, theoretical premises or theoretical statements, Leininger presents a systematic view of the phenomenon of care for purposes of describing, explaining, and predicting these phenomena.

In summary, care is the central concept in the Leininger theory. Care is derived from, and embedded in, the concept of culture with its social structure, worldview, and environmental factors. Care is related to the other components at different levels in the theory: the level of social systems and perceptions of the outside world; the level within individuals, families, groups, and cultures, the level of folk and professional health and nursing systems; and finally, the level of nursing care actions and decisions.

Analysis of Consistency

Leininger has clearly defined the concept of care as a noun and as a phenomenon to document, explain, and predict nursing. She has also distinguished the term *caring* as a verb denoting action, from the phenomenon of care. Not only has she maintained a consistency of definition of care as a phenomenon throughout the various phases of her theory's development, but her definition of the concept of culture has remained consistent from the theory's initial stages. Various levels of abstraction of the concept of care are apparent. Care is included in the three specific nursing care actions and decisions: culture care preservation, accommodation, and repatterning. Leininger introduces the concept of *ethnocare,* another more focused type of care, in her writing.

The concept of care is dominant in the assumptive, theoretical premises underlying the theory. Care is manifested in different aspects of the theory, such as human care, care patterns, caring beings, care values, care acts, transcultural care, nursing care, and folk and professional healthcare systems. Care is also linked to other central concepts in the theory. The theoretical statements developed by Leininger reflect linkages between care and culture, social structure, and health system.

The concept of health systems is consistently defined in terms of the folk, professional, and nursing systems. Leininger has maintained the necessity of including these three systems as integral aspects of the theory and as major structural dimensions of the health systems.

Analysis of Adequacy

Hardy identified the criteria for analyzing the adequacy of a theory as meaning, logical adequacy, and operational or empirical adequacy (1974, p. 105). Leininger, however, believes that "empirical (five senses), logical, experimental evaluations of a theory with operational definitions, hypotheses, and measurement scales are not congruent or appropriate to use with qualitative constructed theories . . . [and that] logical deductions . . . may severely limit knowing" (1991, p. 60). With respect to evaluation of nursing theories, Leininger (1991) disputes the use of traditional criteria:

> Logical adequacy of a theory is usually not of great importance in qualitative studies, and can be detrimental to exploring largely unknown, illogical, subjective, and transcendental data offered by informants. . . . A theory which has logical structure and its own concepts, definitions, and rigid formulations may be quite inappropriate for the culture and social setting being studied. Logic may reside in the researcher's world, but

may not be known or understandable in the informants' conceptual and lived world (p. 62).

Care theory may not be readily apparent because of new ideas that may become "useful" to nursing in the future. Qualitative data may not be meaningful in the present context but the knowledge may be valuable in and of itself (Leininger, 1991, p. 62).

Leininger stresses that "in qualitative, theoretical research, generalizations are not the goal. Instead the goal is to obtain findings that are meaningful to particularized individuals or groups. A theory can be extremely valuable even though it is not generalizable to many people and populations" (1991, p. 62).

The concept of parsimony is not acceptable to Leininger as a criterion for evaluating the scope or complexity of the phenomena in qualitative theory. Leininger has repeatedly addressed the inappropriateness of ". . . a few equations, explanations, or a specific mathematical equation" (1991, p. 63) to enhance understanding of phenomena. Alternatively, Leininger has offered qualitative criteria to analyze and evaluate the soundness of qualitative nursing studies in keeping with the qualitative research paradigm. The following criteria have been developed: *credibility,* or "accuracy, or believability" of findings; *confirmability,* or "repeated direct and documented evidence"; *meaning-in-context,* or data understandable with reference to the informants' environment; *recurrent patterning,* or "repeated instances" recurring over time, *saturation,* or exhaustive occurrences; and *transferability,* or transference of findings to another similar situation (Leininger, 1991, pp. 112–114).

EXTERNAL ANALYSIS

Nursing Research on the Model

Theory can be generated at three levels in the sunrise mode: macro, mid, and micro levels. Knowledge gained from research at the macro level will be applicable beyond nursing in that it will explain the totality of human behavior (Leininger, 1985a, p. 42). Research questions conceptualized within the mid and micro levels of the model will involve smaller domains of inquiry. Studies at these levels will focus on individuals, families, or cultural groups as they enter the folk and professional healthcare systems.

A variety of research methods may be used to test theories derived from the model. To date, the primary methods used have been those of an ethnographic, ethnonursing approach (Leininger, 1992b). Because the theory of culture care diversity and universality has only recently been presented to nurses (primarily because of the lack of a cadre of nurses sufficiently pre-pared to deal with cultural concepts), studies grounded in the theory have only begun to emerge. Leininger utilized the theory to describe, explain, and predict the health and care lifestyles and patterns of 10 cultures in an urban setting (1981–1991). Ray (1984) conducted the first large-scale general hos-pital ethnocare study in nursing using concepts and methods from Leininger's framework. A number of doctoral studies throughout the United States and Canada have conceptualized research questions within the culture care theory (Table 9–1). Cameron (1990) investigated the influence of ex-tended caregiving on the health status of elderly Anglo-Canadian wives. Gates (1988) studied the care and cure meanings and experiences of those who were dying in hospice and hospital settings. Care and cultural context of Lebanese Muslims in an urban community was the focus of Luna's (1989) ethnographic and ethnonursing study. Findings from Rosenbaum's (1990) study revealed the meaning and experience of cultural care, cultural care continuity, cultural health and grief phenomena of older Greek-Canadian widows. Wenger (1988) studied the phenomena of care in a high-context cul-ture with the Old Order Amish. Several master's students have utilized Leininger's theory for conceptualizing research questions (Burns, 1987; Gelazis, 1988; McFarland, 1989; Morgan, 1989; Stasiak, 1991).

Leininger initiated the establishment of the Committee on Nursing and Anthropology and the Transcultural Nursing Society as organizations for nurses interested in transcultural nursing and human care to share their research and other experiences together. In 1988, the International Associ-ation for Human Caring was formed to encourage scholarly exchange of ideas and encourage research (Leininger, 1991, p. 17).

TABLE 9–1 Dissertations on Transcultural Nursing Care Mentored by Professor Leininger (1988–2001)

Author	Title
Edith Morris, PhD, RN (2003)	Culture Care Values, Meanings, Experiences of African-American Adolescent Gang Members
Dorothy Stitzlein, PhD, RN (1999)	The Phenomenon of Moral Care/Caring Conceptualized within Leininger's Theory of Culture Care Diversity and Universality
Betty Horton, DNSc, RN (1998)	Culture Care by Private Practice APRNS in Community Contexts
Joanne T. Ehrmin, PhD, RN (1998)	Culture Care: Meanings and Expressions of African-American Women Residing in an Inner City Transitional Home for Substance Abuse
Tamara George, PhD, RN (1998)	Meanings, Expressions, and Experiences of Care of Chronically Mentally Ill in a Day Treatment Center Using Leininger's Culture Care Theory

TABLE 9–1 *Continued*

Author	Title
Judith Lamp, PhD, RN (1998)	Generic and Professional Culture Care Meanings and Practices of Finnish Women in Birth within Leininger's Theory of Culture Care Diversity and Universality
Rick Zoucha, RN, DNSc, CS (1997)	The Experiences of Mexican Americans Receiving Professional Nursing Care: An Ethnonursing Study
Marguerite R. Curtis, PhD, RN (1997)	Cultural Care by Private Practice APRNS in Community Contexts
June Miller, PhD, RN (1996)	Politics and Care: A Study of Czech Americans within Leininger's Theory of Culture Care Diversity and Universality
Akram Omeri, PhD, RN (1996)	Transcultural Nursing Values, Beliefs, and Practices of Iranian Immigrants in New South Wales.
Anita Berry, PhD, RN (1995)	Culture Care Expression, Meanings, and Experiences of Pregnant Mexican-American Women within Leininger's Culture Care Theory
Marilyn McFarland, PhD, RN (1995)	Cultural Care of Anglo- and African-American Elderly Residents within the Environmental Context of a Long-Term Care Institution
Rauda Gelazis, PhD, RN (1994)	Human, Care, and Well-Being of Lithuanian Americans: An Ethnonursing Study Using Leininger's Theory of Culture Care Diversity and Universality
Joan MacNeil, PhD, RN (1994)	Culture Care: Meanings, Patterns, and Expressions for Baganda Women as AIDS Caregivers within Leininger's Theory
Marjorie Morgan, PhD, RN (1994)	Prenatal Care of African-American Women in Selected USA Urban and Rural Cultural Contexts Conceptualized within Leininger's Cultural Care
Julianna Finn, PhD, RN (1993)	Professional Nurse and Generic Care of Childbirthing Women Conceptualized within Leininger's Culture Care Theory and Using Colaizzi's Phenomenological Method
Zenaida Spangler, PhD, RN (1991)	Nursing Care Values and Caregiving Practices of Anglo-American and Philippine-American Nurses Conceptualized within Leininger's Theory
Teresa Thompson, PhD, RN (1990)	A Qualitative Investigation of Rehabilitation Nursing Care in an Inpatient Rehabilitation Unit Using Leininger's Theory
Cynthia Cameron, PhD, RN (1990)	An Ethnonursing Study of the Influence of Extended Caregiving on the Health of Elderly Anglo-Canadian Wives Caring for Physically Disabled Husbands
Janet Rosenbaum, PhD, RN (1990)	Cultural Care, Cultural Health, and Grief Phenomena Related to Older Greek Canadian Widows within Leininger's Theory of Culture Care
Linda Luna, PhD, RN (1989)	Care and Cultural Context of Lebanese Muslims in an Urban US Community: An Ethnographic and Ethnonursing Study Conceptualized within Leininger's Theory
Marie Gates, PhD, RN (1988)	Care and Cure Meanings, Experiences, and Orientations of Persons Who Are Dying in Hospital and Hospice Settings
Anna Frances Wenger, PhD, RN (1988)	The Phenomenon of Care in a High Context Culture: The Old Order Amish

Nursing Education Based on the Model

As founder and developer of the field of transcultural nursing, Leininger has been instrumental in the establishment of master's and doctoral programs in nursing that espouse transcultural care perspectives. In the early 1960s, she realized that very little care and cultural nursing content existed in nursing curricula. "Clearly nurses without preparation in transcultural nursing would be greatly handicapped when working with people of diverse cultures" (Leininger, 1991, p. 16). The University of Colorado offered the first course in transcultural nursing in 1966–1967, followed by the Universities of Washington (1969) and Utah (1977), and Wayne State University (1981) in Detroit (Leininger, 1984, p. 43). By 1980, about 20 percent of nursing programs accredited by the National League for Nursing incorporated cultural concepts and principles into the undergraduate program and by 1991, 15 percent of graduate nursing programs in the United States had transcultural nursing courses (Leininger, 1989a, 1989b, 1993). Leininger's publications on the culture care theory have played a valuable role in educating nurses about her theory. She held back on the publication of a book on the theory itself until nurses were educated in transcultural nursing, but prepared the way with numerous workshops, presentations, and journal articles. Nursing educators from several countries continue to benefit from Leininger's expert consultation during short-term intensive exchange visits to Wayne State University.

Nursing Practice Based on the Model

Leininger maintains that the coming decade will witness the utilization of transcultural nursing knowledge and research in practice. Because of the dearth of transculturally prepared faculty, much of the potential for the theory of culture care diversity and universality to influence and guide nursing practice has yet to be realized. She maintains that the time has come "... to prevent cultural imposition practices, cultural care negligence, cultural care conflicts, and many other practice" ... 'problems' ... Nurses are now keenly feeling and demanding transcultural care knowledge to help them function in a tense multicultural world" (Leininger, 1991, p. 41).

Nursing Diagnosis and the Model

Leininger holds that there are some major problems and ethical concerns that need to be addressed about the North American Nursing Diagnosis Association (NANDA) cultural movement. Writing in the *Journal of Transcultural Nursing* (1990), she discussed the major views of her position. Her concerns centered on the dominance of the Anglo-American Western value base reflected in the NANDA taxonomy of nursing diagnoses; linguistic insensitivity and translation difficulties for non-Anglicized nurses; absence of culture-specific health and care conditions within different cultural contexts; pronounced medical model focus; little room for transcultural variations within physical and emotional states; and limited attention to ethical and moral issues (Leininger, 1990, pp. 23–24). She firmly believes that ". . . the NANDA diagnostic classificatory system needs to be reevaluated, reconsidered, and refocused, into transculturally relevant, meaningful and useful transcultural nursing perspectives" (Leininger, 1990, p. 24).

Given the position taken by Leininger, it would be inappropriate to derive nursing diagnoses from the culture care theory and to assess their congruence with the existing NANDA nursing diagnoses. Leininger contends that "transcultural nursing specialists are needed to ". . . redirect the NANDA movement into the systematic study of transcultural human care, health, and well-being of different cultures" (1990, p. 24).

SUMMARY

As we move into the future, various societal trends will demand that nurses employ a worldwide vision in responding to clients' cultural needs. State boards of nursing are stipulating the recognition of cultural diversity and soon consumers will be demanding culturally sensitive care. The theory of culture care diversity and universality holds great potential for enhancing quality humanistic and holistic care to people of all cultures.

REFERENCES

Algase, D., & Whall, A. (1993). Rosemary Ellis' views on the substantive structure of nursing. *IMAGE: The Journal of Nursing Scholarship, 25*(1) 69–72.

Bodner, A., & Leininger, M. (1992). Transcultural nursing care values, beliefs, and practices of American (U.S.A.) gypsies. *Journal of Trans-Cultural Nursing, 4,* 17–28.

Burns, G. (1987). *Ethnocare of the homeless in large urban communities.* Unpublished master's field study, Wayne State University, Detroit.

Cameron, C. (1990). *Health status of elderly Anglo-Canadian wives providing extended caregiving to their disabled husbands within Leininger's theory.* Unpublished doctoral dissertation. Wayne State University, Detroit.

Fawcett, J. (1989). *Analysis and evaluation of conceptual models of nursing.* Philadelphia: F. A. Davis.

Fitzpatrick, J., & Whall, A. (1989). *Conceptual models of nursing. Analysis and application.* Bowie, MD: Brady.

Gates, M. (1988). *Care and cure meanings, experiences and orientations of persons who are dying in hospital and hospice settings.* Unpublished doctoral dissertation, Wayne State University, Detroit.

Gelazis, R. (1988). *Well-being and humor in Lithuanian Americans*. Unpublished post-master's field study, Wayne State University, Detroit.

Hardy, M. (1974). Theories: Components, development, evaluation. *Nursing Research, 23* (2), 100–106.

Kloosterman, N. (1991). Cultural care: The missing link in severe sensory alteration. *Nursing Science Quarterly, 4*(3), 119–122.

Leininger, M. (1978). *Transcultural nursing: Concepts, theories, and practices*. New York: Wiley.

Leininger, M. (1984). Transcultural nursing: An essential knowledge and practice field for today. *The Canadian Nurse, 80*(11), 41–45.

Leininger, M. (1985a). *Qualitative research methods in nursing*. New York: Grune & Stratton.

Leininger, M. (1985b). Transcultural care diversity and universality: A theory of nursing. *Nursing and Health Care, 6*(4), 209–212.

Leininger, M. (1988). Leininger's theory of nursing. Culture care diversity and universality. *Nursing Science Quarterly, 1*(4), 152–160.

Leininger, M. 1989a. *Transcultural nursing trends in schools of nursing in U.S.A.* Unpublished manuscript. Wayne State University, Detroit.

Leininger, M. (1989b). Transcultural nursing: Quouvadis (where goeth the field). *Journal of Transcultural Nursing, 1*(1), 33–45.

Leininger, M. (1990). Issues, questions, and concerns related to the nursing diagnosis cultural movement from a transcultural nursing perspective. *Journal of Transcultural Nursing, 2*(1), 23–32.

Leininger, M. (1991). *Cultural care diversity & universality: A theory of nursing*. New York: National League for Nursing.

Leininger, M. (1992a). Strange myths and inaccurate facts in transcultural nursing. *Journal of Transcultural Nursing, 4*(2), 39–40.

Leininger, M. (1992b). Current issues, problems, and trends to advance qualitative paradigmatic research methods for the future. *Qualitative Health Research, 2*(4), 392–403.

Leininger, M. (1993). Assumptive premises of the theory. In C. Reynolds & M. Leininger (Eds.), *Madeleine Leininger: Cultural care diversity and universality theory* (pp. 15–38). Newbury Park, CA: Sage.

Leininger, M. (1994). *Transcultural nursing: concepts, theory, research, and practice* (2nd ed.). Columbus, OH: McGraw-Hill and Greden.

Luna, L. (1989). *Care and cultural context of Lebanese Muslims in an urban U.S. community: An ethnographic and ethnonursing study conceptualized within Leininger's theory*. Unpublished doctoral dissertation, Wayne State University, Detroit.

McFarland, M. (1989). *Culture care theory and ethnonursing mini-study of care experiences in residential nursing homes and Mexican-American communities*. Unpublished post-master's field study. Wayne State University, Detroit.

Morgan, M. (1989). *Ethnonursing: A study of care in a hospital context using Leininger's theory of culture care*. Unpublished post-master's field study, Wayne State University, Detroit.

Ray, M. (1984). The development of a classification system of institutional caring. In M. Leininger (Ed.), *Care: The essence of nursing and health* (pp. 95–112). Thorofare, NJ: Slack.

Reynolds, C., & Leininger, M. (1993). *Madeleine Leininger: Cultural care diversity and universality theory*. Newbury Park, CA: Sage.

Rosenbaum, J. (1990). *The meaning and experience of cultural care, cultural care conti-nuity, cultural health and grief phenomena of older Greek Canadian widows.* Unpub-lished doctoral dissertation, Wayne State University, Detroit.

Spangler, Z. (1991). *Nursing care values and practices of Philippine-American and Anglo-American nurses using Leininger's theory.* Unpublished doctoral dissertation, Wayne State University, Detroit.

Stasiak, D. (1991). *Ethnonursing: A study of Mexican-Americans in urban cities.* Unpub-lished master's field study, Wayne State University, Detroit.

Wenger, A. F. (1988). *Phenomenon of care in a high-context culture: The Old Order Amish.* Unpublished doctoral dissertation, Wayne State University, Detroit.

10

Neuman's Systems Model

Patricia Hinton Walker

Developed in 1970 and first published in 1972, the Neuman systems model (NSM) continues to be used widely by educators, practitioners, and researchers nationally and internationally. "In the early years, the model was primarily used to guide education and practice and as a conceptual framework for some master and doctoral level research" (Lowry, Walker, & Mirenda, 1995, p. 64). Now, after three decades, its growth and utility are well documented by the authors of the most recent book on the NSM (Neuman & Fawcett, 2001). This book not only provides comprehensive documentation of the growing use of the model in textbooks, journal publications, master's and doctoral research, but it provides a comprehensive summary of the use of the model in education, practice, and research.

As expected, the model remains popular as a framework for nursing education across the United States and Canada, as well as in a growing list of other countries internationally. In practice, the model continues to be applied to both general and specialty areas of nursing practice, given that it encompasses a wide variety of clients and client system stressors. Finally, although many of the nursing models have had difficulty breaking through the research barrier, use of the NSM has significantly increased during the last 10 to 12 years from approximately 38 studies in the review conducted by Louis and Koertvelyessy (1989) to the 200 studies in the integrative review conducted by Fawcett and Giangrande (2001).

The NSM represents various important aspects of health care; at the same time it presents nursing as a unique profession from a holistic, comprehensive care approach to client situations (Lowry et al., 1995). According to its author, Betty Neuman (Neuman, 2001) "The NSM helps nurses to organize the nursing field within a broad systems perspective as a logical way of dealing with its growing complexity. Earlier, the NSM was criticized as being too broad, as were other conceptual models of nursing; now, this quality has become the major reason for increasing acceptance of the model and its documented utility" (p. 10). Consequently, it is not surprising that use of this particularly conceptual model continues to expand.

The NSM philosophically encompasses holism, a wellness orientation, client perception, and motivation, with a systems perspective of variable interaction with the environment. Caregivers and clients work in partnership to achieve optimal health retention, restoration, and maintenance (Neuman, 2001 p. 12). The Neuman model focuses primarily upon two components: the nature of a client's response to stressors and the nurse's interventions that assist the client to best respond to the stressors. Thus, although nursing's goal within the model is to assist the client in maintaining an optimal state of wellness, the overall process the caregiver uses to determine and support that wellness state receives more emphasis.

The model was first developed to help University of California, Los Angeles, graduate students in nursing conceptualize a systems approach to health care. It is based upon Neuman's own personal philosophy, teaching, and experience as a consultant in public health and community mental health nursing (Neuman, 2001, p. 327). Thus, it is not surprising that her concepts of *levels of prevention* and *lines of defense* are reminiscent of the emphasis upon disease prevention that was prevalent in the public health literature in the 1950s and 1960s.

The basic nursing phenomena of interest within the Neuman model are the person as a *client* or *client system* and the *related environment* (Neuman, 1989, p. 24; Neuman, 1995, p. 24; Neuman, 2001, p. 22). The client reacts to, or may potentially react to, various stressors within the environment. Stressors are considered inert forces that have the potential to impact the client's steady state (Neuman, 1989, pp. 12, 24; Neuman, 1995, p. 23; Neuman, 2001, pp. 21–22). Thus, they are highly individualized experiences that may require adjustment or change within a client. If stressors are perceived by the client as motivating or strengthening factors, then they typically result in a beneficial outcome. Such stressors may increase one's self-awareness or assist the client in experiencing continued personal growth and development. A stressor can also be viewed as a phenomenon that is to be avoided or mitigated so that a state of stability or balance may be maintained. Encounters with such stressors may result in negative or noxious outcomes such as variances from wellness. Thus, it is very important that the healthcare professional understand how the client perceives and reacts to stressors to identify and implement effective interventions.

One of the primary problems with the application of general systems theory to phenomena of interest to nursing is that the "what" of assessment, intervention, and evaluation is not identified. Neuman (1989) addressed this shortcoming by clearly identifying how the model relates to the nursing process rather than using the less meaningful general systems language of "inputs," "throughputs," and "feedback loops."

In contrast to more lengthy presentations of other nursing conceptual models, the brevity of the Neuman model is the result of stating many relationships in general or user-friendly terms (Lowry et al., 1995, p. 70). One potential advantage to such generality is that the model can be seminal in the production of a variety of creative inferences. Neuman states that the model is "open to creative implementation. Although creative interpretations and implementation of the model are valued, structural changes that could alter its original meaning and purpose are not sanctioned" (Neuman, 2001, p. 31). To this end, Dr. Neuman established the NSM Trustees Group, Inc., in the fall of 1988. The purpose of this Trustees Group is to "preserve, protect and perpetuate the integrity of the model for the future of nursing" (Neuman, 2001, p. 360). These trustees, originally consisting of 22 professional nurses, were personally chosen by Neuman (as of the fall of 2000, there were 21 active Trustees).

BASIC ELEMENTS INCLUDED IN THE MODEL

The model components are organized by the nursing metaparadigm concepts: *person, environment, health,* and *nursing.* These four metaparadigm concepts explicitly or implicitly present in the NSM (Neuman, 1982, 1989, 1995, 2001) and all nursing models. Nursing models also contain additional model-specific concepts that are used to explain the interrelationship of the four metaparadigm concepts as well as other relationships within the model. Thus, although the Neuman model provides a common language for various health professionals, it also addresses nursing's four metaparadigm concepts.

Nursing

Neuman states that nursing is a "unique" profession concerned with the interrelationship of "all variables affecting a client's possible or actual response to stressors" (1989, p. 24). Thus, nursing's uniqueness is related to the way the discipline organizes and utilizes its knowledge (Neuman, 1989).

With this broad perspective and the objective of preventing fragmentation of care, Neuman believes that nurses should serve as coordinators of health care for clients. Through purposeful interventions, nursing can help individuals, families, and groups to "retain, attain, and maintain a maximum level of optimal system wellness" (Neuman, 1989, p. 17; Neuman, 1995, p. 16; Neuman, 2001, p. 25).

The nurse in Neuman's model is seen as an intervener whose goal is either to reduce the client's encounter with certain stressors or to mitigate his or her perceived effect through implementation of appropriate interventions within the three levels of prevention (1989, pp. 17). The nurse may choose to intervene at the primary prevention level by helping the client to strengthen his or her ability to respond to the stressor. This would be accomplished through interventions that expand the flexible line of defense and thereby help the client *retain* system stability. Health promotion is a component of this level of prevention (Neuman, 1989, p. 38; Neuman, 1995, p. 37; Neuman, 2001, p. 26).

Secondary prevention interventions are appropriate when a stressor reaction occurs and are aimed at treatment of symptoms. The outcomes of such interventions are strengthened lines of resistance that protect the basic client structure and help the client to *attain* system stability. After a stressor reaction occurs and some degree of system stability is achieved, tertiary prevention interventions are appropriate to help the client to reconstitute and thereby *maintain* the current level of wellness. Thus, regardless of the outcome of the stressor encounter, the nurse serves as an active participant by supporting the client's defenses and thereby assisting him or her to effectively respond to the stressor.

The nursing process within the Neuman model consists of three components: *nursing diagnosis, goals,* and *outcomes* (Neuman, 1989, p. 40; Neuman, 1995, p. 37; Neuman, 2001, p. 30). A large component of the nursing diagnosis phase of the Neuman nursing process involves nurse assessment of all factors influencing the client. Because the perceptions of client and nurse may vary widely and thereby influence appropriate interventions, active client participation is essential to validate the meaning of a client's experience with the nurse (Neuman, 1989, p. 40; Neuman, 2001, p. 30). This collaborative activity between the nurse and the client is unique to the Neuman nursing process format. Once a problem has been identified, a decision is made about what level of intervention should be implemented. This decision results from the collaborative negotiation of goals between the client and nurse. Actual outcomes are the result of the effectiveness of selected interventions and are evaluated in relation to mutually set goals (Neuman, 1989, p. 20; Neuman, 1995, p. 38; Neuman & Fawcett, 2001, p. 30).

The nurse's role in relation to assessment and intervention varies depending upon the type of intervention (primary, secondary, or tertiary) that is needed. For example, if the stressor had not yet broken through the client's normal line of defense (the primary prevention level), the nurse's assessment might focus on client risk factors, and effective interventions on client education. If the stressor had penetrated the client's normal line of defense (the secondary prevention level), the nurse would focus assessment on the nature of any disease process present and the interventions on maladaptive responses. If the stressor had resulted in residual symptoms (the tertiary prevention level) the nurse may attempt to limit such effects by use of rehabilitative resources.

In summary, the nurse in the Neuman model is an active evaluator and intervener. The client is also viewed as active but in some situations may be less so in comparison with the nurse because of an altered health state. The uniqueness of nursing described by the model is related to the holistic nature of humans and the influence of interacting variables within the client's internal, external, and created environments.

Person

The concept of person in the Neuman model is called *client* or *client system*. Neuman (1989; Neuman, 1995, p. 25; Neuman, 2001, p. 15) explained that she chose this term because of the wellness focus of the model and to indicate the collaborative lateral relationship between clients and caregivers. Clients are composed of a basic structure of survival factors inclusive of the five client system variables and surrounded by various lines of defense and resistance (Neuman, 1989, p. 48; Neuman, 1995, pp. 25–26; Neuman, 2001, p. 17). The client or client system, whether an individual, group, community, or social system, is a dynamic composite of the interrelationships between physiological, psychological, sociocultural, developmental, spiritual, and basic structure variables (Neuman, 1989, pp. 22, 25; Neuman, 1995, p. 28; Neuman & Fawcett, 2001, p. 16).

The spiritual variable was added to the model in 1989 for the purpose of being more congruent with a holistic perspective of humans (Neuman, 1989). Whether or not the client acknowledges or develops his or her spirituality, this variable is considered to be an innate component of every client's basic structure (p. 29). The addition of a 10th assumption to the 1989 version of the model further describes the client as being involved in constant dynamic energy exchange with the environment and therefore an open system (Neuman, 1989, p. 22; Neuman, 1995, p. 28; Neuman & Fawcett, 2001, p. 16).

Neuman's holistic concept of humans is related to the interrelationship of variables that determine the amount of resistance a client has in response to any given stressor. Thus, Neuman's definition of person was originally as a *physiological, psychological, sociocultural, spiritual,* and *developmental being*. The spiritual variable was added in the 2nd edition (1989), but was explicated more in the 3rd edition by Fulton (1995) and

Curran (1995). The fact that there are five variables should not be interpreted as a focus only on selected parts. Her holistic approach to the client is also embedded in the need to assess the perception and meaning of the total experience to the client, as well as the effect of the interrelationship of the five client variables on any given stressor.

The client possesses various lines of *defense* and *resistance* and is viewed as being engaged in varying amounts of activity in relation to stressors. When stressors occur, the client may simply need more information about the experience, or require additional assistance from the nurse, to effectively respond to the stressor. Stressor reactions occur when the flexible line of defense has failed to protect or support the normal line of defense that is considered the client's usual stability state.

One's normal line of defense is dynamic, evolves over time, and contains the client's normal range of responses to stressors, thereby reflecting his or her usual wellness level (Neuman, 1989, p. 17; Neuman, 1995, p. 26; Neuman, 2001, p. 18). It represents the client's ability to adjust to daily environmental stressors. Protecting the normal line of defense and serving as the outer boundary of the client system is the flexible line of defense. Neuman describes this as a reaction system or potential that can be used in the presence of stressors to strengthen existing buffers and thus improve the normal wellness state or prevent stressor reactions to maintain the existing wellness states. The model further maintains that each client also has internal lines of resistance that function to protect the client's basic structure or system integrity. If effective, the lines of resistance help to stabilize the person or bring about balance following reaction to a stressor; if ineffective, system energy depletion and eventually death occur (Neuman, 1989, p. 30, Neuman, 1995, p. 30; Neuman, 2001, p. 18).

An example of how a client's lines of defense and resistance function is presented in the following example. When a client is faced with a stressor, such as a family history of breast cancer, it is the strength of the flexible line of defense that determines whether or not a stressor reaction will occur. In this situation, the client may initiate primary prevention coping behaviors to manage the perceived threat of developing breast cancer. These coping behaviors could include reduction in intake of alcohol, estrogen, dietary fat, or body weight. If the flexible line of defense is adequate, breast cancer symptoms remain absent and the client maintains her usual state of wellness. If the flexible line of defense is inadequate to prevent stressor reaction, the client's normal line of defense is disrupted and symptomatology of breast cancer will occur, resulting in a variance from the client's usual state of wellness. The strength of the client's lines of resistance to deal with this variance from wellness will determine whether or not the client can reconstitute or return to and maintain a state of system stability. If the client's lines of resistance are inadequate, death will occur.

Environment

Conceptualized as all factors affecting or affected by the client system, the environment in the Neuman model consists of the following typology: internal, external, and created (Neuman, 1989, p. 12; Neuman, 1995, p. 31; Neuman, 2001, pp. 18–19). The internal environment is composed of those forces contained only within the defined client boundary and correlate with intrapersonal stressors identified in the model. All forces external to the defined client system, such as inter- and extrapersonal stressors, make up the external environment (Neuman, 1989, p. 31; Neuman, 1995, p. 31; Neuman, 2001, pp. 22–23).

In the 1989 revision of the model, Neuman also added the concept of *created environment*. Like the addition of spirituality to the client variables, this concept is another example of Neuman's efforts to further delineate the holistic approach of the model. The created environment is unconsciously developed by the client (Neuman, 1989, p. 32; Neuman, 1995, pp. 31–32; Neuman, 2001, p. 19) when a threat to the basic structure or system function exists (Reed, 1993a, 1993b). Therefore, created environments can serve to protect the client from intra-, inter-, and extrapersonal stressors and thereby function to maintain system stability by changing the response or possible response of the client to environmental stressors (Neuman, 1989, p. 32; Neuman, 1995, p. 31; Newman, Neuman, & Fawcett, 2001, p. 21). Neuman (1989) further describes it as a "process based concept of perceptual adjustment" (pp. 32–33) that functions to either increase or decrease the client's wellness state by unconsciously shielding the client from the true reality of a situation.

Because the created environment constantly exchanges energy with the internal and external environments, it requires energy from all system variables to maintain it. Such energy is then unavailable for actions that contribute to an improved health state (Lowry & Anderson, 1993).

Stressors, defined as "tension producing stimuli with the potential for causing disequilibrium," occur within the internal and external environments and are classified as being intra-, inter-, or extrapersonal in nature (Neuman, 1989, p. 23; Neuman, 1995, p. 23; Neuman, 2001, p. 23). Intrapersonal stressors occur within the boundary of the client system; interpersonal stressors occur between the client system boundary and one or more other client systems; and extrapersonal stressors are those forces that occur outside the client system boundary (Neuman, 1989, p. 24; Neuman, 1995, p. 23; Neuman & Fawcett, 2001, p. 23). All stressors are considered inert or neutral in and of themselves but result in either a positive or negative outcome (Neuman, 1989, p. 24; Neuman, 1995, p. 23; Neuman, 2001, p. 21).

When stressors are identified, the nurse assesses the client's internal, external, and created environments, as well as the interactions among them. The client's feelings, emotions, and perceptions related to the stressors are assessed to clarify the nature and condition of the environment related to the client as a system. The effect of the stressor in any given environment is mitigated by a variety of factors. These could include the number, nature, and intensity of stressors present at any given point in time; the timing of the stressor occurrence; current client system condition; ability to protect against the stressor; and so forth.

Health

Health is equated with *living energy* and is viewed as a continuum running from greatest negentropic state (wellness) to greatest entropic state (illness) (Neuman, 1989, pp. 33–34; Neuman, 1995, pp. 32–33; Neuman, 2001, p. 23). Health is a condition determined by the degree of harmonious arrangement of the five client variables and the basic structure factors and is reflected in the client's level of wellness (Neuman, 1989, p. 12; Neuman, 1995, p. 12; Neuman, 2001, p. 12). Change is implicit in this definition of health, given that achievement and maintenance of client stability/balance (i.e., having more energy available to the system than is being used) is related to the client's reactions to constant changes in the environment. Therefore, constant energy flow exists between the client system and environment. The degree of client wellness is determined by the amount of energy required to retain, attain, or maintain system stability (Neuman, 1989, p. 13; Neuman, 1995, p. 13; Neuman, 2001, p. 12). Optimal wellness (i.e., the best possible level of health achievable at a given point in time) exists when system needs are met; unmet needs reduce the wellness state (Neuman, 1989, pp. 12, 34; Neuman, 1995, pp. 12, 32; Neuman, 2001, p. 12).

The normal line of defense represents the client's usual wellness level and is the baseline against which variances are measured (Neuman, 1989, pp. 17, 30; Neuman, 1995, p. 30; Neuman, 2001, p. 17). A client's degree of wellness is determined by how effectively client system variables react to environmental stressors. Thus, like the flexible line of defense, the normal line is dynamic in that it too can expand or contract over time. Health, then, in the Neuman model is related to internal, external, and created environmental forces inclusive of genetic factors, past experiences, and current perceptions.

For example, clients who have experienced depression in the past may have a biologic predisposition to this condition. In certain circumstances, their flexible line of defense could be more permeable and thus they would experience a reduced state of health compared with that of another individual without the genetic predisposition. Similarly, a client who experiences an attack of influenza develops antibodies. Such antibodies become components of the client's flexible line of defense and thus serve to protect the client's normal line of defense during future encounters with this stressor.

Another level of wellness is reflected by a client's retention of a reconstitutive state, such as use of a prosthesis after a limb amputation.

In summary, Neuman's definition of health allows for individual client system differences and is not considered a perfect state or some absolute standard. The best possible state of optimal health for a specific client or client system varies at any given point in time.

Interrelationship of Basic Concepts

The client is in constant dynamic interaction with the environment, the outcome of which is corrective or regulative for the client system (Neuman, 1989, p. 31; Neuman, 1995, p. 30; Neuman, 2001, p. 12). The nurse is seen as an active participant and as an external interpersonal environmental influence on the client. Her or his purpose is to assist the client to retain, attain, and/or maintain system stability through implementation of the appropriate level(s) of prevention interventions. By doing so, the nurse creates a link among the four nursing metaparadigm concepts of the model.

Health is dynamic harmony of all five client variables and basic structure components over time, and is optimal when system needs are met (Neuman 1989, p. 12; Neuman, 1995, p. 12). Stressors occur in the internal and external environments. Clients may create environments as a "self-help" method of dealing with internal and external stressors (Neuman, 1990). Before interventions are identified and for them to be effective in returning client stability, the nature of the stressor as perceived by the client needs to be assessed.

In summary, there is a strong interrelationship among the major model concepts. The four nursing metaparadigm concepts are present, fit logically with one another, and are useful to nursing and other healthcare practitioners.

INTERNAL ANALYSIS

Model Origins

The philosophical basis for the Neuman model (1982, 1989, 1995, 2001) began with Neuman's own personal philosophical beliefs as well as from knowledge gained from her work in community mental health nursing and clinical teaching (p. 458). In addition, it represents a synthesis of her knowledge from a variety of other disciplines.

Klir (1972) and von Bertalanffy's (1968) general systems theories as well as the work of other systems thinkers (Miller, 1965; Lazlo, 1972; Gray, Rizzo, & Duhl, 1969), de Chardin's (1955) philosophical views of the wholeness of life, and the notion represented by Marxist philosophy that the whole is greater than the sum of its parts (Cornu, 1957) all form the backbone of the Neuman model. In addition, Gestalt theory, with its focus on the importance of perception (Pearls, 1973), and Edelson's (1970) field theory, which suggests the interrelatedness and interdependency of all parts of the system, are clearly reflected in Neuman's work. Caplan's (1964) work is reflected in Neuman's typology of prevention interventions.

Seyle's (1950) theory of stress and adaptation as well as Putt's (1972) notions of entropy and negentropy, which are reflected in the model's concept of wellness, is in conflict with the overall organismic approach of the model. Entropy is characteristic of only closed systems (von Bertalanffy, 1968). Seyle's mechanistic theory of stress and coping could be replaced by incorporation of Lazarus' (1966) more dynamic views of these concepts. Neuman (personal communication, May 14, 1994) has indicated that her 1995 text revision will address how the work of Lazarus and Folkman (1984) relate to the model.

Also aligned with a more mechanistic view is Neuman's use of the term *stability* to describe the client's steady state. In an open systems model that is experiencing constant change because of a dynamic energy exchange (Neuman, 1989, p. 10; Neuman, 1995, p. 13), such a term seems incongruent. Perhaps more consistent use of the term *balance* rather than *stability* would be a more accurate descriptor for this concept and more congruent with the organismic focus of the model.

Underlying Assumptions

An assumption is defined as a basic premise that is accepted without proof (Stevens, 1979). The major explicit assumptions identified by Neuman in the 1989 book were explicated in the 3rd edition of *Conceptual Models of Nursing* by Fitzpatrick and Whall (1996) and were paraphrased based on the 1989 version (pp. 17, 21–22). Since that time, the 10 assumptions were written as "propositions" in the 1995 book (p. 22–23) and have now been identified as presented below, in the 2001 book as "statements" (p. 14). Assumption number 10 is now number 2 in the 4th edition (2001). The basic assumptions have not changed significantly, but have been more clearly articulated. These "statements" are paraphrased below:

1. Each client or client system is unique, with composite innate characteristics, and possesses a normal range of responses.
2. The client as a system constantly exchanges energy with the environment.
3. There are many types of known, unknown, and universal stressors that may upset a client's equilibrium (normal line of defense). The

interrelationship of the five client variables determines the degree of protection offered by the flexible line of defense.

4. Over time, each individual client or client system develops a normal range of responses called the client's normal line of defense.

5. The cushioning, accordion-like flexible line of defense protects the client against stressors. When it cannot, the stressor upsets the client system equilibrium and interrelationships among the five variables determine the degree of reaction.

6. Wellness is a dynamic composite of the interrelationship of the five client variables and represents a continuum of available system energy.

7. Following a stressor reaction, internal resistance lines attempt to stabilize the client by returning to a normal or enhanced wellness state.

8. Primary prevention assessment and intervention identifies and allays risk factors associated with stressors. Included in primary prevention is health promotion.

9. Secondary prevention relates to symptom identification and implementation of interventions to deal with system disruptions.

10. Tertiary prevention assists client adjustment as reconstitution is initiated and maintenance factors move the client back toward primary prevention.

(Neuman, 2001, p. 14)

Two of these assumptions define and/or describe major model concepts. The remaining eight assumptions reflect the interrelationships of the basic model concepts, focusing on the interaction between the client and environment, and are therefore model propositions rather than assumptions (Fawcett & Downs, 1986). Assumptions implicit to the model can also be inferred. For example, the client's individuality and perceptions are valued, and attempts at retaining, maintaining, or attaining stability are a prime focus for clients and nurses.

Families, communities, and social issues are also referred to in the Neuman model (1982, 1989, 1995, 2001). The current assumptions (statements) have been revised to reflect this group focus through consistent use of the more general terms *client* and *client system*. Neuman's hope that others will expand the assumptions to more clearly address larger client systems is being realized.

For example, in addition to Neuman's (1983) own early work, Reed (1982, 1989, 1993a) has applied the concepts within the Neuman model to the family unit as the client. Building on these initial efforts, Reed (1993b) is currently developing operational definitions of the abstract model concepts for application to families. This step is essential if Reed's objective of theoretical testing of the family-focused Neuman model concepts is to be realized.

Similar work of adapting Neuman model concepts to the community as client was conducted by Anderson, McFarlane and Helton (1986), and Beddome (1989). More recent application of model concepts has been demonstrated by Oklahoma State Public Health Nursing (Frioux, Roberts, & Butler, 1995) and in a Continuing Care Retirement Community in Maryland (Rodriguez, 1995).

Central Components of the Model

The primary model components are *stressors, lines of defense and resistance, levels of prevention,* the *five client system variables* (*basic structure, interventions, internal and external environment,* and *reconstitution*) (Figure 10–1). All of these concepts have been defined by Neuman (1982, 1989, 1995, 2001).

The flexible and normal lines of defense concepts are clearly differentiated from one another. The former serves to protect the latter in the presence of stressors. The definition of the normal line of defense indicates what could be the range of responses developed by an individual over time. For example, one's normal line of defense or usual state of wellness could range from effective coping behaviors to development of psychotic behavior. The lines of resistance are activated once a stressor breaks through the system's normal line of defense. They are defined as forces that attempt to stabilize and return the client to his or her normal line of defense.

In terms of the types of concepts contained in the model, Dubin (1978) would consider most to be relational units. A relational unit is a property characteristic of a concept that can only be determined by examining the relationships among two or more other properties (p. 62). Thus, only when a stressor and client come into contact may one speak of lines of defense or levels of prevention. This is similar to Hill's (1966) discussion of cumulative concepts (i.e., those that build upon each other). Dubin (1978) indicates that relational units sum up the properties of concepts and that other aspects should be ignored because of the summing nature of the units.

The nursing metaparadigm concepts of person, environment, health, and nursing are summative units or concepts that stand for an entire complex of a thing. According to Dubin (1978), summative units are too broad for use in theory-building efforts. However, relational units may be used for such efforts. Thus, Neuman's model, although at a broad level of abstraction, has great potential in terms of derivation of specific theories. In fact, Neuman indicates that she and her colleague, Audrey Koertvelyessy,

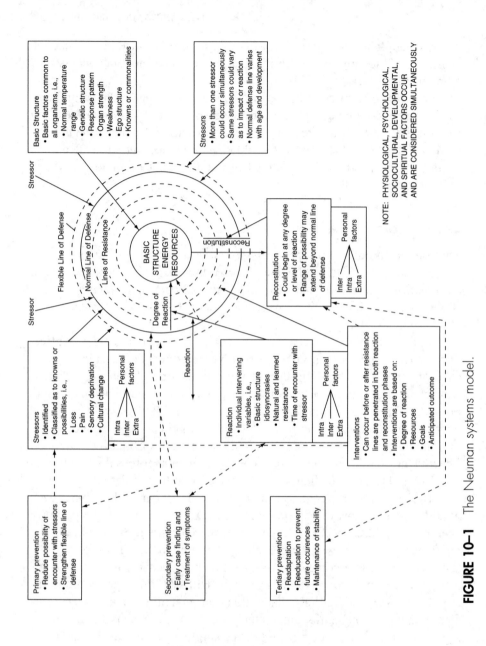

FIGURE 10-1 The Neuman systems model.

have derived the theory of optimal client system stability (Louis & Koertvelyessy, 1989). In addition, Koertvelyessy has suggested the theory of prevention as intervention from the model. Although Koertvelyessy introduced this theory to the participants of the Second Biennial NSM Symposium in 1988, unfortunately, the details of neither theory were not clearly presented in Neuman's 1989 text nor have they been made available in the professional literature since that time. Despite this dearth of information, Mynatt and O'Brien (1993) state that they have used the theory of optimal client system stability as the basis for the prevention efforts delineated in the West Tennessee Nurses' Peer Assistance Program. The function of the program is to prevent chemical dependency.

Ziemer (1983) was the first researcher to publish research that tested hypotheses derived from the Neuman model. Similarly, Lancaster (1992) has derived a middle-range theory of breast cancer prevention from the Neuman model. After assumptions, specific propositional statements, and empirical indicators for key theoretical concepts were identified, the relationships between theory concepts were tested through the research process.

Thus, the model has potentially wide applicability in health care, and is becoming more specific in its directives through the operationalization of key concepts and testing of relationships proposed within it through research.

Analysis of Consistency

Consistency considerations have to do with internal and external events. Neuman's model is internally consistent in that the three types of stressors, environment, levels of prevention, five client variables, and basic structure factors are discussed throughout the model in the same manner. The description of relationships among the concepts remains consistent throughout Neuman's explanation of the model (1982, 1989, 1995, 2001).

External consistency relates to the generality or level of model abstraction (Hill, 1966). Not tied to specific and thus limited situations, the Neuman model (1989) is at a high level of abstraction. It presents a framework from which many client system concerns can be analyzed.

Analysis of Adequacy

Model adequacy is related to assessing whether operational definitions of model concepts can be developed and tested, and how accurately these reflect the theoretical definitions (Hardy, 1974). Hoffman's (1982) initial attempt to develop operational definitions for key model concepts is applauded but falls short in its ability to identify clearly how researchers could measure the concepts through the research process. This attempt was not expanded upon in the books by Neuman published in 1989, 1995, or 2001. Ziemer's (1983) and Lancaster's (1992) works were successful in operationally defining and testing the relationships among Neuman's concepts of stressors, lines of defense, and primary prevention. In addition, Lowry and Anderson (1993) operationally defined and tested relationships among Neuman model concepts of stressors, four intrapersonal client variables, and the interpersonal factor of social support to study the created environment of ventilator-dependent patients.

Contribution to understanding is another point to be considered in terms of model adequacy (Hardy, 1974). Herein lies a major benefit of this model. In addition to its potential to provide a common language for use by various healthcare professionals, the concept of created environment suggests potential new directions for assessing individuals and situations. In addition, the explanatory nature of the model in relation to client stressors and reactions to them remains sound.

However, as with all conceptual models, Neuman's is not at the level of predictability suggested for theory testing. Because pragmatic adequacy has to do with the ability to predict, control, and explain, the pragmatic adequacy of the Neuman model has much potential but remains limited. Prediction and control cannot be addressed until operational definitions of all model concepts are formulated.

EXTERNAL ANALYSIS

The overall goals of the model (i.e., holistic care, prevention, health promotion, and systems concepts) are still congruent with current societal values held by the World Health Organization, the American Nurses' Association (Neuman, 1989, p. 10; Neuman, 2001, p. 32), and the focus on primary prevention and interdisciplinary care being promoted in the healthcare industry today. In addition, given the current complexities of healthcare and the need for healthcare providers to rapidly and easily assimilate change, the expansive characteristic of systems models becomes an essential component of effective practice (Neuman, 1989, p. 5).

Relationship to Nursing Research

As evidenced by the model's increased empirical utilization through research, the NSM is being used as a guide for conceptualization of research problems. The findings of a 1986–1987 survey of graduate nursing programs regarding use of the Neuman model in research identified 38 studies (Louis & Koertvelyessy, 1989). The vast majority of these ($N = 520$) were descriptive in nature and studied adult populations. The only Neuman model concept not being investigated was that of the spiritual variable. Recently, an integrative review of NSM-based research through 1997 was conducted by Fawcett and Giangrande (2001). Through various search methods, these authors identified 200 research reports: "59 journal articles; 2 abstracts published in journals, one of which was published only as an abstract, and the other only as an abstract in English (the full report was published in Chinese); 3 book chapters; 81 master's theses; and 55 doctoral dissertations" (p. 122). A comprehensive analysis was conducted on only 117 research reports published (journal articles, book chapters, and dissertations).

Codebooks developed by the authors were designed to analyze elements related to three areas: general information, scientific merit, and the NSM. In the analysis of general information, the majority of the 200 studies (75%) analyzed focused on clinical nursing topics, whereas 14% focused on nursing administration, 9% on nursing education, and 2% on continuing education. Analysis of the scientific merit revealed that descriptive studies were most frequently used (37%), followed closely by the number of experimental studies (32%). Correlational studies were used in 25% of the research, with approximately 4% designed to develop and test instruments (Fawcett & Giangrande, 2001, p. 124.) Next, elements related to the NSM were analyzed. Development or testing of prevention interventions was most frequently documented, followed closely by interest in the perception of stressors (24%). The next area of interest was the client system variables (9%) with a few studies each (ranging from 1% to 5%) on the lines of defense and/or resistance, the central core, various client system perceptions, coping, the environment, and the nursing process (p. 124). Five percent focused on evaluation of NSM-based education programs, with 2% related to guiding practice in clinical agencies.

A similar review was conducted just on the 62 NSM-based research studies reported in journals and book chapters. Clinical topics were the focus of 44 (72%) of these publications, and 28 (almost one-half were experiments. Twenty-three (37%) focused on the NSM prevention interventions, and of those, a larger number (26%) focused on primary prevention. Conclusions relating to the utility and credibility of the NSM according to Fawcett and Giangrande (2001, p. 125) were evidenced by the result that 30% of the 10 correlational studies and 54% of the 28 experimental studies yielded a combination of statistically significant and nonsignificant results. Furthermore, Fawcett and Giangrande (2001, p. 126) indicated that data analysis procedures were appropriate for the research question in most (89%, $n = 55$) studies. They also reported that in 89% of the studies, all NSM concepts or study variables were linked to empirical indicators (p. 26).

Doctoral dissertations ($n = 55$) have been conducted by students at 17 different universities. Consistent with other analysis data, about three fourths of the dissertations were focused on clinical topics and slightly less (29%) were designed as experiments, with only about one-third of the researchers investigating some aspect of the prevention interventions, and of those a higher percentage focused on primary prevention (50%). Conclusions regarding the utility of the NSM were evident in 91% of the studies. However, related to the issue of credibility, 77% of the 22 correlation studies and 81% of the 16 experimental studies yielded a combination of statistically significant and nonsignificant results. In general, based on the integrative review, Fawcett and Giangrande (2001) found that the sample sizes were adequate for study purposes and the research design. Again, the authors indicated as a result of the analysis that in 93% of the studies, all NSM concepts or study variables were linked to empirical indicators.

The authors of the integrative review summarized recommendations for NSM research, indicating that teams or networks of researchers with complementary skills should study the interrelationships between all of the phenomena encompassed by the NSM. "Cluster studies" were encouraged, using the same sample of study participants. These studies would look at related phenomena—one researcher might study the impact of extrapersonal stressors on some of the five variables, and another researcher could study the impact of interpersonal stressors on the variables. Collaborative research approaches would help in filling in the gaps and extending the knowledge of the NSM through research (Fawcett & Giangrande, 2001, pp. 136–137).

In addition, in the 4th edition (2001), a systematic review of instrumentation used in research guided by the NSM was presented. "The goal of the literature review was to identify instruments used for data collection, the middle-range theory concept measured by each instrument and the NSM as stated in each research report . . . any empirical indicator that was used to measure a middle-range theory concept was regarded as an instrument, including questionnaires, rating scales, visual analog scales, chart reviews, interview schedules, needs assessments, logs, evolution tools, physiological measures and intervention protocols" (Gigliotti & Fawcett, 2001, pp. 150–151). From the 212 research reports applicable for this review, 121 different instruments were identified (some of the instruments were used more than once and were counted only once in the total).

Of those instruments applicable to this analysis, 75 different instruments were explicitly linked to the NSM, with some of the instruments used more than once, sometimes for different purposes. For example, the Beck Depression Inventory was used in three studies: once to measure depression; another time to measure mental health status, and another time for measurement of psychological well-being. Other instruments that were explicitly linked to the NSM in research included the State Trait Anxiety Inventory, the Norbeck Social Support Questionnaire; the Dynamap, the Carter Center Institute Health Risk Appraisal, and the Health Status Questionnaire. Of those analyzed, 26 of the instruments were not explicitly linked to the NSM in research (Gigliotti & Fawcett, 2001).

Regarding middle-range theory, 26 instruments measured concepts related to stressors, 24 measured middle-range theory related to lines of defense and/or resistance, 24 measured client system interactions, and 22 measured middle-range theory concepts representing prevention interventions. Other middle-range theory concepts broadly associated with the NSM were measured by the remaining 16 instruments. Of those instruments, 59 were classified as standardized (having sufficient evidence of validity and reliability testing) and 62 were considered nonstandardized (Gigliotti & Fawcett, 2001, pp. 153–154). Fourteen of the 26 instruments used to measure middle-range theory concepts related to stressors were used to elicit information about the client's perception of specific stressors. These instruments included interview schedules, questionnaires, stressor rating scales, stressor assessment scales, one log, and one needs inventory. In addition, 5 of the 14 instruments were used to measure caregiver's perception of stressors (Gigliotti & Fawcett, 2001, pp. 150–151). This analysis was particularly notable because the NSM places great emphasis on client perception and the need for shared perceptions with caregivers to produce shared goals and outcomes.

Of the remaining instruments used to measure middle-range theory concepts, 24 were used to measure concepts related to client's response to stressors, 19 were used to measure NSM concepts such as lines of defense and/or lines of resistance, and 6 were used to measure diverse NSM concepts such as physiological, psychological, and sociocultural changes, as well as reaction to intrapersonal, interpersonal and extrapersonal stressors. In conclusion, the authors identified recommendations for instrumentation used for NSM research, including give more attention to the validity of existing instrumentation; examine logical congruence with NSM concepts; when there is no existing logically congruent instrument, derive instruments from the NSM; examine the utility of instruments used in NSM-based clinical practice; and identify the research potential of clinical and educational tools, which would help facilitate the integration of research, practice, and education (Gigliotti & Fawcett, 2001, pp. 166–169). A detailed set of tables is included with the instrument analysis that provide excellent information for relationships between middle-range theory concepts and instrumentation (Gigliotti & Fawcett, 2001, pp. 152–160).

Neuman and Fawcett (2001) have included delineation of a compre-hensive set of guidelines for NSM-based research that includes purpose of the research; phenomena of interest; problems to be studied; research methods; study participants; data analysis; contributions to knowledge de-velopment and research and clinical practice. These guidelines are not just designed for nursing, but are designed and explicated in multidisciplinary perspective, encouraging interdisciplinary collaboration in clinical prac-tice and research.

Relationship to Nursing Education

The model was originally designed as a teaching aide and later used as a curriculum guide (Neuman, 1972). Since 1972, the potential of the NSM to guide a curriculum that had implications for use nationally and interna-tionally in nursing was recognized, and subsequently it also has been used to guide the education of other disciplines (Toot & Schmoll, 1995). Guide-lines for NSM-based education for the health professions have been pre-sented by Newman, Neuman, and Fawcett (2001). These represent refinements of the original guidelines that were extracted from the content of the model by Fawcett (1989). The 4th edition provides a detailed expla-nation of each guideline, which is organized according to focus of the cur-riculum, nature and sequence of the content, settings for education for the healthcare professions, characteristics of the learners, and teaching-learning strategies. Subsequently, an ideal NSM-based curriculum for bac-calaureate education, associate's degree (AD) in education, and master's degree (MS) in education is presented in detail (Newman et al., 2001, pp. 199–213).

An integrative review of the NSM and education was conducted by Lowry (2001) using a nonexperimental design in which information was obtained from the literature and systematically categorized and summa-rized. Published articles, book chapters, and three accreditation self-study reports published from 1980 to 2000 focusing on NSM and education were used in this analysis (p. 216). A data collection tool was designed for the integrative review based on items derived from Fawcett's (1989) rules for use of conceptual models in education.

From the review of publications, 52 different programs were identi-fied (61% from the United States and 39% from other countries). The NSM was first used in baccalaureate education, with four schools adopting the model in the late 1970s and eight in the 1980s. Two consortia, each of which encompassed three schools, also adopted the model (Lowry, 2001). For graduate and multilevel programs (having programs at more than one level using the NSM), nine graduate programs have used the model for a specific specialty. Texas Woman's University (TWU) and Northwestern

State University were the first to use the model for advanced practice specialties in 1976. During the 1980s, three other universities used the model for multilevel programming. Four AD programs started using the NSM in the 1980s and three others adopted the NSM as a curricular framework in the 1990s. According to Lowry (2001), currently the NSM is used in nine AD programs. Lowry (2001) provided a number of detailed tables listing each school and/or university, the year of NSM adoption, and current use of the NSM model in education.

Outside the United States, nursing programs began to adopt the NSM in the late 1990s. Documentation in the literature indicates use in 10 programs in Canada; 3 colleges in Sweden, and 1 program in Denmark, and 1 in South Australia have also adopted the model. In addition, the NSM model has been accepted and is in use as a framework for physical therapy (Toot & Schmoll, 1995). The literature also revealed discussions about NSM-based teaching-learning strategies for a variety of courses and populations. The majority of the publications presented and described various teaching-learning strategies: three publications included clinical evaluation tools, three schools reported program evaluation processes and tools using the NSM, and three publications describe ways to introduce faculty and maintain interest in the NSM (Lowry, 2001, p. 224).

In addition to the integrative review from the literature, a telephone or electronic mail survey was conducted to determine current use of the NSM by 45 schools that have been known to use the NSM in education (either from published reports or conference presentations) (Lowry, 2001). Of the 36 respondents, 34 responses were from the United States and two were from other countries. Of the responses from the United States, 17 of the responding programs were described in the literature review and information about 17 other programs had not been published in the literature.

Twenty-three of the programs responding continue to use the NSM in its entirety as a curricular framework and 11 have become more eclectic (Lowry, 2001, pp. 224, 231). The 23 programs continuing to use the NSM include Athens Area Technical Institute, GA (AD); California State University, CA (bachelor of science [BS]/MS); Cecil Community College, MD (AD); Central Florida Community College, FL (AD); Gulf Coast Community College, FL (Practical Nursing [PN]/AD); Fitchburg State College, MA (BS); Holy Names College, CA (BS); Indiana University–Purdue University, IN (AD); Lander University, SC (BS); Loma Linda University, CA (BS/MS); Los Angeles County Medical Center, CA (AD); Louisiana College, Pineville, LA (BS); Mansfield College, PA (BS); Milligan College, TN (BS); Minnesota Intercollegiate Consortium, MN (BS); Neumann College, PA (BS); Santa Fe Community College, FL (PN/AD); Seattle Pacific College, WA (BS); Southern Adventist University, TN (AD); St. Anselm's College, NH (BS); Texas Woman's

University, Houston, TX (BS); University of Nevada, NV (BS/MS); and University of Tennessee, Martin, TN (BS). As evidenced in the list, many small church-related schools continue to use the NSM as a curricular framework. Lowry (2001) indicated that the model is especially favored by church-related institutions because of the inclusion of the spiritual variable.

Relationship to Nursing Practice

Like its application to nursing education, the Neuman model has been applied to a wide variety of nursing practice arenas. Model application has been facilitated through the development and testing tools designed to facilitate incorporation of model terminology and assist in model implementation in the practice arena. Such tools include the Neuman nursing process and the prevention as intervention formats (Neuman, 1989, p. 17).

Like the guidelines for use of the NSM in research and education, new guidelines have also been written to guide NSM-based clinical practice (Freese, Neuman, & Fawcett, 2001). Again, rudimentary guidelines were extracted from the content of the model developed by Fawcett (1989) and were later refined. The guidelines were written and discussed in the context of multidisciplinary practice and include the following elements: purpose of clinical practice, clinical problems of interest, settings for clinical practice, characteristics of legitimate participants in clinical practice, the process of clinical practice, client–caregiver relationship, diagnostic taxonomy, typology of clinical interventions, typology of outcomes, contributions of clinical practice to participant's well-being, and clinical practice and research (Freese et al., 2001, p. 38).

An integrative review of NSM-based clinical practice was conducted by Amaya (2001) from published literature from 1974 to 2000. Of the 115 publications reviewed with practice-related titles, 8 were eliminated because they were in a foreign language or were unrelated to clinical practice. The remaining 107 were reviewed based on the structure of the NSM for client system development, holistic process, and the range and diversity of clinical situations (Amaya, 2001, p. 44).

The NSM is most frequently used in practice with the individual client system, although in the NSM the client may be an individual, family, group, or community. Of the 107 publications, the majority of clinical practice publications were describing the individual as client (44 are listed in the application of the NSM to individual clients, p. 45). Of these, the majority (23 publications) described care related to medical-surgical conditions. Six of the medical-surgical publications described some aspect of NSM-based clinical practice in a critical care or intensive care unit, six were related to pediatric care, six were related to women's health, five focused on psychiatric-mental health clients, and three were related to care of the gerontological client. Clinical diagnosis included, but was not limited to substance and spousal abuse, depression, health promotion, human immunodeficiency virus, leukemia, spinal cord injury, pulmonary conditions, cardiac conditions, cancer orthopedics, and cardiovascular disease such as hypertension.

There were significantly fewer publication related to the family as client and the community as client. Reed (1993a, 1993b) is most frequently referenced regarding the use of the NSM in practice with the family as the client system. Other authors explicating use of the NSM in the context of family-centered care include Cross (1995), who's work related to Hodgkin's disease; Beckingham and Baumann (1990), who integrated crisis management and NSM for family-centered care of the elderly; Goldblum-Graff and Graff (1982), who described the use of the NSM in family therapy practice; and Tomlinson and Anderson (1995), who uniquely described family as a separate entity interacting with the environment.

Amaya (2001) presents a table describing application of the NSM to the community as client. Beddome (1989) promoted the NSM for use in community health nursing. Spradley (1990) described the compatibility of the NSM with community health nursing and the community client system. Other authors explicating various aspects of the community as client include Anderson, McFarlane, and Helton (1986); Benedict and Sproles (1982); Buchanan (1987); and Haggart, (1993). Helland (1995) demonstrated a practical application to formulating a nursing diagnosis for the community as client. Pierce and Fulmer (1995) related the NSM to elders as an aggregate cohort in the community.

Relationship to American Nurses Association (ANA)-Approved Nursing Classification Systems

The focus of nursing within the NSM is the diagnosis and treatment of the client system's response to stressors. Neuman (1989) supports the formulation of holistic, comprehensive diagnostic statements reflective of actual or potential variances from wellness and based on the integration of assessment data with various appropriate theories (pp. 43–44). However, only references to North American Nursing Diagnosis Association (NANDA) and nursing diagnosis were consistently located in relation to the use of the NSM. There was only one reference to the exploration of a relationship between the NSM and the Omaha System and it was found in the "future initiatives" section of the 4th edition. (Neuman, 2001). There was no mention in the literature of the use of other ANA-approved nursing classification systems such as Nursing Intervention Classification (NIC),

Nursing Outcomes Classification (NOC), Home Health Care Classification (HHCC), or the Ozbolt Patient Care Data Set.

A taxonomy for classifying nursing diagnoses based on the Neuman model was developed by Ziegler (1982). Her theoretical definition is congruent with Neuman's discussions of nursing diagnoses and the operational definition of a two-part diagnostic statement indicative of the actual problem and the client's response to the problem joined together with the phrase "related to" is congruent with the NANDA approach to diagnostic statements.

The Neuman model variables provide five major foci for organizing the nursing diagnosis classification system. They include (a) the responding subsystem (i.e., the five client variables); (b) the system being diagnosed (i.e., individual, family, group, or community); (c) the level of response (i.e., primary, secondary, or tertiary); (d) the source of the stressor etiology (i.e., intra-inter-, or extrapersonal system); and (e) type of stressor etiology (i.e., physiological, psychological, or sociocultural) (Ziegler, 1982).

An example diagnostic statement based on Ziegler's work is "potential for altered health maintenance related to lack of seat belt use." This diagnosis involves a potential physiological response related to an extrasystem physiological stressor. The diagnosis of "delayed language development related to lack of adequate stimulation" involves a reconstitutive psychological response due to an intersystem psychological stressor.

Delunas (1990) suggested that clinical nurse specialists use the Neuman (1982) framework to develop diagnoses aimed at preventing elder abuse and maintaining family integrity. She identified 11 diagnoses that could be suggestive of a family system at high risk for elder abuse. Some examples include "potential for ineffective family coping related to history of abusive relationship with parents," and "knowledge deficit related to lack of awareness of available financial resources."

Piazza, Foote, Wright, and Holcombe (1992) used Neuman's assessment and intervention tools to formulate 18 nursing diagnoses related to both primary and secondary prevention interventions for an 8-year-old boy diagnosed with leukemia. Primary prevention diagnoses were related to potential variances from wellness (i.e., "potential for infection related to altered immune status," or "potential alteration in body image related to alopecia, weight loss, bruising, and presence of Hickman catheter.").

The secondary prevention diagnoses were related to actual variances from wellness. These included diagnoses such as "fluid volume deficit related to fever and decreased intake," and "anxiety related to poor prognosis and impending death." Tertiary prevention diagnoses were not appropriate for this client at this time but would relate to promotion of readaptation. They could address the long-term effects of chemotherapy and/or maintaining family stability.

Two major criticisms of the first NANDA nursing diagnosis taxonomy included lack of a wellness/health promotion perspective and its inability to effectively address aggregate groups such as families or communities (Allen, 1989). However, in 1990, the NANDA Taxonomy Committee for Taxonomy II recommended use of a minimum of four axes, which gives the current taxonomy structure a multidimensional focus and addresses these criticisms (Hoskins et al., 1992). For example, the first axis, unit of analysis, has three different categories: individual, family, and community. The third and fourth axes address the wellness versus illness issue, and there is consideration of adding additional axes that would address acuity versus chronicity issues.

Changes such as these enhance the degree of congruence between the current NANDA nursing diagnosis taxonomy and those diagnoses derived from the Neuman model. Of the nine diagnostic patterns identified by NANDA, seven of them are represented by the diagnoses presented by the authors reviewed above. Diagnoses from the remaining two patterns (i.e., relating and valuing) would be congruent with the Neuman model concepts because they deal with concepts such as spirituality, sexuality, and social interactions.

In addition, the focuses of Ziegler's diagnostic taxonomy are congruent with the NANDA efforts. For example, the first focus in Ziegler's taxonomy, the responding subsystem, corresponds to each of the nine NANDA diagnostic patterns. The second focus, the type of system diagnosed, is reflected in NANDA's individual, family, and community diagnoses. Larger groups, such as social systems, are not yet presented in the NANDA taxonomy. Zeigler's level of response focus corresponds with actual (secondary prevention) and high-risk (primary prevention) diagnoses. Example tertiary diagnoses that correlate with NANDA work could include body image disturbance or health-seeking behaviors. The fourth and fifth focuses, source and type of stressor etiology, are reflected in any one of the NANDA diagnoses. In conclusion, either taxonomy is congruent with the Neuman model but Ziegler's work is much more specific to various model concepts.

Neuman expresses concerns (1995) that existing NANDA diagnostic nomenclature does not "fit" the entirety of nursing models. She stated that "though considerable progress has been made in the past few years . . . there is major concern that the NANDA criteria relate only in part to various nursing conceptual frameworks" (Neuman, 1995, p. 37). She subsequently presented a family case study abstract which suggested a "variance from wellness" approach to nursing diagnosis. Torakis (2001) provided an up-to-date example at Children's Hospital of Michigan where the NSM is used as an organizing framework to guide nursing service administration. In this pediatric setting, a Neuman Process Summary was developed to incorporate

NSM nursing process into the nursing documentation system. In this system, NANDA is used to guide the care of both individuals and families, and is congruent with Neuman's definition of the client system, which includes individual, families, and communities.

Relationship to Theory-Driven, Evidenced-Based Practice

Concerns that evidence-based practice may be threatening the foundation of nursing's disciplinary perspective on theory-guided practice are articulated by Walker and Redman (1999). Fawcett, Watson, Neuman, Walker, and Fitzpatrick (2001) wrote that "although multiple patterns of knowing in nursing have been acknowledged at least since the publication of Carper's work (1978), nurses have ignored this disciplinary perspective and reverted to a medical perspective of evidence when discussing evidence-based nursing practice" (p. 115). Carper (1978) described four ways or patterns of knowing in nursing: empirics, ethics, personal, and esthetics. Processes associated with each pattern of knowing were subsequently identified by Chinn and Kramer (1999). Fawcett et al. (2001) take this a step further and raise the question of whether these ways of knowing can be considered as sets of theories or different types of inquiry. When nursing conceptual models such as the NSM are analyzed, one important question is whether the NSM can be used for theory-guided, evidence-based practice in the context of the questions about the four ways of knowing and/or four types of theories.

The NSM can be analyzed as representing all four types of knowing as evidenced by recent publications and the integrative review for research conducted by Fawcett and Giangrande (2001). Clearly, there is demonstration of empirical NSM-based research, with 34% of the research in the literature identified as experimental. In addition, Gigliotti and Fawcett (2001) in their analysis of instrumentation indicated that empirical indicators were identified appropriately for more than 90% in articles, book chapters, and dissertations using the NSM. Consequently, the NSM is beginning to look as if it meets the criteria of being an "empirics theory."

However, also in the integrative review, 37% of the NSM-based studies were descriptive and the authors of the integrative review (Fawcett & Giangrande, 2001) recommend that more work be done to explicate the holistic elements of the NSM, such as the spiritual variable and created environment. Clearly, the ethics way of knowing must be used to examine through inquiry about how the created environment can serve as a protective mechanism, through cultural or spiritual beliefs and/or belief systems (such as hope). The study by Pothiban (2001) from Thailand is a good example of how the NSM could be considered an ethics theory. Pothiban collected data by means of focus groups and in-depth interviews of 30 elderly Thai females and males. In the discussion of the results of her study, she validates how the Buddhist doctrine, particularly the reality of life under the law of kamma, influences beliefs about stress and suffering (p. 184). In addition, sociocultural factors influence the beliefs and descriptions about the meaning of health. These examples and the methodologies used to conduct the research support the proposition that the NSM could be considered an "ethics theory."

Other research conducted and documented by Breckenridge (2001) can make the case that the NSM model is "personal theory." The purpose of Breckenridge's research was to study patient's perceptions from the NSM to determine how, why, and by whom treatment modalities are chosen. Her research was a descriptive theory-generating qualitative study, using the interpretive method of naturalistic inquiry (Breckenridge, 2001). With both renal patients and later with patients who were diagnosed with prostate cancer, Breckenridge was able to identify four themes that represent factors influencing decision making: provider influence, immediate family influence, friends/relatives influence, and information influence. On a later study with prostate cancer patients in another region of the United States, another theme was identified—a spiritual influence. Unfortunately at this time, the research has only looked at patient perceptions; however, it is clear that provider behavior and information influence the patient's goals and outcomes through the decision-making process. Fawcett and Giangrande (2001) in their integrative review strongly recommend that NSM research include the nurses' (or providers') perceptions as well as the patients' perceptions in the future. With the full research agenda conducted for both patient and provider perceptions and behaviors, the NSM could be considered a "personal theory."

The NSM emphasis on assessment of perceptions of both the client system and the caregiver requires much greater attention in NSM-based studies according to Fawcett and Giangrande (2001). Only a few studies could be identified that would demonstrate the possibility of the NSM being an "aesthetic theory." However, the dearth of studies does not mean that this topic (of conducting research on the provider perceptions along with patient perceptions) is not feasible and important for congruence with the NSM approach to care. Studies that could support that the NSM is an aesthetic theory were Puetz's (1990) study of nurse and patient perceptions associated with coronary artery bypass; Gibson's (1989) study of interpersonal trust in the nurse–client relationship; Peoples' (1991) study of the relationship of selected client, provider, and agency variables and the utilization of home care services; Cullen's (1994) study of nurses perceptions of humor as a preventive intervention to promote health of clients;

and Harper's (1993) study of nurses' beliefs about social support and the effect of nursing care on cardiac clients' attitudes in reducing cardiac risk. These research studies demonstrate the potential for the NSM to be considered an aesthetics theory, but clearly much more research needs to be conducted regarding both patient and nurse and their perceptions, beliefs, and behavior to understand how this impacts care.

Finally, consistent with the Fawcett et al. (2001) concerns regarding only the valuing of empirical research, Meleis (1995) also challenged the profession to consider theory validation instead of a rigid notion of theory testing and encourages the use of the term *theory support.* She wrote that the empirics approach alone is limiting and incongruent with the discipline of nursing. She advocates theory support through philosophical analysis, conceptual analysis, and through the conduct of narrative studies based on clinician's experiences as well as assessment of clients' situations and the therapeutics used. After reviewing the literature, the publications related to the NSM and the methodologies used for research, it is the author's perspective that the NSM could be considered in each of the four ways of knowing or as each of the types of theories—empirics, ethics, personal, and aesthetics.

SUMMARY

Neuman has presented a comprehensive and systematic approach for organizing nursing phenomena that is based on tested scientific findings from multiple disciplines. It is a valuable model for understanding relationships between clients and their environments.

Ellis (1968) has noted that the characteristics of significant theories are scope, complexity, testability, generation of information, and usefulness. Although the model is not a specific theoretical structure, these characteristics are relevant because specific theories have been developed from this model. The model has a broad scope and is highly ordered. It demonstrates complexity through its consideration of multiple variables and the relationships among those variables. Middle-range theories derived from the model have been formulated and tested, and have therefore supported the model's usefulness and ability to generate knowledge. Thus, nursing education, practice, and research have all benefited from the application and outcomes of this model. The NSM continues to grow and thrive in a changing healthcare environment, and the Neuman Systems Model Trustees Group, Inc., have had a significant impact on the use of the model for generation and testing of knowledge. With the support and guidance of both Dr. Neuman and the Trustees Group, the NSM is well positioned for the 21st century.

REFERENCES

Allen, C. J. (1989). Incorporating a wellness perspective for nursing diagnosis in practice. In R. M. Caroll-Johnson (Ed.), *Classification of nursing diagnoses: Proceedings of the eighth conference*. Philadelphia: J. B. Lippincott.

Amaya, M. A. (2001). The Neuman Systems Model and Clinical Practice: An Integrative Review, 1974–2000. In B. Neuman & J. Fawcett (Eds.), *The NSM* (4th ed.). Upper Saddle River, NJ: Prentice Hall.

Anderson, E., McFarlane, J., & Helton, A. (1986). Community as client: A model for practice. *Nursing Outlook, 34,* 220–224.

Beckingham, A. C., & Baumann, A. (1990). The aging family in crisis: Assessment and decision-making models. *Journal of Advanced Nursing, 15,* 782–787.

Beddome, G. (1989). Application of the NSM to the community-as-client. In B. Neuman (Ed.), *The NSM* (2nd ed.). Norwalk, CT: Appleton & Lange.

Benedict, M. B., & Sproles, J. B. (1982). Application of the Neuman model to public health nursing practice. In B. Neuman (Ed.), *The NSM: Application to nursing education and practice* (pp. 223–240). Norwalk, CT: Appleton-Century-Crofts.

Breckenridge, D. M. (2001). Using the Neuman Systems Model to guide nursing research in the United States. In B. Neuman & J. Fawcett (Eds.), *The NSM* (4th ed.). Upper Saddle River, NJ: Prentice Hall.

Buchanan, B. F. (1987). Human-environment interaction: A modification of the Neuman Systems Model for aggregates, families and the community. *Public Health Nursing, 4,* 52–64.

Caplan, G. (1964). *Principles of preventive psychiatry.* New York: Basic Books.

Carper, B. A. (1978). Fundamental patterns of knowing in nursing. *Advances in Nursing Science, 1*(1), 13–23.

Chinn, P. L., & Kramer, M. K. (1999). *Theory and nursing: Integrated knowledge development* (5th ed.). St. Louis, MO: Mosby.

Cornu, A. (1957). *The origins of Marxist thought.* Springfield, IL: Charles C. Thomas.

Cross, J. R. (1995). Nursing process of the family client: Application of Neuman's System Model. In P. J. Christensen & J. W. Kenney (Eds.), *Nursing process: Application of conceptual models* (4th ed., pp. 246–269). St. Louis: Mosby-Year Book.

Cullen, L. M. (1994). Nurses' perceptions of humor as a preventive intervention to promote the health of clients in a health care setting. *Master's Abstracts International, 32,* 937.

Curran, G. (1995). The spiritual variable. In B. Neuman (Ed)., *The NSM* (2nd ed., pp. 581–590). Norwalk, CT: Appleton and Lange.

de Chardin, P. T. (1955). *The phenomenon of man.* London: Collins.

Delunas, L. R. (1990). Prevention of elder abuse: Betty Neuman health care systems approach. *Clinical Nurse Specialist, 4*(1), 54–58.

Dubin, R. (1978). *Theory building.* New York: Free Press.

Edelson, M. (1970). *Sociotherapy and psychotherapy.* Chicago: University of Chicago Press.

Ellis, R. (1968). Characteristics of significant theories. *Nursing Research, 17,* 217–222.

Fawcett, J. (1989). *Analysis and evaluation of conceptual models in nursing* (2nd ed.). Philadelphia: F. A. Davis.

Fawcett, J., & Downs, F. S. (1986). *The relationship of theory and research.* Norwalk, CT: Appleton-Century-Crofts.

Fawcett, J., & Giangrande, S. K. (2001). The Neuman Systems Model and research: An integrative review. In B. Neuman & J. Fawcett (Eds.), *The NSM* (4th ed.). Upper Saddle River, NJ: Prentice Hall.

Fawcett, J., Watson, J., Neuman, B., Walker, P. H., & Fitzpatrick, J. J. (2001). On nursing theories and evidence. *Journal of Nursing Scholarship, 33,* 115–119.

Fitzpatrick, J., & Whall, A. L. (1996). *Conceptual Models in Nursing* (3rd ed.). Upper Saddle River, NJ: Prentice Hall.

Freese, B. T., Neuman, B., & Fawcett, J. J. (2001). Guidelines for Neuman Systems Model-based clinical practice. In B. Neuman and J. Fawcett (Eds.), *The NSM* (4th ed.). Upper Saddle River, NJ: Prentice Hall.

Frioux, T. D., Roberts, A. G., & Butler, S. J. (1995). In B. Neuman (Ed.), *The NSM* (3rd ed.). Norwalk, CT: Appleton-Century-Croft.

Fulton, R. A. B. (1995). The spiritual variable: Essential to the client system. In B. Neuman (Ed.), *The NSM* (3rd ed., pp. 77–91). Norwalk, CT: Appleton & Lange.

Gibson, D. E. (1989). A Q-analysis of interpersonal trust in the nurse-client relationship. *Dissertation Abstracts International, 50,* 493B.

Gigliotti, E., & Fawcett, J. (2001) The Neuman Systems Model and research instruments. In B. Neuman & J. Fawcett (Eds.), *The NSM* (4th ed.). Upper Saddle River, NJ: Prentice Hall.

Goldblum-Graff, D., & Graff, H. (1982). The Neuman model adapted to family therapy. In B. Neuman (Ed.), *The NSM: Application to nursing education and practice,* Norwalk, CT: Appleton-Century-Crofts.

Gray, W., Rizzo, N. D., & Duhl, F. D. (Eds.). (1969). *General systems theory and psychiatry.* Boston: Little Brown.

Haggart, M. (1993). A critical analysis of Neuman's Systems Model in relation to public health nursing. *Journal of Advanced Nursing, 18,* 1917–1922.

Hardy, M. (1974). Theories: Components, development, evaluation. *Nursing Research, 23*(2), 100–107.

Harper, B. (1993). Nurses' beliefs about social support and the effect of nursing care on cardiac clients' attitudes in reducing cardiac risk status. *Master's Abstracts International, 31,* 273.

Helland, W. Y. (1995) Nursing diagnosis: Diagnostic process. In P. J. Christensen & J. W. Kenney (Eds.), *Nursing process: Application of conceptual models* (4th ed., pp. 120–138). St. Louis: Mosby-Year Book

Hill, R. (1966). Contemporary developments in family theory. *Journal of Marriage and Family, 28,* 3–6.

Hoffman, M. K. (1982). From model to theory construction: An analysis of the Neuman health care systems model. In B. Neuman (Ed.), *The NSM.* Norwalk, CT: Appleton-Century-Crofts.

Hoskins, L. M., Fitzpatrick, J. J., Warren, J. J., Carpenito, L. J., Jakob, D., & Mills, W. C. (1992). Axes for NANDA Taxonomy II. In R. M. Carroll-Johnson (Ed.), *Proceedings of the Tenth NANDA Conference.* Philadelphia: J. B. Lippincott.

Klir, G. J. (1972). Preview: The polyphonic general systems theory. In G. J. Klir (Ed.), *Trends in general systems theory.* New York: Wiley.

Lancaster, D., R.N. (1992). Coping with appraised threat of breast cancer. Primary prevention coping behaviors utilized by women at increased risk. *Dissertation Abstracts International, 53*(1), 202B.

Lazarus, R. S. (1966). *Psychological stress and coping response.* New York: McGraw-Hill.

Lazarus, R. S., & Folkman, S. (1984). *Stress, appraisal, and coping.* New York: Springer.

Lazlo, E. (1972). *The systems view of the world: The natural philosophy of the new development in the sciences.* New York: Braziller.

Louis, M., & Koertvelyessy, A. (1989). The Neuman model in nursing research. In B. Neuman (Ed.), *The NSM* (2nd ed., pp. 93–113). Norwalk, CT: Appleton & Lange.

Lowry, L. W. (2001). The Neuman Systems Model and education: An integrative review. In B. Neuman and J. Fawcett (Eds.), *The NSM* (4th ed.). Upper Saddle River, NJ: Prentice Hall.

Lowry, L. W., & Anderson, B. (1993). Neuman's framework and ventilator dependency: A pilot study. *Nursing Science Quarterly, 6,* 195–200.

Lowry, L. W., Walker, P. H., & Mirenda, R. (1995). In B. Neuman (Ed.), *The NSM* (3rd ed., pp. 63–75). Norwalk, CT: Appleton & Lange.

Meleis, A. I. (1995). Theory testing and theory support: Principles, challenges and a sojourn into the future. In B. Neuman (Ed.), *The NSM* (3rd ed., pp. 447–458). Norwalk, CT: Appleton & Lange.

Miller, J. (1965). Living systems: structure and process. *Behavioral Science, 10,* 337–379.

Mynatt, S. L., & O'Brien, J. (1993). Partnership to prevent chemical dependency in nursing: Using Neuman's systems model. *Journal of Psychosocial Nursing, 31*(4), 27–34.

Neuman, B. (1972). The Betty Neuman model: A total person approach to viewing patient problems. *Nursing Research, 21,* 264–269.

Neuman, B. (Ed.). (1982). *The NSM: Application to nursing education and practice.* New York: Appleton-Century-Crofts.

Neuman, B. (1983). Family intervention using the Betty Neuman health-care systems model. In I. Clements & F. Roger (Eds.), *Family health: A theoretical approach to nursing care* (pp. 161–176). New York: John Wiley.

Neuman, B. (Ed.) (1989). *The NSM* (2nd ed.). Norwalk, CT: Appleton & Lange.

Neuman, B. (1990). Health as a continuum based on the NSM. *Nursing Science Quarterly, 3,* 129–135.

Neuman, B. (1995). The NSM. In B. Neuman (Ed.), *The NSM* (3rd ed., pp. 3–62). Norwalk, CT: Appleton & Lange.

Neuman, B. (2001). The Neuman Systems Model. In B. Neuman & J. Fawcett (Eds.), *The Neuman Systems Model* (4th ed.). Upper Saddle River, NJ: Prentice Hall.

Neuman, B., & Fawcett, J. (Eds.). (2001). *The Neuman Systems Model* (4th ed.). Upper Saddle River, NJ: Prentice Hall.

Newman, D. M., Neuman, B., & Fawcett, J. (2001). Guidelines for Neuman Systems Model-based education for the health professions. In B. Neuman & J. Fawcett (Eds.), *The NSM* (4th ed.). Upper Saddle River, NJ: Prentice Hall.

Pearls, F. (1973). *The Gestalt approach: Eyewitness to therapy.* Palo Alto, CA: Science and Behavior Books.

Peoples, L. T. (1991). The relationship between selected client, provider, and agency variables and the utilization of home care services. *Dissertation Abstracts International 51,* 3782B.

Piazza, D., Foote, A., Wright, P., & Holcombe, J. (1992). NSM used as a guide for the nursing care of an eight-year-old child with leukemia. *Journal of Pediatric Oncology Nursing, 9*(1), 17–24.

Pierce, A. G., & Fulmer, T. (1995). Application of the Neuman Systems Model to gerontological nursing. In B. Neuman (Ed.), *The NSM* (3rd ed., pp. 293–308). Norwalk, CT: Appleton & Lange.

Pothiban, L. (2001). Using the Neuman Systems Model to guide nursing research in Thailand. In B. Neuman & J. Fawcett (Eds.), *The NSM* (4th ed.). Upper Saddle River, NJ: Prentice Hall.

Puetz, R. (1990). Nurse and patient perception of stressors associated with coronary artery bypass surgery. Unpublished thesis, University of Nevada, Las Vegas.

Putt, A. (1972). Entropy, evolution and equifinality in nursing. In J. Smith (Ed.), *Five years of cooperation to improve curricula in western schools of nursing.* Boulder, CO: Western Interstate Commission for Higher Education.

Reed, K. (1982). The NSM: A basis for family psychosocial assessment and intervention. In B. Neuman (Ed.), *The NSM* (pp. 188–193). Norwalk, CT: Appleton-Century-Crofts.

Reed, K. S. (1989). Family theory related to the NSM. In B. Neuman (Ed.), *The NSM* (2nd ed., pp. 385–395). Norwalk, CT: Appleton & Lange.

Reed, K. S. (1993a). *Betty Neuman: The NSM.* (Notes on nursing theories Monograph No. 11.) Newbury Park, CA: Sage.

Reed, K. S. (1993b). Adapting the NSM for family nursing. *Nursing Science Quarterly, 6*(2), 93–97.

Rodriguez, M. L. (1995). The Neuman Systems Model adapted to a continuing care retirement community. In B. Neuman (Ed.), *The NSM* (3rd ed., pp. 431–442). Norwalk, CT: Appleton & Lange.

Seyle, H. (1950). *The physiology and pathology of exposure to stress.* Montreal: ACTA.

Spradley, B. W. (1990). *Community health nursing: Concepts and practice* (3rd ed., pp. 72–74). Glenview, IL: Scott, Foresman/Little Brown Higher Education.

Stevens, B. J. (1979). *Nursing theory: Analysis, application, and evaluation.* Boston: Little Brown.

Tomlinson, P. S., & Anderson, K. H. (1995). Family health and the Neuman Systems Model. In B. Neuman (Ed.), The *NSM* (3rd ed., pp. 231–246). Norwalk, CT: Appleton & Lange.

Toot, J. L., & Schmoll, B. J. (1995). The Neuman Systems Model and physical therapy education curricula. In B. Neuman (Ed.), *The NSM* (3rd ed., pp. 231–246). Norwalk, CT: Appleton & Lange.

Torakis, M. L. (2001). Using the Neuman Systems Model to guide administration of nursing services in the United States: Redirecting nursing practice in a freestanding pediatric hospital. In B. Neuman & J. Fawcett (Eds.), *The NSM* (4th ed.). Upper Saddle River, NJ: Prentice Hall.

von Bertalanffy, L. (1968). *General systems theory.* New York: George Braziller.

Walker, P. H., & Redman, R. (1999). Theory-guided, evidence-based reflective practice. *Nursing Science Quarterly, 12,* 298–303.

Ziegler, S. M. (1982). Taxonomy for nursing diagnosis derived from the NSM. In B. Neuman (Ed.), *The NSM.* Norwalk, CT: Appleton-Century-Crofts.

Ziemer, M. (1983). Effects of information on postsurgical coping. *Nursing Research, 32,* 282–287.

11

King's Conceptual System and Theory of Goal Attainment

Maureen A. Frey

Imogene King has a long history of support for and contributions to advancing nursing science. This includes advocacy for a distinct perspective of nursing as a science and specification of the structure and process for developing that body of knowledge. King received a diploma in nursing from St. Johns Hospital in St. Louis, Missouri (1945), a bachelor's of science in nursing education (1948) and master's of nursing in nursing (1957) from St. Louis University, and a doctorate of education (EdD) from Teacher's College (1961), Columbia University, New York. She has served as professor of nursing at Loyola University, Ohio State University, and the University of South Florida. In addition, she was the Director of the Department of Nursing at Ohio State University. Although formally retired as Professor Emerita in 1990, she continues to be active in the nursing theory movement, encouraging the testing of theory in research and practice mentoring second generation theorists, and providing professional leadership.

Initially, King's interest in theory was to develop a conceptual framework for a nursing curriculum. Writings in the mid-1960s (King, 1964) expressed ideas about the need for focus, organization, and use of nursing's knowledge base. In 1968, King wrote of a conceptual frame of reference for nursing based on the concepts of perception, communication, interpersonal relationships, health, and social institutions. A conceptual framework for nursing, the interrelationship between personal, interpersonal, and social systems was developed and included the concepts of perception, information, energy, interpersonal relationships, communication, social organization, role, and status was published in *Toward a Theory for Nursing* (1971). The goal in developing the framework was to address the essence of nursing and move toward a general system theory for nursing (King, 1971, 1975).

Refinements and changes were made during the 1970s, a very productive period for nursing theory in general. *A Theory for Nursing: Systems, Concepts, Process* was published in 1981. In that text, King reformulated the metaparadigm concepts of person and environment, refined the open systems orientation, and expanded concepts for understanding systems and their interactions, resulting in a more formalized conceptual framework. Concepts relating primarily to the personal system were perception, self, growth and development, body image, time, and space. Concepts relating primarily to the interpersonal system were human interaction, communication, transaction, role, and stress. Concepts related primarily to social systems were organization, authority, power, status, and decision making.

In the 1981 text, King presented the theory of goal attainment derived from the personal and interpersonal systems. The theory of goal attainment addressed how nurses interact with clients to achieve health goals. The 1981 text has served as the primary source for learning about, studying, and critiquing King's work for more than two decades.

Although there have been no major changes to the framework or theory of goal attainment since the 1981 text, King has provided explanation, clarification, and expansion of concepts through numerous publications and presentations. Changes include addition of the concepts of learning and coping, addition of the word *spiritual* to the assumptions about human beings, and use of the term *conceptual system* rather than conceptual framework, model, or paradigm (King, 2001). King has addressed questions and concerns raised by others (Gonot, 1986; Fawcett, 1989; Magan, 1987; Meleis, 1991), explicated the philosophical and ethical basis of the conceptual system and theory of goal attainment, and affirmed a strong belief in the enduring nature of her perspective over time and for the 21st century (King, 1995, 2001). King has specifically addressed such contemporary themes as expanding technology, changes in organization and delivery of health care, nursing informatics, and nursing languages.

In 1995, Frey and Sieloff published *Advancing King's Systems Framework and Theory for Nursing,* the first comprehensive volume on advancing and extending King's work. The process of publishing that text also served to identify and pull together a cadre of nurses working within King's conceptual system. In 1997, the King International Nursing Group (KING) was founded. The organization has sponsored several theory conferences and offers mentoring and networking opportunities in order to further knowledge development. This fourth edition provides an excellent opportunity to indicate the use of King's conceptual system, the use of the transaction process model in her theory of goal attainment, and highlight recent contributions to nursing science. For depth and understanding, readers are encouraged to read King's original books and articles.

BASIC PARADIGM CONCEPTS INCLUDED IN THE CONCEPTUAL SYSTEM

Definition and Description of Person

Persons are defined as *personal systems*. Characteristics of persons are found in the philosophical assumptions of the conceptual system. When personal systems interact, interpersonal systems are formed. Accordingly, understanding personal systems is foundational to nursing (King, 1981). Personal systems, because they are a basic component of the conceptual system, will be reviewed and discussed in subsequent sections of this chapter.

Definition and Description of Environment

King's (1971, 1981, 1990a) perspective of environment is drawn from general systems theory. Systems have both internal and external environments through which there is exchange of energy, matter, and information. According to king, environments are multiple, changing, and integral to health. The importance of the cultural, social, community, and professional environment in individual and group behavior has been an early and consistent theme of King's work. The emphasis on multiple systems and environments reflects an ecological perspective although King does not generally use that term in reference to her work.

Definition and Description of Health

Health is an essential concept and clearly identified as the goal for nursing. "Health is defined as dynamic life experiences of a human being, which implies continuous adjustment to stressors in the internal and external environment through optimum use of one's resources to achieve maximum potential for daily living" (King, 1981, p. 5). King (1990b) reaffirmed that definition in 1991.

Although formally defined, King's perspective of health is better understood through her discussions of the concept. For example, health is multidimensional; it is genetic, subjective, relative, dynamic, environmental, functional, cultural, and perceptual (King, 1981, 1990b). Health has different meanings for different persons and is influenced by past experiences, standards of living, culture, perceptions, disease and illness, and transactions with the environment. King identifies that measurement of health is problematic and often expressed by morbidity and mortality data. She suggests that indicators of health should include developmental processes and the attributes essential to function in roles. Although defined for the individual, or personal system, the concept of health can be applied to interpersonal, and social systems (Evans, 1991; King, 1990b).

King's perspective of health has been viewed by others as on a continuum with illness (Fawcett, 1989). This conclusion might have been drawn from statements such as, "The polarity between health and illness is almost a thing of the past," and "Illness is a deviation from normal, that is, an imbalance in a person's biological structure or in his psychological make-up, or a conflict in a person's social relationship" (King, 1981, p. 5). More recently, King has provided clarification of the concept and deleted language that would suggest in any way that health is on a continuum, is linear, or is static (King, 1989a, 1990b).

Definition of Nursing and Nursing Activity

King views nursing as a scientific, professional discipline. Although the knowledge base draws from other disciplines, its structure, content, and use are distinct. The structure is identified as an open, interacting framework of personal, interpersonal, and social systems. Various concepts, synthesized and redefined by King (1981), are used to identify relevant knowledge for understanding systems and their interactions. Knowledge of the concepts is used (applied) to help nurses function in their roles and to meet the goal of health for individuals and groups. The focus of nursing is the care of human beings in the domain of health promotion, health maintenance and/or restoration, care of the sick or injured, and care of the dying (King, 1990b). The unit of analysis is human behavior or acts. Strategies used by nurses include *teaching, supporting, counseling, guiding,* and *motivating* (King, 1981).

Nursing and nursing process are strong and consistent elements of King's work. Nursing is formally defined as "a process of human interactions between nurse and client whereby each perceives the other and the situation; and through communication, they set goals, explore means, and agree on means to achieve goals" (King, 1981, p. 144). The process of nursing is represented in the *interaction-transaction process model,* which operationalizes one concept in the theory of goal attainment (King, 1981, 1989a). King makes explicit links between the processes of nursing and nursing process as a method whereby nurses assess, plan, implement, and evaluate nursing care (King 1989a, 1990a). Both the processes of nursing and nursing process are firmly grounded in decision making. In a 1971 publication, a diagram entitled "Methodology for the study of nursing process" specifically included the terms *analyze, synthesize, verify,* and *interpret* (Daubenmire & King, 1973). Norris and Frey (2002) used this diagram to demonstrate that *critical thinking,* a topic that has received considerable attention in nursing for only about the past decade, was a foundational element in King's conceptual approach to nursing and the transaction process.

Interrelationships Among the Metaparadigm Concept

The metaparadigm concepts of person, environment, health, and nursing are explicitly linked: "The focus of nursing is human beings interacting with their environment leading to a state of health for individuals, which is an ability to function in social roles" (King, 1981, p. 143). This statement serves as a basic underlying assumption upon which the conceptual system is based.

INTERNAL ANALYSIS AND EVALUATION

Assumptions

Worldviews are distinguished from each other by basic assumptions about human nature, ontology, and epistemology. These philosophical assumptions link directly to methodology: how research should proceed and the methods and techniques for collecting evidence (Harding, 1987).

King (1981, 1990a, 1991b, 2001) identifies the origin of her philosophical perspective as both personal and derived from general systems theory. Recall that when introduced, general systems theory was a new way of thinking about living systems that was in direct opposition to the traditional, positivistic orientations that had long dominated science. King selected systems theory because it reflected perspectivism and wholeness, rather than reductionism.

Assumptions about human beings and nurse-client interactions are explicit. Human beings are spiritual, social, sentient, rational, reacting, perceiving, controlling, purposeful, action oriented, and time oriented (King, 1981, 1990a). Assumptions about nurse-client interactions follow:

- Perceptions of nurse and of client influence the interaction process.
- Goals, needs, and values of nurse and client influence the interaction process.
- Individuals have a right to knowledge about themselves.
- Individuals have a right to participate in decisions that influence their life, their health, and community services.
- Health professionals have a responsibility to share information that helps individuals make informed decisions about their health care.

- Individuals have a right to accept or reject health care.
- Goals of health professionals and goals of recipients of health care may be incongruent (King, 1981, pp. 143–144; 1990a, p. 77).

These assumptions, which address personal and interpersonal systems, characterize persons as capable of processing information and symbols rather than simply adapting to events and situations. Assumptions about social systems are not explicit but could be extrapolated given the extent of discussion about and importance of social systems and the social world to human behavior.

An understanding of the ontological and epistemological foundation of King's conceptual system can be inferred based on Morgan and Smircich's (1980) discussion of subjectivity and objectivity within the social sciences and Whelton's (1999) examination of King's work from the perspective of classical philosophy. Morgan and Smircich viewed subjectivity and objectivity on a continuum rather than by discrete categories. Systems theory tends to be toward the objectivist extreme, which is associated with positivist science. However, King seems to view reality (ontology) somewhat more subjectively than as a concrete process, and closer to symbolic discourse and a contextual field of information. For example, the relationship between human action, interaction, and change is based on individual perception and interpretation. Additional evidence of subjectivity is the role of information processing in patterns of change and adjustment. Furthermore, changes and adjustments are capable of changing the whole in fundamental ways.

The epistemology of systems theory suggests that knowledge about the social world is based on studying relationships among elements of the structure (Morgan & Smircich, 1980). King (1990b) identifies that her conceptual system specifies structure and function for the discipline. However, knowing is not limited to empirical analysis of concrete relationships, a description that reflects positivism (Morgan & Smircich, 1980). King's epistemological stance stresses patterns and context. However, despite moderate subjectivism, King clearly states that the goal of theory is to describe, explain, and predict phenomena, which suggests a more objective perspective of science.

Whelton (1999) identified that the core of King's conceptual system and theory of goal attainment was consistent with the teachings of the classic Greek philosopher Aristotle. In doing so, Whelton cited King's use of systems theory, emphasis on human nature, and assumptions about human beings. The influence of Aristotle's 2,300-year-old reflection of human life is not surprising given the links between Aristotle, Thomas Aquinas, and King's Jesuit education.

In summary, this author places King's perspective of ontology, human nature, and epistemology in the "middle of the road" in relation to the subjective-objective continuum and, based on the work of Whelton, effectively bridges classic philosophy and nursing. Because classical philosophy preceded the quantitative emphasis of the scientific revolution, both qualitative and quantitative methodologies would be consistent with King's underlying world view. King's view that theory may be derived from conceptual frameworks, that hypotheses from theories are tested for research, and that research may identify theories and so on (King, 1991a) tends to lend more to quantitative methods, although it should be noted that King used inductive approaches to developing concepts in her conceptual system.

Overall, philosophical-theoretical-methodological consistency is very important in developing science. King's perspective demonstrates both pre- and postpositivist science orientations in that it clearly demonstrates, stresses, and respects subjectivity, perception, self-definition, values, and the dignity of humans (Whall, 1989). These are reflected throughout the framework, but are particularly evident in the definition of health, perspective of human beings, complexity of multiple system variables and human behavior, mutuality in nurse-client interactions, the role of personal and professional values, and the process orientation of communication and nursing.

Concepts and Components of the Framework

Concepts are critical to knowledge development in that they describe structure and provide building blocks of conceptual frameworks and theories (King, 1988, 1991b). King's process of concept development is one of synthesis and reformulation using inductive and deductive processes, critical thinking, empirical observations, as well as extensive reviews of the nursing and other literature. *Personal systems,* or individuals, are best understood by the concepts of perception, self, growth and development, body image, learning, time, personal space, and coping (King, 1981). When two or more personal systems interact, *interpersonal systems* are formed. An interpersonal system could be a dyad, triad, or small group. Concepts important to understanding interpersonal systems are *interaction, communication, role stress/stressors,* and *transaction. Social systems* are larger groups that serve to meet the needs, wants, and goals of individuals and groups and reflect political, social, cultural, and economic influences. Concepts useful for understanding social systems are *organization, authority, power, status,* and *decision making.* Although grouped by system, King (1988) identifies that concepts have meaning and can be used across systems. Systems and concepts are shown in Table 11–1.

BOX 11-1 CONCEPTUAL DEFINITIONS

Perception: "Process of organizing, interpreting, and transforming information from sense data and memory" (King, 1981, p. 24).

Self: "The self is a composite of thoughts and feelings which constitute a person's awareness of his/her individual existence, his/her conception of who and what he/she is. A person's self is the sum total of all he/she can call his/hers. The self included, among other things, a system of ideas, attitudes, values and commitments. The self is a person's total subjective environment. It is a distinctive center of experience and significance. The self constitutes a person's inner world as distinguished from the outer world consisting of all other people and things. The self is the individual as known to the individual. It is that to which we refer when we say 'I'" (Jersild, 1953, in King, pp. 9–10).

Growth and development: "The processes that take place in an individual's life that help the individual move from potential capacity for achievement to self actualization" (King, 1981, p. 31).

Body image: "An individual's perceptions of his/her own body, others' reactions to his/her appearance which results from others' reactions to self" (King, 1981, p. 33).

Learning: "A process of sensory perception, conceptualization, and critical thinking involving multiple experiences in which changes in concepts, skills, symbols, habit and values can be evaluated in observable behaviors and inferred from behavioral manifestations" (King, 1986, p. 24).

Time: "Duration between the occurrence of one event and occurrence of another event" (King, 1981, p. 44).

Personal space: "Existing in all directions and is the same everywhere" (King, 1981, p. 37).

Coping: "The constantly changing cognitive and behavioral efforts to manage specific external and internal demands that are appraised as taxing or exceeding the resources" (Lazarus & Folkman, 1984, p. 141). (Note: King added concept but did not define. Use of Lazarus & Folkman's definition is suggested by Molewyk Doornbos, 1993).

Interaction: "Acts of two or more persons in mutual presence" (King, 1981, p. 85).

Communication: "Information processing, a change of information from one state to another" (King, 1981, p. 69).

Role: "Set of behaviors expected when occupying a position in a social system" (King, 1981, p. 93).

Stress: "Dynamic state whereby a human being interacts with the environment to maintain balance for growth, development, and performance which involves an exchange of energy and information between the person and the environment for regulation and control of stressors" (King, 1981, p. 98).

Transaction: "A process of interaction in which human beings communicate with environment to achieve goals that are valued" (King, 1981, p. 82).

Organization: "A system whose continuous activities are conducted to achieve goals" (King, 1981, p. 119).

BOX 11–1 *Continued*

Authority: "Transactional process characterized by active, reciprocal relations in which members' values, backgrounds and perceptions play a role in defining, validation, and accepting the [directions] of individuals within an organization" (King, 1981, p. 124).

Power: "Capacity to use resources in organizations to achieve goal"; "process whereby one or more persons influence other persons in a situation"; capacity or ability of a group to achieve goals" (King, 1981, p. 124).

Status: "The position of an individual in a group or a group in relation to other groups in an organization" (King, 1981, p. 129).

Decision making: "Dynamic and systematic process by which a goal-directed choice of perceived alternatives is made, and acted upon, by individuals or groups to answer a question and attain a goal' (King, 1981, p. 132).

TABLE 11–1   Concepts by System

Personal	Interpersonal	Social
Perception	Interaction	Organization
Self	Communication	Authority
Growth and development	Role	Power
Body image	Stress/stressors	Status
Learning	Transactions	Decision making
Time		
Personal space		
Coping		

Concepts are related both within and between systems. King provides many examples. The following statements illustrate a few such examples: perception is a basis for developing a concept of self-reflected in patterns of growth and development; knowledge of self and growth and development helps one understand body image; body image is an integral component of growth and development that in turn influences a concept of self. Spatial-temporal dimensions of the environment are presented as influencing perceptions, self, body image, and growth and development (King, 1981, pp. 24–47). Quoting King, ". . . If this sounds circular, it is because they are facets of human experience" (p. 142). King identifies that perception, interaction and organization are comprehensive concepts for personal, interpersonal, and social systems, respectively (King, 1989a).

Relationships between systems are inherent in systems theory. Personal systems form, and therefore are part of interpersonal systems. Social systems interact and influence both personal and interpersonal systems.

BOX 11-2 THEORETICAL DEFINITIONS

Perception: "Each person's representation of reality; awareness of persons, objects, and events" (King, 1981, p. 146).

Communications: "Process whereby information is given from one person to another either directly in face-to-face meeting or indirectly through telephone, television, or the written word" (King, 1981, p. 146).

Interaction: "Process of perception and communication between person and environment and between person and person, represented by verbal and nonverbal behaviors that are goal-directed" (King, 1981, p. 145).

Transaction: "Observable behaviors of human beings interacting with their environment" (King, 1981, p. 147).

Growth and development: "Continuous changes in individuals at the cellular, molecular, and behavioral levels of activities" (King, 1981, p. 148).

Time: "Sequence of events moving onward to the future" (King, 1981, p. 148).

Personal space: "The immediate environment in which nurse and client interact and move to goal attainment" (King, 1981, p. 129). King does not specify theoretical [less abstract] definitions for self, role, coping, or stress/stressors.

These influences include behavior, attitudes, beliefs, values, and customs (King, 1981). For example, the concept of role is aligned with the interpersonal system because interpersonal systems are two or more persons and role is defined in relation to a counterpart. Yet role is also related to personal systems because an individual's behavior is influenced by the concepts of self and perception. Role also has relevance within social systems when considering the role expectations inherent in assuming a position in a formal organization. The concept of health offers another example because health can be defined for individuals, families, and communities. However, it is very likely that indicators and measures of concepts would be different for each system. This is especially true when considering personal systems in contrast with interpersonal and social systems, given that characteristics of individuals are different than characteristics of groups.

The Theory of Goal Attainment

King's *theory* of *goal attainment* (1981, 1991a) is derived from concepts in the personal and interpersonal systems. The focus of the theory is nurse–client interactions that lead to transactions and goal attainment. The theory is based on philosophical assumptions about human beings and interactions. Concepts in the theory of goal attainment are perception, interaction, communications, transaction, growth and development, self, role, coping, stress/stressors, time, and personal space (King, 1981, 1991a).

Model of Transaction and Classification System

In addition to the conceptual system and theory of goal attainment, King (1981) also presented a model of transaction. The distinction among these three elements (conceptual system, theory of goal attainment, and model of transaction) is not always recognized by persons when referring to King's work (King, 1989a). The model of transactions was developed by King based on a descriptive study of nurse-patient interactions. The results of the study were also used to develop a classification system of observable behaviors in nurse-patient interactions that lead to transactions (King, 1981, 1990a, 1991a). Observable behaviors are action, reaction, disturbance, mutual goal settings, explore means to achieve goals, agree on means to achieve goals, and transactions. Mutual goal setting is a critical variable in the process.

Goal-Oriented Nursing Record

King's (1981) goal-oriented nursing record (GONR) was developed to record the process and outcome of nursing. The major elements of the GONR are the database, nursing diagnosis goal lists, nursing orders, flow sheets, progress notes, and discharge summary. King (1981, 1991a, 1994) has linked use of the GONR to continuity of care, systematic data retrieval, and quality assurance.

Analysis of Consistency

Examination of consistency involves consideration of definitions, logic, implications, and adequacy of concepts and relationships as well as underlying assumptions. These concerns are a prerequisite to consideration of external analysis. Taken together, they provide a basis for determining the actual and potential contribution to development of knowledge.

Several concepts have been added since the theory was first published in comprehensive form in 1981. First is the addition of the concept of learning for the personal system (King, 1986). Second is the addition of the concept of coping. Coping was first used in discussing application of the theory of goal attainment to family health (King, 1983). King stated, ". . . a theory of goal attainment is useful for nurses when called to assist families to maintain their health or to cope with problems or illness" (King, 1983, p. 182). In 1990, coping was included as a concept in the theory of goal attainment. Placement of the concept of coping by system was not made explicit by King (1990c). As noted, concepts in the theory of goal attainment are drawn from both personal and interpersonal systems. This author chose to list the concept of coping with the personal system. Despite a statement to the contrary (Hawks, 1991), the concept of control has not been formally added to the framework (King, personal communication, 1994). Several concepts have been clarified. Stress and stressors are considered together, and the concept of space refers to personal space. Over and above the clarification, refinement, and additions as noted, assumptions, concepts, and relationships have been very consistent over time.

Fawcett (1989) stated that propositions and statements of relationships among concepts of conceptual frameworks were often very broad and general. This is certainly true of King's framework. It follows, however, that definitions of concepts and relationships among them would be more specifically stated in theories derived from the conceptual system and, furthermore, that operational definitions would be stated for variables tested in research. Conceptual definitions are given for all concepts. Some concepts, but not all, have been defined at the theoretical level. Although different, theoretical definitions remain fairly abstract. King (1981) has offered an operational definition of transaction.

Analysis of Adequacy

The final area to consider is analysis of adequacy. According to Ellis (1968) adequacy depends on scope, complexity, and usefulness. The conceptual framework has both depth and complexity for understanding the nature of the systems and their interactions. Usefulness refers to clinical practice. Two questions need to be asked: Is the framework applicable to all nursing situations? and Has adequate knowledge been derived to provide direction for practice?

King fully intended the conceptual system to be suitable for all nursing situations. However, broad applicability of King's conceptual system has been challenged in critiques by Meleis (1991), Austin and Champion (1983), and Jonas (1987). One limitation is use with clients who are not able (i.e., unconscious adults or newborns) to fully participate in care. Carter and Dufour (1994) specifically addressed this limitation drawing from neuroscience. They recommend interaction with the interpersonal and social systems of patients with neurological impairments, and delegated authority that allows nurses to "make decisions that guide the actions of self and others" (King, 1981, p. 122) when all other avenues are closed.

Another limitation that has been cited is cultural utility. That is, use of the framework and/or theory in situations in which participation in decision making, importance of the self, and attitudes toward the sick role might be different from those found in Western culture. Others, however, including Spratlen (1976), Rooda (1992), Frey, Rooke, Sieloff, Messmer, and Kameoka (1995), Richard-Hughes (1997), Porteous and Tyndall (1994), and Carter and Dufour (1994), offer excellent examples of use of the concepts with diverse cultures. King (1993, 1994) has always maintained that her conceptual system and theory of goal attainment were acultural.

Additional evidence of adequacy is that the conceptual framework and theory of goal attainment can be used with different units of analysis. Examples include the family (Frey, 1993; Doornbos, 1993; Rawlins, Rawlins, & Horner, 1990; Symanski, 1991), other groups (Brooks & Thomas, 1997; Murray & Baier, 1996), community (Hanchett, 1990), and nursing departments (Jolly & Winkler, 1995; King, 1986; Sieloff, 1996).

EXTERNAL ANALYSIS

Relationship to Research and Practice

According to King (1988), knowledge of concepts and relationships in the conceptual system guides research, education, and practice. Prior to 1988, application and extension of the conceptual system was limited. Silva (1986) did not include King's framework in her review of research testing nursing theory because it did not meet the inclusion criteria of six published studies (Silva, 1987).

There has been a considerable increase in publications on theory development, testing, and practice based on King's conceptual system and theory of goal attainment in the last decade. In addition to reviewing publications based on the conceptual system and theory of goal attainment, Sieloff, Frey, and Killeen (2001) reviewed and classified publications based on concept development; instrument development; clients across the life span; personal, interpersonal, and social systems; client concerns; nursing specialties; nursing work settings; nursing process and related languages; and applications to health care beyond nursing. Overall, King's conceptual system and theory of goal attainment have wide appeal and utility. Both have been used with more than 40 client concerns, including autonomy, health promotion, illness management, risky behaviors, and smoking, to name a few.

Several hospitals have implemented practice based on King's conceptual framework and theory of goal attainment in patient care departments or units. These include the Centenary Hospital in Scarborough, Ontario, Canada (Coker & Schreiber, 1990); Tampa General Hospital, Tampa, FL (Messmer, 1995); and Hamilton Civic Hospitals, Hamilton, Ontario, Canada (Fawcett, Vaillancourt, & Watson, 1995). A summary of the scope, number, and publication dates from the review by Sieloff et al. (2001) are listed in Table 11–2. Despite evidence of increased use in research and practice, there is not a large body of empirical evidence in support of King's

TABLE 11–2 Summary of King-Related Publications

Areas of applicability	Number of publications	Years of publications
Application of King's conceptual system	37	1978–1995
Application of theory of goal attainment	44	1983–1997
Client concerns (40 concerns identified)	65	1982–1996
Client populations		
Infants	3	1991–1997
Children	7	1981–1998
Adolescents	6	1983–1995
Adults	33	1978–1996
Adults, mature	13	1982–1995
Adults, young	1	1995
Health care beyond nursing	5	1994–1996
Client systems		
Personal	18	1982–1997
Interpersonal	31	1978–1997
Social system	30	1973–1996
Concept development	12	1983–1995
Instrument development	4	1988–1998
Middle-range theory developed	6	1993–1998
Multicultural applications	6	1976–1997
Nursing process and related languages	7	1984–1997
Nursing specialties (25 specialties)	67	1973–1998
Work settings (10 settings)	46	1978–1998

conceptual system or derived theories. Unfortunately, many of the practice applications are "conceptualized within" the conceptual system and/or theories, but the propositions that guide nursing care and evaluation are lacking. Evaluation data from hospitals and other agencies that base practice on the conceptual system is lacking as well. In terms of research, the conceptual system and/or theory is often used to "guide" the project, but linkages between concepts, variables, measures, and hypotheses are not explicit. In addition, validity studies with the theory of goal attainment, which could be used in so many practice areas, are very limited. Clearly, these areas represent the focus for future work. Developing a knowledge base for nursing using King's theory of goal attainment and theories derived from her conceptual system is the primary focus of the KING.

Education

King's early work in theory was closely tied to curriculum development. King expanded on these ideas in *Curriculum and Instruction in Nursing: Concepts and Process,* published in 1986. The text demonstrates the use of the conceptual system to organize courses, identify objectives, plan instruction, and conduct evaluation. Additional examples of utility of the conceptual system for curriculum are provided by Gulitz and King (1988). The Ohio State University has based its baccalaureate curriculum on King's framework. Daubenmire (1989) published many of those materials. The framework has also been applied to continuing nursing education (Brown & Lee, 1980).

Nursing Classification Systems

Classification systems in nursing are directed toward identification of a common language for practice, minimum data set use, computerized patient records, determination of the cost of nursing care, and for education and research (Gordon, 1998). Classification systems include nursing diagnoses, interventions, and outcomes. The American Nurses Association (ANA) has recognized numerous classifications systems. However, there is a great deal of variability among the classification systems in terms of method of development, extent of development, scope of nursing practice, use in nursing practice, and testing in nursing practice. Because none of the classification systems were derived or developed from a nursing framework or theory, relationships between classification systems and existing nursing frameworks and theories is a matter of "fit." For the purpose of this chapter, fit will be considered in terms of assumptions and orientation of King; the structure and function of the conceptual system, theory of goal attainment, and other derived theories; and the essential features and ease of use.

Overall, King has been a long-time advocate for a common nursing language to identify nursing's essential data (King, 1998). The conceptual basis of classification systems closely parallels King's emphasis on the importance of concepts and the role concepts play in organizing, applying, and communicating knowledge (King, 1988). The structure and purpose of the theory of goal attainment focused on nursing interventions and outcomes prior to the efforts to develop intervention and outcome classification systems in the 1980s and 1990s. Early on, King (1981) stated: "This theory [of goal attainment], derived from the conceptual framework, includes organized elements of the process of nurse-client interactions that result in outcomes, that is goals attained" (p. 143). Furthermore, "Goal attainment results in outcomes that are measurable events in nursing situations" (p. 145).

The "oldest" component of classifications systems is nursing diagnosis. When asked if nursing diagnosis fit with her conceptual framework, King replied, "It certainly does" (Smith, 1988, p. 83). A major reason given by King for supporting nursing diagnosis was the need for development of a professional language. The GONR system calls for diagnoses rather than problem statements. King stated, however, that "What nursing [diagnosis] means to me probably is not the same as what it means to the people in the [taxonomy] movement. It means clinical judgment on the basis of the assessment data gathered" (Smith, 1988, p. 83). As identified previously and discussed in Norris and Frey (2002), King's perspective of diagnosis as interpretation and decision making predated the nursing diagnosis movement that gained momentum in the 1970s. However, it would be consistent with King's perspective to reject the many inductive approaches to nursing diagnosis and, instead, advocate for a deductive approach based on the concepts, relationships, and nursing perspective identified in *her* framework and the theories derived from it. However, deriving distinct nursing diagnoses does not support a system of common diagnostic language because no nursing framework is in universal use.

Given the explosion of diagnostic labels, classification systems, and the methods of developing both, it is likely that many will be useful for practice and research from King's conceptual system. The use of King's conceptual system, theory of goal attainment, and other derived theories is further facilitated because the concepts identified by King as representing essential knowledge about systems (e.g., stress, growth and development, organizations, and role) are not unique to nursing. However, to date there are no published reports systematically examining the relationship between King's conceptual system and the ANA-approved classification systems.

Byrne-Coker et al. (1990), reported North American Nursing Diagnosis Association's (NANDA's) lists of taxonomy as useful when working with King's framework. Using definitions and defining characteristics, these investigators were able to categorize 94% of the NANDA diagnoses with concepts from personal, interpersonal, and social systems. However, several modifications were necessary. For example, the concept of growth and development was divided to accommodate various body systems. In addition, several diagnoses were categorized under more than one concept. Diagnoses were considered categorized if they were linked to the same concept by 70% of the participating nurses after two rounds. A study conducted with practicing nurses indicated that use of the categorization tool, along with inservice education, facilitated the diagnostic process.

Of the existing classification systems on nursing interventions, Killeen (2001) identified considerable congruency between King's conceptual system and the Nursing Intervention Classification System (NIC) developed by Johnson and Maas (1997). From King's perspective of nursing process and transaction process, nurses and clients identify and make decisions about goals, which are mutually set, and make decisions about actions to meet goals (Norris & Frey 2002). Mutual goal setting is a critical variable in the transaction process that leads to goal attainment (King, 1981). Implementation of actions to meet goals is transactions made, which are inferred from interactions. The NIC includes mutual goal setting and collaboration with patients to identify, prioritize, and plans to achieve goals as an established nursing intervention.

Again, the theory of goal attainment clearly reflects King's historical emphasis on identification and measurement of nursing outcomes. According to King (1981), outcomes are goals achieved and can be used to evaluate the effectiveness of care. Overall, nursing outcome classifications have been less controversial than diagnostic classifications (Gordon, 1998). The domains of outcomes identified by the Nursing Outcomes Classification (NOC) (Johnson & Maas, 1997), functional, physiological, and psychosocial health, knowledge, behavior, perceived health, and family health, are all very consistent with King's conceptual system and theory of goal attainment given the emphasis she places on health and perceptions. Goal attainment nursing would certainly strengthen the missing but critical link between diagnosis, interventions as mutually set goals or expected outcomes, and actual outcomes or goals attained (Killeen, 2001; Sieloff et al., 2001).

Relationship to Theory-Driven, Evidence-Based Practice

The need to establish an empirical basis for practice is well recognized within the discipline of nursing. Evidenced-based practice is defined as "the conscientious and judicious use of current best evidence to guide health care decisions" (Titler, 1998, p. 1). Clearly, evidence in support of practice from a particular nursing frame of reference will only result from testing, applying, and retesting propositions from that frame of reference. Frey's program of research (1989, 1993, Frey et al., 1995) with children and adolescents is well on the way to this goal. After several empirical tests and revisions, her multisystem theory of health and illness serves as the basis for a multidisciplinary randomized intervention trial with adolescents with diabetes in very poor metabolic control. The work of Killeen (1996) with client-consumers and Sieloffs (1996) with nurse caregivers and nurse administrators is ready for application and subsequent retesting.

Recently, Fawcett, Watson, Neuman, Walker, and Fitzpatrick (2001) challenged nurses to move beyond the gold standard of randomized trials as evidence for theory-guided, evidence-based nursing practice. The authors drew from Carper's (1978) classic work on patterns of knowing, Stein, Corte, Colling, and Whall's (1998) analysis of Carper's patterns of knowing, and Chinn and Kramer's (1999) discussion of integrated knowledge. According to Chinn and Kramer, empiric, ethical, personal, and aesthetic patterns of knowing should not be used in isolation from each other. Fawcett et al. (2001) contend that each pattern of knowing represents a type of theory, mode of inquiry, and source of data for evidence-based nursing practice.

Although these ideas are too new to determine how these theories might be developed, there is considerable evidence that ethical, personal, and aesthetic ways of knowing are embedded in King's conceptual system and will contribute to knowledge development over time, as will the empirical way of knowing. For example, King (1999) has described and identified the relationship of ethical principles to nursing with particular emphasis on the conceptual system and theory of goal attainment. Evidence of ethical principles is explicit in the assumptions of persons, nurse–client interactions, and decision making. Norris and Frey (2002) demonstrated how ethical decision making is related to the transaction process, critical thinking process, and King's view of the nursing process.

Personal knowing is described as the quality and authenticity of the interpersonal process between nurse and patient (Fawcett et al., 2001). The interpersonal process between nurse and patient is the theory of goal attainment. Modes of inquiry resulting in knowledge of nurse--client interpersonal processes could be implemented. Likewise, aesthetic knowledge could be discovered through examination of perception in interpersonal interactions. Essential components of the transaction process involve perception, judgment, action, and reaction of the nurse and patient. Congruent perception between the nurse and patient is the first step toward mutual goal setting (King, 1981). Overall, ethical, personal, and aesthetic ways of knowing will contribute to knowledge generated from use of the theory of goal attainment. If they do not, it would raise questions about whether or not goal attainment was really occurring.

SUMMARY

King's conceptual system demonstrates a high degree of internal analysis and evaluation, external analysis, staying power over time, and utility for keeping pace with nursing in the 21st century. King has responded to questions and issues raised by others, which has provided clarification, refinement, and several additions to her concepts. There has been increased use of the conceptual system and theory of goal attainment by others, although identification of core knowledge for practice is in its infancy. However, there is a core of theorists, researchers, practitioners, and an international organization dedicated to that end.

REFERENCES

Austin, J. K., & Champion, V. L. (1983). King's theory for nursing: Explication and evaluation. In P. L. Chinn (Ed.), *Advances in nursing theory development* (pp. 49–61). Rockville, MD: Aspen Systems Corporation.

Brooks, E. M., & Thomas, S. (1997). The perception and judgement of senior baccalaureate student nurses in clinical decision making. *Advances in Nursing Science, 19*(3), 50–69.

Brown, S. T., & Lee, B. T. (1980). Imogene King's conceptual framework: A proposed model for continuing nursing education. *Journal of Advanced Nursing, 5*(5), 467–473.

Byrne-Coker, E., Fradley, T., Harris, J., Tomarchio, D., Chan, V., & Caron, C. (1990). Implementing nursing diagnoses within the context of King's conceptual framework. *Nursing Diagnosis, 1*(3), 107–114.

Carper, B. A. (1978). Fundamental patterns of knowing in nursing. *Advances in Nursing Science, 1*(1), 13–23.

Carter, K. F., & Dufour, L. T. (1994). King's theory: A critique of the critiques. *Nursing Science Quarterly, 7*(3), 128–133.

Chinn, P. L., & Kramer, M. K. (1999). *Theory and nursing: Integrated knowledge development* (5th ed.), St. Louis, MO: Mosby.

Coker, E. B., & Schreiber, R. (1990). Implementing King's conceptual framework at the bedside. In M. E. Parker (Ed.), *Nursing theories in practice* (pp. 85–102). New York: National League for Nursing.

Daubenmire, M. J. (1989). A baccalaureate nursing curriculum based on King's conceptual framework. In J. Riehl-Sisca (Ed.), *Conceptual models for nursing practice* (pp. 167–178). Norwalk, CT: Appleton & Lange.

Daubenmire, M. J., & King, I. M. (1973). Nursing process: A systems approach. *Nursing Outlook, 21,* 512–517.

Doornbos, M. M. (1993). *Family health in the families of the young chronically mentally ill.* Unpublished doctoral dissertation. Wayne State University, Detroit.

Ellis, R. (1968). Characteristics of significant theories. *Nursing Research, 17,* 217–222.

Evans, C. L. (1991). *Imogene King: A conceptual framework for nursing.* Thousand Oaks, CA: Sage Publications.

Fawcett, J. (1989). *Analysis and evaluation of conceptual models of nursing.* Philadelphia: F.A. Davis.

Fawcett, J., Watson, J., Neuman, B., Walker, P. H., & Fitzpatrick, J. J. (2001). On nursing theories and evidence. *Journal of Nursing Scholarship, 33,* 115–119.

Fawcett, J., Vaillancourt, V., & Watson, A. (1995). Integration of King's framework into nursing practice. In M. A. Frey & C. L. Sieloff (Eds.), *Advancing King's framework and theory for nursing* (pp. 176–191). Thousand Oaks, CA: Sage Publications.

Frey, M. A. (1989). Social support and health: A theoretical formulation derived from King's conceptual framework. *Nursing Science Quarterly, 2,* 138–148.

Frey, M. A. (1993). A theoretical perspective of family and child health derived from King's conceptual framework for nursing: A deductive approach to theory building. In S. L. Feetham, S. B. Meister, J. M. Bell, & C. L. Gilliss (Eds.), *The nursing of families* (pp. 30–37). Newbury Park, CA: Sage Publications.

Frey, M. A., Rooke, L., Sieloff, C., Messmer, P. R., & Kameoka, T. (1995). King's framework in Japan, Sweden, and the United States. *IMAGE: Journal of Nursing Scholarship, 277*(2), 127–130.

Frey, M. A., & Sieloff, C. (1995). *Advancing King's framework and theory for nursing.* Thousand Oaks, CA: Sage Publications.

Gonot, P. W. (1986). Family therapy as derived from King's conceptual model. In A. Whall (Ed.), *Family therapy theory for nursing: Approaches.* Norwalk, CT: Centrury-Crofts.

Gordon, M. (1998). Nursing nomenclature and classification development. *Online Journal of Issues in Nursing, 3*(2) http://www.nursingworld.org/ojin/xpc7. Retrieved Feb. 20th 2004.

Gulitz, E. A., & King, I. M. (1988). King's general systems model: Application to curriculum development. *Nursing Science Quarterly, 1*(3), 128–132.

Hanchett, E. S. (1990). *Nursing frameworks and community as client: Bridging the gap.* Norwalk, CT: Appleton & Lange.

Harding, S. (1987). Is there a feminist model? In S. Harding (Ed.), *Feminism and methodology.* Bloomington, IN: Indiana University Press.

Hawks, J. H. (1991). Power: A concept analysis. *Journal of Advanced Nursing, 16,* 754–762.

Johnson, M., & Maas, M. (1997). *Nursing Outcomes Classifications (NOC).* St. Louis, MO: Mosby.

Jolly, M. L., & Winkler, C. K. (1995). Theory of goal attainment in the context of organizational structure. In M. A. Frey & C. L. Sieloff (Eds.), *Advancing King's framework and theory for nursing* (pp. 305–316). Thousand Oaks, CA: Sage Publications.

Jonas, C. (1987). King's goal attainment theory: Use in gerontological nursing practice. *Perspectives, 11*(4), 9–12.

Killeen, M. B. (1996). *Patient-consumer perceptions and responses to professional nursing care: Instrument development.* Unpublished doctoral dissertation. Wayne State University, Detroit.

Killeen, M. B. (2001, January). *Extensions of King: Measurable outcomes and expanded nursing process.* Paper presented at King's Framework and Related Theories in the New Millennium, Tampa, FL.

King, I. M. (1964). Nursing theory—problems and prospect. *Nursing Science, 2,* 394–403.

King, I. M. (1968). A conceptual frame of reference for nursing. *Nursing Research, 17*(1), 27–31.

King, I. M. (1971). *Toward a theory for nursing.* New York: John Wiley & Sons.

King, I. M. (1975). A process for developing concepts for nursing through research. In P. J. Verhonick (Ed.), *Nursing research I* (pp. 25–43). Boston, MA: Little Brown.

King, I. M. (1981). *A theory for nursing: Systems, concept, process.* Albany, NY: Delmar.

King, I. M. (1983). King's theory of Nursing. In I. W. Clements & F. B. Roberts (Eds.), *Family health: A theoretical approach to nursing care.* New York: John Wiley & Sons.

King, I. M. (1986). *Curriculum and instruction in nursing: Concepts and process.* Norwalk, CT: Appleton-Century-Crofts.

King, I. M. (1988). Concepts: Essential elements of theories. *Nursing Science Quarterly, 1*(1), 22–25.

King, I. M. (1989a). King's general systems framework and theory. In J. P. Riehl-Sisca (Ed.), *Conceptual models for nursing practice* (pp. 149–158). Norwalk, CT: Appleton & Lange.

King, I. M. (1990a). Health as the goal for nursing. *Nursing Science Quarterly, 3*(3), 123–128.

King, I. M. (1990b). King's conceptual framework and theory of goal attainment. In M. E. Parker (Ed.), *Nursing theories in practice* (pp. 73–84). New York: National League for Nursing.

King, I. M. (1990c, July). *The theory of goal attainment: An update.* Paper presented at Wayne State University, College of Nursing 6th Annual Summer Research Conference, Detroit, MI.

King, I. M. (1991a). King's theory of goal attainment. *Nursing Science Quarterly, 5*(1), 19–26.

King, I. M. (1991b). Nursing theory 25 years later. *Nursing Science Quarterly, 4*(3), 94–95.

King, I. M. (1993, June). *King's conceptual system and theory of goal attainment.* Paper presented at the meeting of the Signa Theta Tau International Sixth International Nursing Research Congress, Madrid, Spain.

King, I. M. (1994). Quality of life and goal attainment. *Nursing Science Quarterly, 7*(1), 29–32.

King, I. M. (1995). A systems framework for nursing. In M. A. Frey & C. L. Sieloff (Eds.), *Advancing King's systems framework and theory of nursing* (pp. 14–22). Thousand Oaks, CA: Sage Publications.

King, I. M. (1998). Nursing informatics: A universal nursing language. *The Florida Nurse, 46,* 1–3, 5.

King, I. M. (1999). A theory of goal attainment: Philosophical and ethical implications. *Nursing Science Quarterly, 12,* 292–296.

King, I. M. (2001). Theory of goal attainment. In M. Parker (Ed.), *Nursing theories and nursing practice* (pp. 276–286), Philadelphia: F. A. Davis.

Lazarus, R.S., & Folkman, S. (1984). *Stress, appraisal and coping.* NY: Springer Publishing.

Magan, S. J. (1987). A critique of King's theory. In R. R. Parse (Ed.), *Nursing science major paradigms, theories, and critiques.* Philadelphia: W. B. Saunders.

Meleis, A. (1991). *Theoretical nursing: Developments and progress* (2nd ed.). Philadelphia: J. B. Lippincott.

Messmer, P. R. (1995). Implementation of theory-based nursing practice. In M. A. Frey & C. L. Sieloff (Eds.), *Advancing King's framework and theory for nursing* (pp. 294–304). Thousand Oaks, CA: Sage Publications.

Morgan, G., & Smircich, L. (1980). The case for qualitative research. *Academic Management Review, 5*(4), 491–500.

Murray, R. L. E., & Baier, M. (1996). King's conceptual framework applied to a transitional living program. *Perspectives in Psychiatric Care, 32*(1), 15–19.

Norris, D. M., & Frey, M. A. (2002). King's systems framework and theory in nursing practice. In M. R. Alligood & A. Marriner-Tomey (Eds.), *Nursing theory: Utilization and application* (2nd ed., pp. 173–196). New York: Mosby.

Porteous, A., & Tyndall, J. (1994). Yes, I want to talk to the OR. *Canadian Operating Room Nursing, 12*(2) 15–16, 18–19.

Rawlins, P. S., Rawlins, T. D., & Horner, M. (1990). Development of the family needs assessment tool. *Western Journal of Nursing Research, 12*(2), 201–214.

Richard-Hughes, S. (1997). Attitudes and beliefs of Afro-Americans related to organ and tissue donation. *International Journal of Trauma Nursing, 3*(4), 119–123.

Rooda, L. A. (1992). The development of a conceptual model for multicultural nursing. *Journal of Holistic Nursing, 10*(4), 337–347.

Sieloff, C. L. (1996). *Development of an instrument to estimate the actualized power of a nursing department.* Unpublished doctoral dissertation. Wayne State University, Detroit.

Sieloff, C. L., Frey, M. A., & Killeen, M. B. (2001). Application of King's work to practice. In M. Parker (Ed.), *Nursing theories and nursing practice* (pp. 287–313). Philadelphia: F. A. Davis.

Silva, M. C. (1986). Research testing nursing theory: State of the art. *Advances in Nursing Science, 9,* 1–11.

Silva, M. C. (1987). Conceptual models of nursing. In J. J. Fitzpatrick & R. L. Tanunton (Eds.), *Annual review of nursing research* (Vol. 5, pp. 229–246). New York: Springer.

Smith, M. J. (1988). Perspectives on nursing science. *Nursing Science Quarterly, 1*(2), 80–85.

Spratlen, L. P. (1976). Introducing ethnic-cultural factors in models of nursing: Some mental health care applications. *Journal of Nursing Education 15*(2), 23–29.

Stein, K. F., Corte, C., Colling, K. B., & Whall, A. (1998). A theoretical analysis of Carper's ways of knowing using a model of social cognition. *Scholarly Inquiry for Nursing Practice, 12,* 43–60.

Symanski, M. E. (1991). Use of nursing theories in the care of families with high-risk infants: Challenges for the future. *Journal of Perinatal Neonatal Nursing, 4*(4), 71–77.

Titler, M. G. (1998, June). *Evidence based practice and research utilization: One and the same?* Paper presented at the ANA Council for Nursing Research's 1998 Pre-Convention Research Utilization Conference, Evidence-Based Practice, San Diego, CA.

Whall, A. (1989). The influence of logical positivism on nursing practice. *IMAGE: Journal of Nursing Scholarship, 21*(4), 243–245.

Whelton, B. J. B. (1999). The philosophical core of King's conceptual system. *Nursing Science Quarterly, 12*(2), 158–163.

12

Martha Rogers' Model:
Science of Unitary Beings

Jean Croce Hemphill and Stephanie I. Muth Quillin

Martha E. Rogers, the woman responsible for modern nursing's focus on the person as a unified whole, died March 13, 1994. She was 79 years of age. Although nurses mourned, many outside of nursing also were touched by her passing. Her picture and major accomplishments were printed in the *New York Times* obituary section days after her death (Tomasson, 1994). She shares her birth date, May 12, with Florence Nightingale (Hektor, 1989). History may judge that the two had comparable influences on the development of nursing as a profession.

Martha E. Rogers began college in 1931 at the University of Tennessee, studying science for 2 years before switching to nursing. She earned a diploma from Knoxville General Hospital School of Nursing in 1936 and completed her nursing preparation with a bachelor's of science degree from George Peabody College in 1937. She earned a master's degree in public health nursing from Teacher's College, Columbia University, in 1945. She held numerous leadership positions in public health nursing. In 1952, she earned a master's degree in public health at Johns Hopkins University. In 1954, she earned her doctorate, also from Johns Hopkins University. In the same year, she went to New York University, where she became professor and head of the Division of Nurse Education (Safier, 1977). She headed that program until her retirement in 1975, whereupon she became Professor Emeritus (Malinski, 1986). She continued to write and lecture, explaining and refining her model nearly until her death. Her last article appeared in the Spring 1994 issue of *Nursing Science Quarterly.*

Rogers received numerous awards, honors, and citations both nationally and internationally, including three honorary doctorates. Her colleagues consider her to be one of the most original thinkers in nursing. For example, Levine stated that Rogers' "view of human beings . . . is a philosophic position of over-whelming importance for nursing" (1988, p. 16). Her contributions to the nursing literature are extensively cited. That Rogers valued education, clear and creative thinking, and service to individuals and society is reflected in her writings. Her abstract conceptual model, and more specific theories for nursing, grew from her effort to define, defend, and promote the growth of nurses as learned professionals, capable of unique and responsible service to humankind. In her clear delineation of the scientific focus for nursing, Rogers had a most significant influence upon scientific inquiry in nursing and professional nursing practice.

Rogers' abstract conceptual model was first published in 1970 in her book, *An Introduction to the Theoretical Basis of Nursing,* although its antecedents may be found in prior published works (Rogers, 1961). After its publication in 1970, Rogers made major clarifications as the conceptualizations were further refined. These changes can be found in Rogers' chapter in *Conceptual Models for Nursing Practice* (Rogers, 1980a); in her series of six videotapes, entitled *The Science of Unitary Man* (Rogers, 1980b); in *Family Health, A Theoretical Approach to Nursing Care* by Clements and Roberts (Rogers, 1983); in Violet Malinski's book, *Explorations on Martha Rogers' Science of Unitary Human Beings* (1986); in two articles in *Nursing Science Quarterly* (Rogers, 1988, 1992); and in a chapter in E. A. M. Barrett's *Visions of Rogers' Science-Based Nursing* (1990). Rogers also explained, discussed, and responded to questions about her conceptual model during her presentations at the annual Rogerian Conferences and the Discovery International Nurse Theorist Conferences (Huch, 1991; Smith, 1988), and to students and faculty across the country. The model has served as the basis for explication of other nursing conceptualizations, including those of Newman, Parse, and Fitzpatrick, discussed in this volume and in its previous editions.

Much of Rogers' work has been collected under one cover: *Martha E. Rogers: Her Life and Her Work,* by V. M. Malinski and E. A. M. Barrett. Their book was released a few months after Rogers' death in 1994. Another book released at the same time is *Rogers' Scientific Art of Nursing Practice,* edited by M. Madrid and E. A. M. Barrett. This second new book contains insights regarding nursing practice based on Rogers' science of nursing and personal accounts by nurses using Rogers' model in the art of nursing.

BASIC CONSIDERATIONS INCLUDED IN THE MODEL

The metaparadigm of nursing, person, health, environment, referred to as "commonplaces of the discipline" by Levine (1988), are necessary in any description of nursing. Rogers' definitions of these concepts will be presented first, with emphasis on Rogers' view of the nursing profession, after which other elements unique to Rogers' abstract conceptual model will be discussed. Rogers defines the model's concepts or "building blocks" as energy fields, openness, pattern, and pandimensionality, and defines "principles of homeodynamics" as resonancy, helicy, and integrality. The central focus of Rogers' life process model is unitary human beings in mutual process with their environments. Theories derived from Rogers' model include ones she specifically identified and ones others derived from her principles. Rogers explains two of her theories—the theory of accelerating evolution and the theory of paranormal. She describes the theory of accelerating evolution as one that can be used to study higher frequency wave patterns of growing diversity, sleep-wake periods, and blood pressure levels (Rogers, 1986). Her theory of paranormal phenomena provides the framework for alternative, noninvasive healing modalities such as therapeutic touch (Rogers, 1986, pp. 7–8). Much of the research is framed by her three principles of homeodynamics: the principle of resonancy, the principle of helicy, and the principle of integrality (Bultemeier, 1997).

Definitions of Nursing

Rogers states that the science of nursing is "the science of unitary human beings" (1983). She believed that nursing was unique in that no other science studies the person as a unitary energy field. The word nursing, used as a noun, is a basic science that encompasses a unique body of knowledge. The purpose of the practice of nursing is "to promote human betterment wherever people are" (1992, p. 33).

Description of Nursing Practice

Rogers (1970) saw nursing practice as creative and imaginative, rooted in abstract knowledge, intellectual judgment, and compassion. She emphasized the use of the nurse's own self and the safe utilization of the nursing skills and technology. Rogers (1992) emphasized the use of noninvasive modalities that are compatible with her model, such as therapeutic touch and meditation, as well as modalities that may be developed, such as color, sound, motion and humor. She saw nurses as independent practitioners taking the lead in community-based health centers, with hospitals or "sick" centers providing support services. Rogers' conceptual model specifies the person's innovative development and rhythmical complexity. Nursing practice is based upon the wholeness of human beings and "derives its safety and effectiveness from a unified concept of human functioning" (1970, p. 124). Nurses help people "design ways to fulfill their different rhythmic patterns" (1992, p. 33).

The nursing process becomes dynamic when viewed within Rogers' framework. Instead of a static process wherein the nurse sets time-limited goals for the person, Rogers proposed that nursing be a continuously evolving process that includes the nurse as an environmental component (Rogers, 1980b). Nurses help individuals, families, and groups wherever they are (including space as space exploration continues) to achieve maximum well-being within their potential (Rogers, 1992).

Definition and Description of Person

Critical to Rogers' discussion of the element of the person is the statement that ". . . the whole cannot be understood when reduced to particulars" (1970, p. 44). Person is understood within her conceptual model as a whole that is more than and different from the sum of its parts (1970, p. 91). This unified view of person has been part of nursing history, but Rogers explicitly defined this concept in scientific terms. Person is defined by Rogers as an open system, that is, "an irreducible, indivisible, pandimensional energy field identified by pattern and manifesting characteristics that are specific to the whole and which cannot be predicted from knowledge of the parts" (1992, p. 29). She states that the person's fundamental unit is not the cell but the human energy field.

Rogers cautioned against confusing her view of unitary human beings with other contemporary views of holism, which are really the summation of greater numbers of parts. Persons are to be viewed optimistically, taking into account their capacity to change and their ability to participate knowingly and creatively (although not always wisely) in the process of change (Rogers, 1983, 1992).

Definition and Description of Environment

In Rogers' view, each unique human field is embedded in its unique environmental field. Person and environment are integral with each other and coextensive with the universe. The boundaries of environment become nonexistent in Rogers' model because they extend to infinity. She defined environment as "an irreducible, pandimensional energy field identified by pattern and integral with the human field" (1992, p. 29). Through extensive study, Rogers concluded that the most logical conceptualization is that of a pandimensional universe without spatial or temporal attributes that expresses the idea of a unitary whole (Rogers, 1990, p. 7).

Definition and Description of Health

Rogers often used the word *health* but she declines to give a specific definition. She came to understand that illness and health are value words, broadly defined by each culture "to denote behaviors that are of high value and low value" (1980b). Rogers conceptualized health and illness as expressions of the human life process. The life process is inseparable from the environmental field, challenging the prevailing understanding of health as only an illness manifestation of the physical body. Her own use of the word in sentences is semantically compatible with definitions connoting well-being and positive health promotion.

Rogers raised an interesting point when she observed that processes we consider pathological on earth may "signify health for the spacebound" (1992, p. 27). She specifically mentions physiologic norms, and we speculate that she refers to vital signs such as blood pressure, which might be altered in space. We also know that weightlessness alters calcium content and density of bone. Perhaps certain ailments such as osteoporosis or arthritis would not be considered afflictions in an environment of constant weightlessness. We may further speculate that cancer can have a positive role in the evolution of "homo spacialis," as Rogers (1992) referred to future human beings evolving in space, given that cancer cells have metabolic rates and temporal qualities different from those of other body cells. Rogers may also have had in mind that people who function best with very short, long, or otherwise unusual sleep patterns on Earth would be well suited for certain functions in space travel or space living.

Interrelationships Among Concepts of Person, Environment, Health, and Nursing

Rogers viewed nursing as a "learned profession" with full professional status (1980a, 1980b). This means that nursing not only has a practice component but is also a science. Figure 12–1 illustrates an interpretation by the author of Rogers' view of nursing, including interrelationships among person, environment, health, and nursing. Rogers defines the relationship of the environmental and human energy fields as "integral" because they are considered an inseparable whole (1992, p. 30). As shown, concepts derived from study and observations about human beings provide a basis for the conceptual model. The conceptual model provides a stimulus for and gives

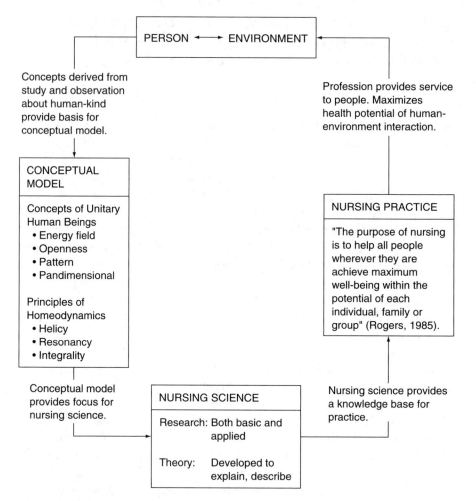

FIGURE 12–1   An interpretation of Rogers' view of nursing, including interrelation among person, environment, health, and nursing.

direction to nursing science. Knowledge generated through model-based research provides a base for practice to maximize health potential. Rogers perceives service as rendered in all settings and appropriate for all people.

Description of Concepts Unique to the Model: Energy Fields, Openness, Pattern, Pandimensionality

Energy fields. Rogers (1980a, 1980b) noted that current literature indicated that the fundamental unit of all living and nonliving things is the energy field. Things do not have energy fields, rather they *are* energy fields. *Fundamental unit* connotes the representative unit of a thing, that if examined, will thoroughly reveal its character or nature. The cell was thought to be the fundamental unit of living things, but current research notes that the sum of all of the information about the functions and inter-actions of cells does not reveal the full nature of the organism. By de-scribing the energy field as the fundamental unit, Rogers hoped to avoid the "summing of parts" in nursing's study of human beings. Such sum-ming, according to Rogers, results in views of humankind that are not help-ful to nurses, such as models in which the body is likened to a machine or closed system (mechanistic models), or models in which the mind and body are viewed separately. Rather, she hoped to promote a conceptual-ization of person, which captures the essence of being in its entirety. Ac-cording to Sarter (1989), Rogers' concept of an irreducible whole as the primary unit of existence is aligned with the philosophy of Teilhard de Chardin, in which consciousness is seen as coextensive with the universe and persons are seen as centers of energy within the overall pattern. Rogers does not use the term consciousness, possibly because such a usage could imply a mind–body dualism.

Openness. Rogers (1980a, 1980b) used *openness* to refer to the qual-ities exhibited by an open system as opposed to a closed system. Open sys-tems (energy fields) are conceptualized as extending to infinity and as integral with one another. Von Bertalanffy (1968) postulated that living sys-tems are open systems displaying negative entropy (negentropy). In other words, living systems do not run down but instead display increasing di-versity or heterogeneity. Rogers expands this view in her conceptual model to include "a universe of open systems" (1992, p. 29). Sarter (1989) states that Rogers denies existence of closed systems. If all systems were open then the concept of openness would extend to the inanimate.

Pattern. *Pattern* (formerly pattern and organization) is perhaps the most abstract of Rogers' concepts. Rogers stated that it is an abstraction, a single wave that identifies the given energy field (1986, p. 5). The wave pattern is ever changing as an expression of the given unitary human be-ing becoming or evolving. The pattern of the wave form is unique to each individual or group and identifies the uniqueness of each individual or group unfolding, integral with the respective environment.

Pandimensional. Rogers said that *pandimensionality* is a "nonlinear domain without spatial or temporal attributes" (Rogers, 1992). Rogers at first used the term "four-dimensionality" (1980a, 1980b) then later pre-ferred multidimensionality (1990), and finally pandimensionalality (1992) as better capturing her meaning. She stated that words in our language are not sufficient to fully explain this concept. Rogers' concept of pandimen-sionality in her model of person and environment was similar to a theory proposed by Albert Einstein. Neither Einstein nor Rogers view time separately from the three dimensions of space. Rogers explained that the concept has to do with nonlinear time and nonstatic space, which Einstein called *spacetime* (Rogers, 1980b). Rogers explained the relevance of this concept to the model many times. She said that human and environmental energy fields and all reality are pandimensional and that change emerges continuously, evolutionally, and unpredictably from nonlinear and nonspatial coordinates (1980a, 1992).

For a discussion of differences and similarities that may be present in Rogerian and Einsteinian worldviews, the reader is referred to Sarter's 1989 article. Nonlinearity describes the pandimensional universe that Rogers envisioned. Nonlinear is also a mathematical term describing formulas for events that are sometimes unpredictable. Any present point in Rogers' view is relative, which has implications for the explanation of previously unexplained phenomena (1980a), sometimes referred to as paranormal events. Rogers model is antithetical to the verificationist perspective of the logical positivists. As described by Whall (1989), the verificationists valued propositions based on observable phenomena and discounted statements or propositions based on less observable phenomena. Conversely, Rogers' model encourages us to seriously examine ideas and theories that lack observable "objective" data or connections but may be reported or entertained as reality by clients and others. Although some may criticize Rogers' concepts on this basis, it is worth noting that "mainstream" scientists are also breaking away from the verificationist perspective. For example, the conservative journal, *Scientific American,* published an article explaining how quantum physics does not negate time travel (Deutsch & Lockwood, 1994).

Relationship of Energy Fields, Openness, Pattern, and Pandimensionality to Person, Environment, Health, and Nursing

The four concepts—energy fields, openness, pattern, and pandimensionality— when synthesized by Rogers, comprise "unitary human beings." Figure 12–1 illustrates how Rogers' four concepts are derived from study and observation of people (person-environment), and form the basis of nursing's abstract conceptual model, which is ultimately related to nursing and health. Internal analysis and evaluation of the model will deal with analysis of Rogers' abstract conceptual system, displayed in Figure 12–2.

Roger's (1970, 1980a) definition of nursing is a reflection of her humanistic rather than mechanistic concept of person and nursing (Rogers, 1983). The focus of nursing is compassionate concern for maintaining and promoting health, preventing illness, and caring for and rehabilitating the sick and the disabled (1970, p. vii). Rogers was committed to nursing as

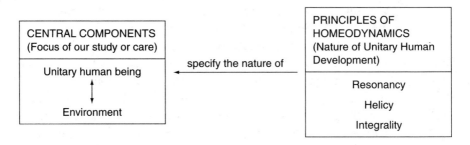

FIGURE 12–2   Central components in Rogers' abstract conceptual system.

both a science, with its abstract body of knowledge, and an art, which uses the science's body of knowledge. Professional practice in nursing "seeks to promote symphonic interaction between man and environment, to strengthen the coherence and integrity of the human field, and to direct and redirect patterning of the human and environmental fields for realization of maximum health potential" (1970, p. 122). Smith (1990) interpreted this person-environmental relationship as meaning that the nurse becomes a coparticipant with the client in repatterning the energy field for maximum health potential. Although Rogers used "repatterning" in her 1970 book, it was not used as a transitive verb (p. 97–98). Rogers did not use the term *repattern* in her 1992 article, perhaps because the prefix "re-" is inconsistent with the principle of helicy, in which rhythmicities are nonrepeating. Barrett (1988, 1990) discusses Rogerian nursing practice as "pattern manifestation appraisal and deliberative mutual patterning" (1990, p. 33).

INTERNAL ANALYSIS

Underlying Assumptions

Rogers (1970) listed five assumptions underlying her conceptual model. However, these assumptions were subsumed and restated in later years in other writings and other parts of her model. Rogers often used the term *man* to refer to human beings in publications prior to 1983; after which she began using the term *unitary human beings*.

1. Man is a unified whole possessing his own integrity and manifesting characteristics that are more than and different from the sum of his parts (1970, p. 47). This was restated as the definition of unitary human being "an irreducible, indivisible, pandimensional energy field identified by pattern and manifesting characteristics that are specific to the whole and which cannot be predicted from knowledge of the parts" (1992, p. 29).

2. Man and environment are continuously exchanging matter and energy with one another (1970, p. 54). The concept of *openness,* in which the fields extend to infinity and are integral with one another, and the principle of *integrality,* describing "continuous mutual human field and environmental field process" (Rogers, 1992, p. 31) replaces the terms *exchanging matter* and *energy.*

3. The life process evolves irreversibly and unidirectionally along the space-time continuum (1970, p. 59). This is now the principle of *helicy:* "continuous, innovative, unpredictable, increasing diversity of human and environmental field patterns (1992, p. 31), removing the terms *irreversible* and *unidirectional,* thereby avoiding any misinterpretation of time as linear.

4. *Pattern and organization* identify man and reflect his innovative wholeness (1970, p. 65). Pattern and organization became the singular concept *pattern,* in which the pattern is an abstract concept of a single wave that identifies the energy field and is ever changing as an expression of the given human being evolving in mutual process with the environment (1986, p. 5).

5. Man is characterized by the capacity for abstraction and imagery, language and thought, sensation and emotion (1970, p. 73).

The fifth assumption, describing persons as sentient beings capable of abstract imagery and thought, remains as Rogers' statement that hers is not a mechanistic model and that human beings are set apart from other living things. Although she did not restate it in later publications, neither did she recant it. Rogers made an explicit assumption regarding human beings in her 1992 article when she wrote that the principles of homeodynamics (p. 14–22) "have validity only within the science of unitary human beings" (p. 30). This is an important statement to note because the energy field is stated to be the fundamental unit of the living and nonliving. The principles of homeodynamics are specific to Rogers' theory regarding human beings and are not meant to be lifted out of this context for the study of other entities or energy fields.

Another statement by Rogers that may be viewed as an assumption is that persons are knowing participants in health care and that they are able to make choices (Rogers, 1990, p. 13).

Central Components

The central components of the model are *unitary human being* and the *environment* engaged in the *life process.* The components are derived from the synthesis of Rogers' four building blocks and comprise, in Rogers' view, nursing's abstract conceptual system. The components are defined earlier in the chapter but are repeated here for clarity:

- *Unitary human being:* "An irreducible, indivisible, pandimensional energy field identified by pattern and manifesting characteristics that are different from those of the parts and cannot be predicted from knowledge of the parts" (1992, p. 5).
- *Environment:* "An irreducible, pandimensional energy field identified by pattern and manifesting characteristics different from those of the parts. Each environmental field is specific to its given human field" (1986, p. 5).

From the abstract conceptual system, Rogers derived the three other components of the model, which she called principles of homeodynamics. They are broad generalizations that postulate the nature and direction of unitary human development (1980a, p. 333).

- *Resonancy:* The continuous change from lower frequency to higher frequency wave patterns in human and environmental fields (Rogers, 1986, p. 6).
- *Helicy:* The continuous innovative, unpredictable increasing diversity of human and environmental field patterns (1992, p. 31) characterized by nonrepeating rhythmicities (Rogers, 1986, p. 6).
- *Integrality:* The continuous, mutual human field and environmental field process (Rogers, 1992, p. 31).

Analysis of Consistency

According to Dubin, "the argument about the adequacy of the theoretical model is always and only an argument about the logic employed in constructing it" (1978, p. 12). Fawcett (1995) also considers logical congruence with philosophical origins as a measure of consistency. Rogers often described her theory as emerging out of creative synthesis (1986) or as "emergent" (1992, p. 28). Rogers invited critique of her model and remained open to change. She progressively refined it for clarity and succinctness. The definitions are clear. There are no flaws in logic and the conceptual content is derived directly from Rogers' philosophical claims. Concepts are used in consistent ways throughout the model. A possible problem might be the use of the word *system.*

Although Rogers (1986) refers to von Bertalanffy (1968) in describing the concept of openness among different systems and the environment, Cowling (1993) illustrates differences in the systems and unitary perspectives. Systems theory is based upon separate but interrelated parts that have boundaries, but that are interdependent. Unitary perspective views temporal and spatial dimensions, not interdependently, but as integral to one another. Phenomena interrelate in mutual process. Rogers continued to use the term *open systems* to describe the integrality of energy fields through 1992, but Rogers' intended focus is on manifestations of wholeness, moving beyond general systems concepts. Therefore, reduced precision may result with continued use of the word *systems,* which when used by scholars other than Rogers, connotes interdependence in a nonpandimensional manner.

Nurse scholars have identified probable philosophical roots of Rogers's model. Sarter (1989) mentions Ludwig von Bertalanffy, Pierre Teilhard de Chardin, Bertrand Russell, Michael Polanyi, Kurt Lewin, Theodosins Dobzhansky, and Albert Einstein. Reeder (1993) compares and contrasts Rogers' views with those of Wilhelm Dilthey and Jurgen Habermas. Hanchett (1992) compares Eastern philosophy as exemplified in Tibetan Buddhist philosophy with several of Rogers' concepts and principles, finding areas of similarity. Rogers emphasized the noncausal nature of change. Rogers stated that the term *unpredictable* "transcends the term probability" and mentioned chaos theory as also transforming our thinking (1990, p. 7; 1992, p. 32). Unpredictability is compatible with the creativity Rogers viewed as inherent in all development, change, and evolution. This creativity is emergent, different from what went before, and neither a sum nor combination of parts. In chaos theory the emergent may be dependent on initial conditions, but is not predictable from initial conditions. In addition, simple systems may breed complexity, and that complexity may yield observable patterns (Gleick, 1987). Central tenets of chaos theory that are similar or compatible with Rogers' theory are complexity, pattern, unpredictability, and creativity. Meleis (1991) states that the model's "view of humanity and environment and the lack of separation between mind and body is congruent with the Eastern view" (p. 322). She says that the model is "understandable in the international arena" (p. 322) and that its use and influence will spread more than expected in the future.

These quests for deeper understanding testify at once to the model's innovativeness, sophistication, and uniqueness. Rogers' model is based on concepts that are difficult to understand. However, once these concepts are clearly understood, the model itself is simple and elegant.

Analysis of Adequacy

Conceptual models are assessed in a variety of ways. Hardy (1974, 1978) and Ellis (1968) suggest examining scope, complexity, and usefulness. Rogers' model is broad in scope and centered on the life process of human beings. In fact, Rogers (1985) and others (Malinski, 1986) referred to the model as a worldview. According to Ellis, the broader the scope, the greater the significance of a theory. Ellis states that another characteristic of significant theories is that they have complexity; they treat multiple variables, and identify multiple relationships or complexity within a single variable (1968, p. 219).

Testability is another desirable characteristic of significant theories (Hardy, 1974; Ellis, 1968). Rogers derived several theories from the abstract conceptual system: the theory of accelerating evolution states that change (evolution) is becoming more and more rapid. Rogers cited increasingly complex technology and changing sleep patterns (1980a, 1992). In her theories of paranormal events, Rogers explained that when human fields are viewed as pandimensional, the relative present for one person is different from that of someone else. This could offer explanations for such phenomena as the well-documented instances of precognition, déjà vu, and clairvoyance (1980a, 1992).

The theory of paranormal events is the basis for the derived theory of therapeutic touch developed by Dolores Krieger (Rogers, 1986). Therapeutic touch is a practice mode that has been formalized and shown to be efficacious by Krieger (Rogers, 1983; Krieger, 1981; Meehan, 1993; Quinn & Strelkauskas, 1993). Therapeutic touch has been defined as a cognitive and a conative way of knowing, both of which encompass knowing in the widest sense (Hayes & Cox, 1999, p. 1252), and as a rhythmic continuous mutual patterning process of nurse and client (Smith & Reeder, 1998). However, therapeutic touch, as a paranormal nursing intervention, has received criticism as a pseudoscience because it has been studied using methods that include aesthetic and personal patterns of discovery (Raskin, 2000). For example, Meehan (1990) uses case report methodology to evaluate therapeutic touch techniques in one participant with metastatic cancer. The reported subjective effects included reduced chronic pain and increased sleep periods Replication of the therapeutic touch using experimental intervention studies involving persons with acute surgical pain resulted in no significant differences in pain relief (Meehan, 1993). In contrast, Lin and Taylor (1998) tested elders in a randomized three-group design and found significant decreases in chronic pain perception and anxiety.

The manifestation of field patterning theory specifies that wave patterns include sleep-wake patterns, patterns of human field motion, and the developmental process of living and dying. These patterns are characterized by increasing complexity and increasing diversity (Rogers, 1980a, 1992). Bultemeier (1997) derived the theory of perceived dissonance from the principles of resonancy and integrality to study patterns within human rhythmic cycles.

Relationships among components. Unitary human being appears to be the most important component. Rogers emphasizes that unitary human being is the focus of nursing's research and practice (Figure 12–2). Within the conceptual model the concept human being is defined as an energy field, inseparable from the environment and interchangeable with the life process. In this sense, human being is the only component in the conceptual model;

the principles have action definitions that describe human being (Figure 12–2). Rogers formerly stated that the derived theories were intended to explain, describe, and predict. When she replaced probability with unpredictability in the helicy definition, she then said that theories and research could provide "description, explanation and vision" (1992, p. 33).

Issues identified in use of the model are the complexity of its language, the need for those using the model to develop a noncausal mind-set, and the need to measure the life process of human beings without resorting to measuring parts. Theories are also significant if they are useful for clinical practice (Ellis, 1968), which Rogers' model is. Use of Rogers' model in research and practice are examined in the following external analysis section.

EXTERNAL ANALYSIS

Relationship to Nursing Research

Ways of knowing. Fawcett, Watson, Neuman, Walker, and Fitzpatrick (2001) contend that "any form of evidence has to be interpreted and critiqued by each person who is considering whether the theory can be applied in a particular practice situation" (p. 117). They suggest that evidence-based practice must be generated from studies that use diverse patterns of knowing, rather than just empirical knowing, so that the uniqueness of nursing science can be elucidated. They consider Carper's (1978) ways of knowing, which include ethical, personal, and aesthetic, and empiric knowing, as types of nursing knowledge necessary for evidence-based nursing practice (Table 12–1). Rogers' focus on unitary human beings evolving integrally with their environments is congruent with the call for nursing knowledge to be developed in each of the patterns of knowing. Ethical, aesthetical, and personal knowledge are essential, otherwise patients would be compelled to only consult robots with databases. Figure 12–3 incorporates the patterns of knowing, evidence-based care, and examples from the literature that demonstrate the eloquence of Rogers' framed research and how diverse ways of knowing are used.

Various data sets have been developed that organize care. The American Nurses Association (ANA) recognizes several classifications, including those by the North American Nursing Diagnosis Association (NANDA), the Omaha System, the Georgetown Home Health Classification, the Nursing Interventions Classification System, and the Nursing Outcomes Classification System (Bulechek & McCloskey, 1999; Carpenito, 1992; Johnson, Maas, & Moorhead, 2000; McCloskey & Bulechek, 2000; Saba, 1996; NANDA, 2001). How does the Rogerian model fit these identified nursing

TABLE 12–1 Integration of Carper's Patterns of Knowing, Rogerian Research, and Evidence-Based Care

Evidence-based care[a]	Carper's patterns of knowing[b]	Rogerian research exemplars of knowledge patterns
Best research evidence: randomized or controlled	Empirics: studies, organized classifications, control, prediction	Leddy (1999) Lin and Taylor (1998) Nursing Data Sets: Bulechek and McCloskey (1999); Carpenito, 1992; Johnson, Maas, and Mead (2000); Saba (1996); NANDA (2001)
Clinical expertise: clinical skills used to examine, diagnose, determine health status, health state, and identify patient's personal values	Esthetics: Art; expressive but resistant to projection into discursive language	Bultemeier (1997)
Patient values: preferences, concerns, expectations, that are integrated into clinical decisions	Personal knowledge: knowledge of a person as unique; different for each person	Donahue and Alligood (1995) Meehan (1990)

[a]Sackett, Straus, Richardson, Rosenberg, and Haynes (2000).
[b]Carper (1978).

data sets that describe and organize nursing activities and care? These systems were developed purposefully to provide definition to nursing actions and interventions, and to identify significant patient outcomes. More practically, they were developed for reimbursement coding, a function independent of theory development. The classifications could be considered middle-range theory because they were derived descriptively and qualitatively from nursing care activities and observation. These data sets provide the initial taxonomy of nursing practice in varied settings framed within a biomedical model. The taxonomies are a blueprint of nursing actions; hence, they represent empirical and personal knowledge as patterns of knowing. However, Rogers' model is unitary and different from the biomedical model. Future testing and interpretation of the taxonomies identified within Rogers' nursing model will determine which actual evidence (or way of knowing) is appropriate for use by the nurse and patient to guide decisions or choices about the most appropriate nursing intervention and expected results.

Rogers originally supported the use of nursing diagnosis, specifically mentioning diagnosis, in her 1970 book (p. 5, 86, 102, 124), for example.

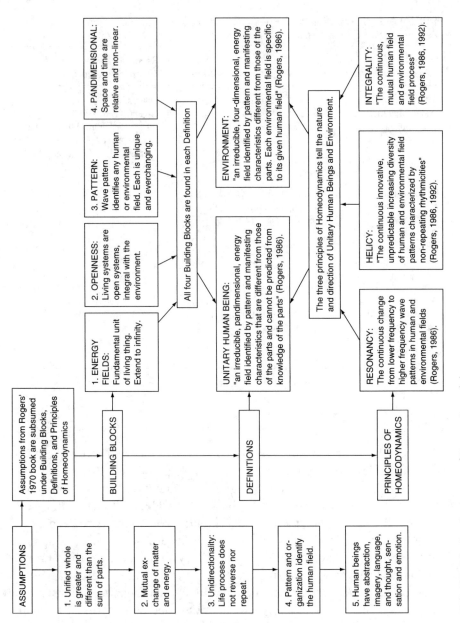

FIGURE 12-3 Summary of Rogers' model.

She stated that nursing diagnosis was a goal of nursing (1970, p. 102). In 1977, she participated in a task force of nurse-theorists to identify a conceptual framework for nursing diagnoses. By the end of the 1980s, Rogers had dropped her support of and use of the term *nursing diagnosis*. She eschewed the term as too static and time limited (Smith, 1988). Further reasons for Rogers' lack of acceptance of the term *nursing diagnosis* may be the presence of logical inconsistencies that appeared between her model and the nursing diagnostic terms themselves (England, 1989). For example, as England points out, the problem-oriented labels are inconsistent with the human response patterns, and the concept of etiology is inconsistent with the concept of multiple and probabilistic contributions to human field patterns. The human response patterns function more as adjectives that may describe a pattern than as categories into which patterns would fall.

Although several problems of logical adequacy exist in the nursing diagnostic taxonomy, nursing as a profession is finding that giving name and structure to its process is adding stature to nursing professionally in many countries. Rogers alludes to methods of "learning skills and techniques" as different from her organized science but nonetheless "important" (1994, p. 34).

Relationship to nursing research: Evidence-based practice using Rogers' model. As the Rogerian body of research continues to grow, examination of hypotheses and results are allowing support and modification of the model. Whether or not the interpretation of linkages between the model and real life is "correct" based upon research outcomes is still a judgment made either by the investigator or by the scientific community as research continues. As shown in Figure 12–1, Rogers' abstract conceptual model is directly related to research and theory development in nursing science. The conceptual model provides the stimulus and direction for these scientific activities. Rogers' model offers a way of looking at reality that is unique to the nursing profession. Rogers' delineation of the science of unitary human beings provides a unique and substantive focus for the discipline. Rogers expected the theory emerging from her model to ultimately describe and explain phenomena (1992). There is a need for both basic and applied research (Rogers, 1980a, 1986, 1992). The model is not testable itself nor is it meant to be. Rather, theories and hypotheses derived from the model are subjected to scientific investigation.

The derivation of testable theories or hypotheses from the model requires understanding and the ability to infer. Some early examples of research related to Rogers' conceptualization include that of Newman (1978), Fawcett (1975), Fitzpatrick (1980), Floyd (1983), and Cowling (1985), as well as several presenters (Moore, Engle, Johnston, and Fromm) at the ANA Council of Nurse Researchers symposium entitled

"Research Related to Rogers' Conceptual Model." Studies by Rawnsley, Ference, Alligood, Gueldner, and Barrett, as well as some of the above, appear in Malinski's *Explorations on Martha Rogers' Science of Unitary Human Beings* (1986).

The number of studies being done and published using Rogers' model is increasing. Twenty studies were reviewed and analyzed by Dykeman and Loukissa (1993). These included only published studies using Rogers' revised three principles of homeodynamics (after 1980) and specifically using Rogers' model as the conceptual framework. Most of these studies contained more than one hypothesis. Overall, less than half of the hypotheses were supported. According to Dykeman and Loukissa (1993), this is most likely a result of measurement problems.

There have been increasing numbers of instruments designed specifically within Rogers' model. Ference (1986) developed the first one, the "human field motion test," in 1978 to study the correlates of human development, later called manifestation of patterning by Rogers (1992). The instrument is based on the semantic differential technique. It has been used in several studies framed within Roger's model, but there have been conceptual and practical difficulties with its use, particularly with elders (Gueldner, 1986).

The second instrument to be developed was Barrett's "human field power test" in 1983, (Ference, 1986), later refined and called the power as knowing participation in change test (Dykeman & Loukissa, 1993). The third was Paletta's temporal experience scales (Dykeman & Loukissa, 1993). Leddy (1995, 1996, 1999) developed the person-environment participation scale, and the Leddy healthiness scale, both based upon unitary patterns. The person-environment participation scale, based upon human-environmental mutual processes, measures perceived ease and expansiveness of participation as a measure of health, and has been repeated with good content validity and reliability. The Leddy healthiness scale derives from the concept of health as unitary patterning of person-environment mutual process (p. 432). Three components of health were revealed: purpose, power, and connections. All of the above tests are paper-and-pencil tests, which require verbal facility of the client.

Young children and certain other clients cannot use paper-and-pencil tests to tell us about themselves. Studies of young infants have mainly relied on weight, sleep patterns, and/or vital signs to identify pattern manifestation or expression of the unitary energy field. An interesting concept, applicable to all clients, is energy and energy flow in relation to therapeutic touch (Krieger, 1981).

Some instruments not designed to measure Rogers' concepts may in fact measure something other than the investigator intended. For example, the personal orientation inventory (POI) was used in three studies to measure actualization or self-actualization. However, the POI measures self-actualizing value(s) held by the testee (Shostrom, 1966). The POI may not correspond to the self-actualization that Rogers described as people fulfilling life's potentials.

Theorists who have extended Rogers' model are Fitzpatrick (1983), Newman (1979), and Parse (1981). These theorists have particularly explained the understanding of health in the model, and Parse added a specific research methodology. Parse's theory of human becoming (Parse, 1995) and Newman's theory of expanding consciousness (Desai et al., 1998) are middle-range theories derived from Rogers' conceptual model of unitary humans.

The theory of accelerating change has been studied by a number of nurse researchers and its name has evolved depending upon the focus of the researcher. It has evolved into the theory of accelerating change in a study of creativity and empathy (Alligood, 1991), the theory of accelerating diversity in a study of time sleep and activity patterns (Alligood & McGuire, 2000), and evolving patterning of human life (Donahue & Alligood, 1995). Alligood's study of creativity, actualization, and empathy found statistically significant relationships of the constructs derived from helicy and integrality. Benedict and Burge (1990) studied the relationship between wavelength light and human field motion but the hypothesis was not supported. Schorr (1993), however, found that music as patterned, environmental resonance decreased pain perception. The theory of power as knowing participation in change was derived by Barrett (1988) in studies of adults in therapy. The theory of power as participation in change has been repeated and supported in a study of women in recovery from a mental health crisis (Rush, 2000). Rush found significance correlations between power and sobriety in women in recovery of at least 1 year.

Relationship to Nursing Education

In 1963, Rogers called for the rebuilding of undergraduate and graduate programs in nursing to reflect the evolution of nursing science (Rogers, 1963). Consistent with her definition of nursing as a learned profession, Rogers called for placement of all nursing education in institutions of higher learning. A learned profession must claim a unique body of knowledge. In 1964, she outlined a doctoral program in nursing at New York University consistent with the science of unitary human beings (Rogers, 1964).

The strength of Rogers' model in education is that it conceptualizes nursing as a theory-based science. This conceptualization mandated university-based education for nurses and paved the way for the development of the doctor of philosophy degree in nursing. Mathwig, Young, and Pepper (1990) designed nursing curricula using Rogers' conceptual model. Content in both was centered on the homeodynamic principles, and Rogers' conceptualization of the nursing metaparadigm. Hanley (1990) developed a concept integration game to teach baccalaureate nursing students Rogers' concepts of energy, pattern, and change. Rogers sees nursing more closely related to the liberal arts college than to any of the other colleges of the university. The science of unitary human beings mandates inclusion of courses in physics and philosophy as well as those in the biological and social sciences. Education that follows Rogers' framework prepares a generalist in nursing who views person and environment as interacting and ever changing.

Relationship to Professional Nursing Practice

The model emphasizes the need for individualized nursing care based on the unique situation of any person or group and the unique environment. Malinski (1986) notes seven trends that occur in practice with the use of Rogers' model: (a) empowering both nurse and client (p. 28); (b) accepting diversity as the norm (p. 28); (c) becoming attuned to patterning (p. 29); (d) recognizing and using wave modalities such as light, music, and movement as integral to the patterning process and thus to health and healing (p. 29); (e) viewing change as positive (p. 29); (f) expanding the assessment phase of the nursing process (p. 30); and (g) accepting the integral connectedness of life (p. 30).

Rogers does not relate her model to the nursing process format (assessment, diagnosis, intervention, and evaluation). Barrett (1988) used the terms *pattern appraisal* and *deliberative mutual patterning* to describe a nursing process in using Rogers' model. Cowling (1993) explicates these concepts. An important point is that pattern appraisal requires an inclusive perspective of what counts as pattern information. He speaks of using the aspects of human existence that are experience, perception, and expression in appraising client patterns. Assessment is focused and guided by what the client wants from the encounter with the nurse. Assessment is not restricted to one modality but includes all that are appropriate. Some of these are observation, language, recognizing recurring themes, intuitive inquiry, sharing between nurse and client, physical examination, and reporting of sensations. Pattern appraisal guides deliberative mutual repatterning. Cowling (1993) calls this mutually derived purposive strategies. (The term *intervention* has been dropped in many arenas because it implies action by the nurse that may not include the client in the exploratory and decision-making process.)

The nurse practicing within the Rogerian model will realize that "appraisal" and "mutual patterning" are themselves only arbitrarily separated for discussion. The nurse is part of the client's environment during appraisal and thus the patterning will alter. Of course, in addition, observation and appraisal go on continuously through purposive repatterning. Fawcett extracted elements of the nursing process from Rogers' publications and related these to the nursing process (1984, p. 223). Some of the suggestions, such as assessing "subsystem pathology" are no longer congruent with Roger's model. Aggleton and Chalmers also did this, providing a brief overview of nursing practice consistent with Rogers' model (1984, p. 38). Whall (1981) elaborates the assessment of families using Rogers' model. Although clearly derived from the assumptions, building blocks, and principles in Rogers' model, Whall focuses on assessment and does not attempt to force an outline of the nursing process from the model. Whall's and later Johnston's (1986) assessment guidelines are very usable, and are related explicitly to terminology and middle-range theories already present in the literature on family functioning. Falco and Lobo (1980) use helicy, resonancy, and complementarity to derive a care plan, however misguided, (assessment, diagnosis, implementation, and evaluation) for a specific individual.

As depicted in Figure 12–1, Rogers' conceptual model is useful in research and theory development. It is the responsibility of the researcher and theorist to further develop and refine the specific knowledge base for practice. The practitioner uses the knowledge creatively in each client care situation. Other types of knowledge are not discarded but are viewed differently. As Newman points out, "disease conditions can no longer be considered as entities unto themselves but must be regarded as manifestations of the total pattern of the individual in interaction with the environment" (1979, p. 21).

Rogers (1980a, 1980b, 1983) envisions changes in nursing practice based on the theories evolving from her model. She gives several examples. The aging process is perceived not as a running down of the individual, but as a growing diversity in field pattern; thus many characteristics of older persons, such as changing sleep patterns, cease to be viewed as abnormal or in need of intervention. Other changes she envisions are that dying be viewed as a developmental process rather than an event; and that nursing care becomes even more individualized to specific persons in their own unique situations.

SUMMARY

Rogers' abstract conceptual model is broad in scope. It addresses the complexity of the single variable, a unitary human being. The model is not meant to be testable, but theories drawn from it are so. It provides a substantive base for research and theory development that provides the knowledge base for practice. For Rogers, professional practice flowed from the application of nursing knowledge. The model generates information by increasing our understanding of human beings and the life process and by encouraging theory development and the delineation of testable hypotheses. Terminology is clear, although the new words sometimes seem difficult. These new words avoid confusion with terms from other fields. The sophisticated concepts and linkages are viewed as recondite by many and require study and understanding.

Many of us walk two steps behind such thinking and perhaps think that we need many more courses in philosophy and physics to even enter these discussions. Nonetheless, many nurses at all levels find an immediate intuitive connection to the implications of the theory in that they have seen people and/or patients who have, or have themselves, experienced phenomena (sometimes described as paranormal) that are accounted for in Rogers' theory but not in other theories. Rogers' theory allows us to examine phenomena that other theories and worldviews encourage us to ignore.

Rogers' model is an optimistic and evolving one. Implicit and explicit values in Rogers' view of nursing are a high respect for individuals, and respect for values and characteristics of individuals and groups that "deviate" in the sense of "not with the average (norm)." Rogers' model challenges the researcher, the educator, and the practitioner to meet their societal obligations in creative ways. Martha Rogers was instrumental in moving nursing to full professionalization. Her conceptual model of unitary human beings presents a clear, direct statement about the unique focus of nursing, and a visionary perspective of nursing as a science and an art.

REFERENCES

Aggleton, P., & Chalmers, H. (1984). Rogers' unitary field model. *Nursing Times, 80*(50), 35–39.

Alligood, M. R. (1991). Testing Rogers' theory of accelerating change: The relationship among creativity, actualization, and empathy in persons 18 to 92 years of age. *Western Journal of Nursing Research, 13,* 84–96.

Alligood, M. R., & McGuire, S. L. (2000). Perception of time, sleep patterns, and activity in senior citizens: A test of a Rogerian theory of aging. *Visions: The Journal of Rogerian Nursing Science, 8*(1), 6–14.

American Nurses Association (ANA). (1981, September). *Research related to Rogers' conceptual model.* ANA Council of Nurse Researchers, Washington, DC.

Barrett, E. A. M. (1988). Using Rogers' Science of Unitary Human Beings in nursing practice. *Nursing Science Quarterly, 1*(2), 50–51.

Barrett, E. A. M. (Ed.). (1990). *Visions of Rogers' science-based nursing.* New York: National League for Nursing.

Benedict, S. C., & Burge, J. M. (1990). The relationship between human field motion and preferred visible wavelengths. *Nursing Science Quarterly, 3,* 73–80.

Bulechek, G. M., & McCloskey, J. C. (1999). *Nursing interventions: Effective nursing treatments* (3rd ed.). Philadelphia: W. B. Saunders.

Bultemeier, K. (1997). Rogers' science of unitary human beings in nursing practice. In M. R. Alligood & A. Marriner-Tomey (Eds.), *Nursing theory: Utilization and application.* (pp. 153–174). St. Louis: Mosby.

Carpenito, L. J. (1992). *Nursing diagnosis: Application to clinical practice* (4th ed.). Philadelphia: J. B. Lippincott.

Carper, B. A. (1978). Fundamental patterns of knowing in nursing. *Advances in Nursing Science, 1*(1), 13–23.

Cowling, W. R., III. (1985). Relationship of mystical experience, differentiation, and creativity. *Perceptual Motor Skills, 61,* 451–456.

Cowling, W. R., III. (1993). Unitary knowing in nursing practice. *Nursing Science Quarterly, 6*(4), 201–207.

Desai, S., Keffer, M. J., Hensley, D. M., Kilgore-Keever, K. A., Langfitt, J. V., & Peterson, L. (1998). In A. M. Tomey & M. R. Alligood (Eds.), *Nursing theorists and their work* (4th ed., pp. 496–515). Baltimore: Mosby.

Deutsch, D., & Lockwood, M. (1994). The quantum physics of time travel. *Scientific American, 270,* 68–74.

Donahue, L., & Alligood, M. R. (1995). A description of the elderly from self-selected attributes. *Visions: The Journal of Rogerian Nursing Science, 3*(1), 12–19.

Dubin, R. (1978). *Theory building.* New York: The Free Press.

Dykeman, M. C., & Loukissa, D. (1993). The science of unitary human beings: An integrative review. *Nursing Science Quarterly, 6*(4), 179–188.

Ellis, R. (1968). Characteristics of significant theories. *Nursing Research, 17*(3), 217–222.

England, M. (1989). Nursing diagnosis: A conceptual framework. In J. J. Fitzpatrick & A. L. Whall (Eds.), *Conceptual models of nursing* (2nd ed.). Norwalk, CT: Appleton & Lange.

Falco, S. M., & Lobo, M. L. (1980). Martha E. Rogers. In Nursing Theories Conference Group & J. B. George (Eds.), *Nursing theories: The base for professional nursing practice.* Englewood Cliffs, NJ: Prentice-Hall.

Fawcett, J. (1975). The family as a living open system: An emerging conceptual framework for nursing. *International Nursing Review, 22*(4), 113–116.

Fawcett, J. (1984). *Analysis and evaluation of conceptual models of nursing.* Philadelphia: F. A. Davis.

Fawcett, J. (1995). *Analysis and evaluation of conceptual models of nursing* (3rd ed.). Philadelphia: F. A. Davis.

Fawcett, J., Watson, J., Neuman, B., Walker, P. H., & Fitzpatrick, J. J. (2001). On nursing theories and evidence. *Journal of Nursing Scholarship, 33,* 115–119.

Ference, H. M. (1986). The relationship of time experience, creativity traits, differentiation, and human field motion. In V. M. Malinski (Ed.), *Explorations on Martha Rogers' science of unitary human beings* (pp. 95–105). Norwalk, CT: Appleton-Century-Crofts.

Fitzpatrick, J. J. (1980). Patients' perceptions of time: Current research. *International Nursing Review, 27*(5), 148–153.

Fitzpatrick, J. J. (1983). A life perspective rhythm model. In J. J. Fitzpatrick & A. L. Whall (Eds.), *Conceptual models of nursing: Analysis and application* (pp. 295–302). Bowie, MD: Brady.

Floyd, J. A. (1983). Research using Rogers' conceptual systems: Development of a testable theorem. *Advances in Nursing Science, 5*(2), 37–48.

Gleick, J. (1987). *Chaos: Making a new science.* New York: Penguin Books.

Gueldner, S. H. (1986). The relationship between imposed field motion and human field motion in elderly individuals living in nursing homes. In V. M. Malinski (Ed.), *Explorations on Martha Rogers' science of unitary human beings* (pp. 161–171). Norwalk, CT: Appleton-Century-Crofts.

Hanchett, E. S. (1992). Concepts from Eastern philosophy and Rogers' science of unitary human beings. *Nursing Science Quarterly, 5*(4), 164–170

Hanley, M. A. (1990). Concept-integration: A board game as a learning tool. In E. A. M. Barrett (Ed.), *Visions of Rogers' science-based nursing* (pp. 335–344). New York: National League for Nursing.

Hardy, M. E. (1974). Theories: Components, development, evaluation. *Nursing Research, 23,* 100–107.

Hardy, M. E. (1978). Perspectives on nursing. *Advances in Nursing Science, 1,* 37–48.

Hayes, J., & Cox, C. (1999). The experience of therapeutic touch from a nursing perspective. *British Journal of Nursing, 8,* 1249–1254.

Hektor, L. M. (1989). Martha E. Rogers: A life history. *Nursing Science Quarterly, 2*(2), 63–73.

Huch, M. H. (1991). Perspectives on health. *Nursing Science Quarterly, 4*(1), 33–40.

Johnson, M., Maas, M., & Moorhead, S. (Eds.). (2000). *Iowa outcomes project: Nursing Outcomes Classification (NOC)* (2nd ed.). St. Louis: Mosby.

Johnston, R. (1986). Approaching family intervention through Rogers' conceptual model. In A. L. Whall (Ed.), *Family therapy for nursing: Four approaches* (pp. 11–32). East Norwalk, CT: Appleton-Century-Crofts.

Krieger, D. (1981). *Foundations for holistic health nursing practices: The Renaissance nurse.* Philadelphia: J. B. Lippincott.

Leddy, S. K. (1995). Measuring mutual process: Development and psychometric testing of person-environment participation scale. *Visions: The Journal of Rogerian Nursing Science, 3*(1), 20–31.

Leddy, S. K. (1996). Development and psychometric testing of the Leddy healthiness scale. *Research in Nursing & Health, 19,* 431–440.

Leddy, S. K. (1999). Further exploration of the psychometric properties of the person-environment participation scale: Differentiating instrument reliability and construct stability. *Visions: The Journal of Rogerian Nursing Science, 7*(1), 55–57.

Levine, M. E. (1988). Antecedents from adjunctive disciplines: Creation of nursing theory. *Nursing Science Quarterly, 1*(1) 132–141.

Lin, Y., & Taylor, A. G. (1998). Effects of therapeutic touch in reducing pain and anxiety in an elderly population. *Integrative Medicine, 1,* 155–162.

Madrid, M., & Barrett, E. A. M. (Eds.). (1994). *Rogers' scientific art of nursing practice.* New York: National League for Nursing.

Malinski, V. M. (Ed.) (1986). *Explorations on Martha Rogers' science of unitary human beings.* Norwalk, CT: Appleton-Century-Crofts.

Malinski, V. M., & Barrett, E. A. M. (Eds.). (1994). *Martha E. Rogers: Her life and her work.* Philadelphia: F. A. Davis.

Mathwig, G. M., Young, A. A., & Pepper, J. M. (1990). Using Rogerian science in undergraduate and graduate nursing education. In E. A. M. Barrett (Ed.), *Visions of Rogers' science-based nursing* (pp. 319–334). New York: National League for Nursing.

McCloskey, J., & Bulechek, G. (Eds.). (2000). *Nursing interventions classification (NIC): Iowa intervention project* (3rd ed.). St. Louis: Mosby-Year Book.

Meehan, T. C. (1990). The science of unitary human beings and theory-based practice: Therapeutic touch. In E. A. M. Barrett (Ed.), *Visions of Rogers' science based nursing.* (pp. 67–81). New York: National League for Nursing.

Meehan, T. C. (1993). Therapeutic touch and postoperative pain: A Rogerian research study. *Nursing Science Quarterly, 6,* 69–78.

Meleis, A. I. (1991). *Theoretical nursing: Development and progress* (2nd ed.). Philadelphia: J. B. Lippencott.

Newman, M. A. (1978). *Application of theory in education and service.* Paper presented at the Nurse Educator Conference at New York University, New York.

Newman, M. A. (1979). *Theory development in nursing.* Philadelphia: F. A. Davis.

North American Nursing Diagnoses (NANDA): Definitions & classifications. (2001). Philadelphia: North American Nursing Diagnosis Association.

Parse, R. R. (1981). *Man-living-health, a theory of nursing.* New York: Wiley & Sons.

Parse, R. R. (Ed.). (1995). *Illuminations: The human becoming theory in practice and research.* New York: National League for Nursing.

Quinn, J. F., & Strelkauskas, A. J. (1993). Psychoimmunologic effects of therapeutic touch on practitioners and recently bereaved recipients: A pilot study. *Advanced Nursing Science, 15,* 13–26.

Raskin, J. (2000). Rogerian nursing theory: A humbug in the halls of higher learning. *The Skeptical Inquirer, 5,* 30–35.

Reeder, F. (1993). The Science of Unitary Human Beings and interpretive human science. *Nursing Science Quarterly, 6*(1), 13–24.

Rogers, M. E. (1961). *Education's revolution in nursing.* New York: Collier MacMillan.

Rogers, M. E. (1963). Building a strong educational foundation. *American Journal of Nursing, 63*(6), 94–95.

Rogers, M. E. (1964). *Reveille in nursing.* Philadelphia: F. A. Davis.

Rogers, M. E. (1970). *An Introduction to the theoretical basis of nursing.* Philadelphia: F. A. Davis.

Rogers, M. E. (1980a). A science of unitary man. In J. P. Riehl & C. Roy (Eds.), *Conceptual models for nursing practice* (2nd ed.). New York: Appleton-Century-Crofts.

Rogers, M. E. (Speaker). (1980b). *The science of unitary man.* [Videotape]. New York: Media for Nursing.

Rogers, M. E. (1983). Science of unitary human beings: A paradigm for nursing. In I. W. Clements & F. B. Roberts (Eds.), *Family health: A theoretical approach to nursing care.* New York: Wiley & Sons.

Rogers, M. E. (Speaker). (1985). *The science of unitary human beings.* [Audiocassette recording from the Discovery International Conference in Pittsburgh, PA]. Louisville, KY: Meetings Internationale.

Rogers, M. E. (1986). Science of Unitary Human Beings. In V. M. Malinski (Ed.), *Explorations on Martha Rogers' science of unitary human beings* (pp. 3–8). Norwalk, CT: Appleton-Century-Crofts.

Rogers, M. E. (1988). Nursing science and art: A prospective. *Nursing Science Quarterly, 1*(3), 99–102.

Rogers, M. E. (1990). Nursing: Science of unitary, irreducible, human beings: Update 1990. In E. A. M. Barrett (Ed.), *Visions of Rogers' science-based nursing* (pp. 5–11). New York: National League for Nursing.

Rogers, M. E. (1992). Nursing science and the space age. *Nursing Science Quarterly, 5*(1), 27–34.

Rogers, M. E. (1994). The science of unitary human beings: Current perspectives. *Nursing Science Quarterly, 7*(1), 33–35.

Rush, M. M. (2000). Power, spirituality, and time from a feminist perspective: Correlates of sobriety in a study of sober female participants in Alcoholics Anonymous. *Journal of the American Psychiatric Nurses Association, 6,* 196–202.

Saba, V. K. (1996). *Home health care classification (HHCC): Nursing diagnoses & interventions* (HCFA Publication No. 17C-98983/3) [On-line]. Available: http://www.sabacare.com. Retrieved February 20, 2004.

Sackett, D. L., Straus, S. E., Richardson, W. S., Rosenberg, W., & Haynes, R. B. (2000). Evidence-based medicine: How to practice and teach EBM (2nd ed.). Philadelphia: Churchill Livingstone.

Safier, G. (1977). *Contemporary American leaders in nursing: An oral history.* New York: McGraw-Hill.

Sarter, B. (1989). Some critical philosophical issues in the science of unitary human beings. *Nursing Science Quarterly, 2*(2), 74–78.

Schorr, J. A. (1993). Music and pattern change in chronic pain. *Advances in Nursing Science, 15,* 27–36.

Shostrum, E. L. (1966). *Personal orientation inventory manual.* San Diego: Educational and Industrial Testing Service.

Smith, M. C. (1990). Pattern in nursing practice. *Nursing Science Quarterly, 3*(2), 57–59.

Smith, M. C. (1988). Perspectives on nursing science. *Nursing Science Quarterly, 1*(2), 80–85.

Smith, M. C., & Reeder, F. (1998). Clinical outcomes research and Rogerian science: Strange or emergent bedfellows? *Visions: The Journal of Rogerian Nursing Science, 6,* 27–38.

Tomasson, R. E. (1994, March 18). Martha Rogers, 79, an author of books on nursing theory. *The New York Times,* p. B8.

von Bertalanffy, L. (1968). *General system theory.* New York: George Braziller.

Whall, A. L. (1981). Nursing theory and assessment of families. *Journal of Psychiatric Nursing and Mental Health Services, 19*(1), 30–35.

Whall, A. L. (1989). The influence of logical positivism on nursing practice. *IMAGE: Journal of Nursing Scholarship, 21*(4), 243–245.

13

Newman's Theory of Health

Veronica F. Engle and Emily J. Fox-Hill

Margaret Newman's first book describing her theory of health, *Theory Development in Nursing,* was published in 1979. A second book that elaborated on her theory of health, *Health as Expanding Consciousness,* was subsequently published in 1986. A second edition appeared in 1994 and was re-released in 2000. Newman has written extensively for nursing journals, focusing on health as expanding consciousness, pattern of the whole, and the unitary-transformative paradigm. She has also described a model of differentiated nursing practice, formulated methodology for research as praxis, and advanced a focus for the discipline of nursing.

The emphasis of Newman's scholarly activities gradually evolved from theory development and elaboration to include theory application in research and practice. A corresponding emphasis by nurse researchers using Newman's theory of health took place, from the initial quantitative study of the theory's major concepts (consciousness, movement, space, and time) to more qualitative examinations of health as expanding consciousness and pattern of the whole (Engle, 1996).

Margaret Newman's early professional and personal activities, as described by Engle (1983, 1989, 1996), appear fundamental to the development of her theory. She has subsequently maintained a sustained focus on theory elaboration and application. She retired from active teaching in 1995 and is Professor Emeritus of nursing at the University of Minnesota. The Margaret A. Newman Collection is located at the library of the University of Tennessee Health Science Center in Memphis, TN (Nollan, 2000).

BASIC CONSIDERATIONS INCLUDED IN THE MODEL

Newman's (1979, 1986, 1994a) theory of health focuses on health as expanding consciousness and on the relationships among the concepts of consciousness, movement, space, and time, as they interact as a *pattern of the whole.* Consequently, less emphasis is placed on the other commonly accepted concepts of nursing theories: person, environment, and nursing. This focus on health is consistent with Newman's (1979) belief that nursing theories should focus on the life process, aspects of the life process related to health, and actions facilitating health. Discussion of the major paradigm concepts found in nursing models—health, person, environment, and nursing—will be presented first, followed by discussion of the concepts of pattern, consciousness, movement, space, and time.

Definition of Health

Newman's (1979, 1986) definition of health is the most complex and fully developed of all of her concepts. This emphasis on health is consistent with Newman's (1979, p. 55) stated purpose of defining the focus of nursing via "a precise conceptualization of the nature of health—in order to specify theory which relates to that phenomenon." Newman has defined both *health,* a "pattern of evolving, expanding consciousness regardless of the form or direction it takes" (Newman, 1986, p. 3), and *manifest health,* the health one manifests at any given time as "the explication of the underlying *pattern* of person-environment" interaction (Newman, 1994a, p. 11). Manifest health is linked to Bohm's (1973, 1980) theory of implicate order, which states that there is an invisible pattern of implicate order within the universe from which all tangibles, such as rigid objects and sounds, are unfolded or explicated. Thus one perceives explicated objects as primary via our senses; according to quantum physics, objects are secondary manifestations of patterns of energy and space rather than solid, separate constructions. All energy fields ultimately merge imperceptibly to form one unified whole or implicate order (Bohm, 1973, 1980). Thus, health reflects the larger pattern of the whole, the underlying pattern of person-environment interaction, and health encompasses both disease and nondisease (Newman, 1983b). The two antithetical concepts of disease and nondisease are fused, eliminating the current dichotomy between health and illness, because the "pattern of the individual that eventually manifests itself as pathology is primary and exists prior to structural or functional changes" (Newman, 1979, p. 57).

Newman's conceptualization of health as *expanding consciousness* appears to be a synthesis from Bentov (1977) on consciousness, Young (1976) on human evolution and choice, and Rogers (1970) and Bohm (1973, 1980) on energy field patterns and implicit wholeness. Bentov

(1977, p. 95) defined consciousness as "the capacity of a system to respond to stimuli." Newman reconceptualized Bentov's (1977) work by overlaying an information processing component and defining consciousness as "the informational capacity of the system: the capacity of the system to interact with its environment" (Newman, 1986, p. 33). Information is necessary for choice, and Young's (1976) theory postulated that, through choice, human beings move from potential freedom to real freedom. Newman (1986) applied Young's (1976) framework, depicting humans as moving from a point of potential conscious through time and space, into infinite space and timelessness, toward absolute consciousness. The movement of humans toward absolute consciousness is in accord with Rogers' (1970) description of the life process as evolving unidirectionally and negentropically, and with Bohm's (1973, 1980) implicate order, out of which all field patterns emerge. Therefore, health is defined as expanding consciousness, a process that is facilitated through *pattern recognition.*

Definition of Person and Environment

Newman (1979) implicitly describes person and environment within the context of the life process. Although there is limited discussion of the *life process* in Newman's (1979, 1986, 1994a) books, the reader may assume that Newman uses life process in a manner consistent with Rogers' (1970) model for nursing. Both Newman and Rogers emphasize *open systems, pattern, wholeness,* and *space-time relativity* (Sarter, 1988; Newman, 1997a), as well as organization, rhythmicity, and unidirectionality. Within the context of the life process, person and environment are defined as coextensive energy fields that evolve simultaneously, moving toward increasing complexity and diversity that is manifested by rhythmic patterns along the dimensions of space and time (Rogers, 1970). All aspects of the person and environment are explicated out of the implicate order and form an unbroken whole of interfacing energy fields (Bohm, 1973, 1980). Person is defined as consciousness (Newman, 1994a), and an individual is identified by his or her pattern. "It is not the substance of our bodies that identifies the person; it is the pattern that identifies the person. . . pattern. . . can be identified across space and time" (Newman, 1990c, p. 132). Consciousness is a quality both of persons and of the environment: "Matter is the vibrating, changing component of pure consciousness" (Newman, 1994a, p. 36).

Definition of Nursing

Nursing was described briefly as nursing theory, nursing science, nursing action, and nursing goal in Newman's (1979) first book, reflecting the theory's early stage of development. Newman's theory of health subsequently defined nursing practice as a process of mutual nurse-client interaction for the purpose of pattern identification and augmentation (Newman, 1986), and the essence of nursing practice as the expansion of consciousness (Newman, 1997a). In contrast to the definition of health in Newman's theory, Newman, Sime, and Corcoran-Perry (1991, p. 3) defined the focus of the discipline of nursing as "the study of caring in the human health experience".

Newman (1990c) focuses on the process of nursing assessment rather than on nursing intervention, stressing the importance of assessment that is nondirective and that involves the client as a coparticipant in the process of pattern identification. The nurse assists in identifying the client's pattern (Newman, 1990c) and, as part of this process, enhances the client's pattern by bringing it into focus (Newman, 1983a). The nurse moves inward and focuses on his or her bodily feelings and inner experiences that mirror the client's inner experiences, thus gathering information about the client via the interference pattern of coextensive energy fields representing the nurse-client interaction (Newman, 1989b). The interaction of nurse and client fields is conceived to be similar to the interference pattern of light rays creating a hologram and is illustrated by sets of overlapping concentric circles around both the nurse and client.

Intervention becomes an extension of the holographic assessment process, with the patterns of the nurse and of the client interfacing in such a way that both individuals are transformed. As a manifestation of a person's overall pattern, disease may assist individuals in becoming aware of the nature of their patterns. As part of the nursing assessment process, Newman (1990c, p. 137) later stated: "We have to be able to allow the clients to make decisions that may go against the predominant values of the medical system . . . we have to learn to let go of our own agenda and get in touch with where they are in this process of expanding consciousness and allow them to make their own choices and follow their own directions." Thus, nursing practice departs from the allopathic paradigm of goals, interventions, and outcomes.

Definitions of Other Concepts

Newman (1979, 1986) presented four concepts (*consciousness, movement, space, time*) that provide a framework from which to view health in her two theory books, emphasizing the concept of consciousness. In her second theory book, *pattern* was included as a fifth concept (Newman, 1986). Although not depicted as a component of Newman's original framework, pattern serves as the context for her theory. The four concepts were described by the following relational propositions, which provide a general focus to orient the reader rather than serving as specific definitions:

1. Time and space have a complementary relationship.
2. Movement is a means whereby space and time become a reality.
3. Movement is a reflection of consciousness.
4. Time is a function of movement.
5. Time is a measure of consciousness

(Newman, 1979, p. 60).

Newman (1979) previously used a tetrahedron to illustrate the relationships among the four concepts. The figure, however, only partially illustrated the complexity of her definition of health and the emphasis on health as expanding consciousness. Newman's (1986) second theory book clarified the relationship of health to consciousness, with greater articulation of movement, space, and time in relationship to each other and as manifestations of expanding consciousness and pattern of the whole. She related her theory to Young's (1976) theory of human evolution such that, through choice, one moves from the constraints of time and space into infinite space and timelessness toward absolute consciousness. Newman (1986, p. 46) stated that we "come into being from a state of potential consciousness, are bound in time, find our identity in space, and through movement learn the 'law' of the way things work and make choices that ultimately take us beyond space and time to a state of absolute consciousness." A final state of absolute consciousness is the state of unconditional love. The concepts of pattern, consciousness, movement, space, and time will be discussed, in turn.

Pattern. In Newman's (1979) first theory book, pattern was identified from the Rogerian perspective that "pattern and organization identify man and reflect his innovative wholeness" (Rogers, 1970, p. 65). An ongoing pattern of person-environment interaction was considered to exist prior to the structural and functional changes that mark the manifestation of physical pathology. In her second theory book, Newman (1986) used Bohm's (1973, 1980) theory of implicate order to support her earlier articulation of the nature of pattern and of the relationship of disease to nondisease within the pattern of the whole. *Pattern* was defined as having the characteristics of *relatedness, movement, diversity,* and *rhythm* (Newman, 1986). Patterning occurs through person-environment interaction and as a result of the interpenetration of human energy fields, leading to transformation (Newman, 1994a).

Consciousness. In her first book, Newman (1979) defined the concept of consciousness in relation to the brain's left and right hemispheres, energy fields, and development over time. Different dimensions of consciousness were illustrated by the left brain hemisphere's "analytical, sequence-perceiving processes [and the right brain hemisphere's] synthesis-oriented, symbolic intuitive modes" (Newman, 1979, p. 65).

Newman's definition reflected the neuropsychological literature of the day, which was beginning to address brain function in relation to consciousness (Pribram, 1976; Sperry, 1969). Bentov's (1977) index of consciousness, the ratio of subjective time to objective time, was used to measure consciousness.

In Newman's (1986) second book, consciousness becomes one of the most fully developed of the four concepts. She explicitly defines consciousness as "the informational capacity of the system: the capacity of the system to interact with its environment" (Newman, 1986, p. 33). Consciousness may be observed in the quantity and quality of responses to stimuli, and is related to health as the capacity to perceive alternatives and to respond to stimuli in a variety of ways (Newman, 1983b). Consciousness includes not only cognitive and affective awareness, but is also a body awareness that interconnects systems within living organisms, such as growth processes, the endocrine system, and the immune system (Newman, 1990a). The pattern of consciousness for mind and for matter differs only by the speed and intensity of energy waves.

Expanding consciousness, the process of evolving person-environment interaction, is the process of health. Person-environment interaction takes place within a network of consciousness that is coextensive with the greater consciousness of the universe. Newman states that expansion of consciousness may come in intuitive leaps (Newman, 1990b) or in fluctuations that catapult individuals to a higher level of organization and functioning (Newman, 1990a). She suggests that as higher levels of consciousness develop over time, there will be more interpenetration of the energy fields and "jumps in consciousness [will occur that] will be manifest as the ability to perceive and interact with phenomena not apparent to everyone" (Newman, 1983b, p. 168). Although these phenomena have been viewed traditionally as "paranormal," energy transfer from one system to another system is consistent with energy therapies such as therapeutic touch, Reiki, and Qi Gong; Aikido and other martial arts; and forms of meditation and yoga (Yamashita & Tall, 1998).

Movement. The definition of the concept of movement in Newman's (1979, 1986) first and second books is less well developed than the concepts of health and consciousness. Movement is "an essential property of matter [that both expresses] awareness of self [and serves as] a means of communication" (Newman, 1979, p. 62). *Movement patterns* take place at the quantum level (e.g., atomic and subatomic particles), microscopic level (e.g., nerve action potentials), or at the macroscopic level (e.g., everyday activities). Without movement, no physical objects could exist. Each individual has a unique pattern of movement, and this pattern is a holistic measure of person-environment interaction. Patterns of movement take place within a space-time matrix, and movement is a reflection of consciousness within the context of a larger consciousness. At an empirical level, movement reflects the organization of the individual's cognitive and emotional processes (Newman, 1979). Thus, there are patterns of physical movement, such as personal tempo (Newman, 1986), as well as movement patterns within the psychological and social domains. A movement in consciousness represents a choice point (Newman, 1997a, p. 23), when an individual recognizes that "the 'old rules' don't work anymore" and a choice must be made to transcend present life situations.

Space. Newman's (1979) definition of the concept of space is the least well developed of the four concepts of her theory of health. According to the theory of relativity, space and time have a complementary relationship such that the energy of motion and matter may be transformed into one another. The world actually consists of "a complicated network of interrelated changing events, as patterns of activity, with space aspects and time aspects" (Newman, 1979, p. 61). The complementarity of space and time at the quantum level may be applied to everyday events in which the "highly mobilized person lives in a world of expanded space and compartmentalized time" (Newman, 1983b, p. 167). Thus, in addition to three-dimensional space, space is also referred to as life space, personal space, and inner space.

Time. Newman's (1979, 1986) definition of the concept of time is also less well developed than the concepts of health and consciousness. Subjective time was defined as a function of the relationship of *awareness* of events, influenced by emotional state and attention to task, to *content* of events, influenced by external events, body movement, and metabolism (Newman & Gaudiano, 1984). Newman (1986) expanded the discussion of time in her second book to include time constraints of the hospital environment on clients' biologic rhythms, and perception of and control over the use of time. She stressed recognizing and respecting both the unique timing of clients, and their cultural differences in relating to time. For example, the linear model of objective time is dominant in Western culture and uses a 24-hour clock in which the past, present, and future follow one another in sequence. In contrast, the spatial model of subjective time is characteristic of Eastern culture and views the past, present, and future as a timeless whole of the ever-present present, emphasizing the continuity of time. The relationship between objective time and subjective time was demonstrated in Newman's initial quantitative evaluation of health patterns using objective time, of necessity; she later assessed health with qualitative methods.

INTERNAL ANALYSIS

The internal analysis of Newman's theory addresses assumptions, central concepts, consistency, adequacy, and significance. Each will be addressed in turn.

Assumptions

Many of the assumptions of Newman's theory of health (1979, 1986, 1994a) about wholeness, pattern, and increasing complexity are derived from Rogers' (1970) theory of nursing, and assumptions about life as a process of expanding consciousness are derived from Bentov (1977). Rogers defines person and environment as energy fields that are open systems, coextensive with the universe. The person is a unified whole, capable of abstraction, thought, sensation, and emotion, with the person's characteristics greater than the sum of his or her parts. Both the person and environment are continuously, mutually, and simultaneously interacting with each other, characterized by pattern and organization, rhythmicity, unidirectionality, and increasing diversity and complexity. These assumptions are most evident in Newman's (1979, 1986, 1994a) discussion of the concepts of health, consciousness, movement, space, time, and nursing.

Newman (1997a, p. 22) articulates the following assumptions of her theory:

- Health encompasses conditions known as disease.
- Disease can be considered a manifestation of the underlying pattern of the person.
- The pattern of the person that manifests itself as disease is primary and exists prior to structural and functional changes.
- Health is the expansion of consciousness.

Newman (1994a) assumes a relational paradigm for nursing practice rather than the instrumental paradigm of allopathic medicine, and application of the complementarity of space and time at the quantum level to everyday events. When describing the process of nursing assessment, she assumes that clients want to copartner with the nurse, clients will gain insight from pattern recognition, and clients will evolve through pattern recognition. More recently, she has acknowledged that clients may not recognize patterns or may not wish to act on insights gained from pattern recognition (Jonsdottir, 1998; Newman, 1989b; Newman & Moch, 1991). Newman assumes that nurses are skilled at pattern identification, and that there may not be reimbursement or time constraints on practice. She also assumes that persons develop expanding consciousness as part of the aging process (Newman, 1987), and that a person's consciousness expands rather than contracts throughout the lifespan (Silva, 1988).

Central Concepts

The central concepts of Newman's theory are *health* as *expanding consciousness* and *pattern of the whole*. Newman's theory of health as expanding consciousness is a grand theory, having relatively abstract concepts and propositions that cannot as readily generate or be tested empirically (Fawcett, 1995). Such theories are typically developed "through thoughtful and insightful appraisal of existing ideas or creative leaps beyond existing knowledge" (Fawcett, 1993, p. 19). Grand theories that are derived from conceptual models are capable of generating mid-range theories (Fawcett, 1999; Young, Taylor, & McLaughlin-Renpenning, 2001) because their global perspectives "serve as guides and heuristics for the phenomena of special concern at the middle-range level of theory" (Walker & Avant, 1988, p. 12). Newman's theory is integrally tied to and flows organically out of the conceptual framework in her first theory book (Newman, 1979; 1997a). Thus, there is potential to derive mid-range theories from Newman's theory of health.

Analysis of Consistency

External consistency is achieved if there is a shared worldview with other disciplines and with nursing (Fitzpatrick & Whall, 1996). Newman's theory is externally consistent with theoretical, philosophical, and scientific sources (Fawcett, 1993; Sarter, 1988) that emphasize pattern of the whole. Newman integrated concepts and propositions from the diverse disciplines of nursing (Krieger, 1979; Rogers, 1970); medicine (Moss, 1981); neuroscience (Pribram, 1986); anthropology (Bateson, 1979); biology (Sheldrake, 1981); chemistry (Prigogine, 1976; Prigogine, Allen, & Herman, 1977); physics (Bohm, 1973, 1980; Capra, 1982); philosophy (de Chardin, 1959; Young, 1976); and popular literature (Bentov, 1977). Capra (1982) supports the importance of this transdisciplinary integration by nursing. It is necessary to read works from these disciplines, however, to fully understand Newman's theory.

Although Newman's theory is not aligned with the scientific perspective of logical empiricism, it is externally consistent with the postmodern perspectives of pluralism, relativism, and diversity (Litchfield, 1999). Newman's theory also is externally consistent with nursing because the theory is linked to nursing's metaparadigm by the shared concept of health. The unitary-transformative paradigm of Newman's theory is externally consistent with nursing models of Rogers (1970, 1990), Leininger (1985, 1995), Parse (1981, 1998), Patterson and Zderad (1976, 1988), and Fitzpatrick (Fitzpatrick, 1983; Pressler, 1996).

Internal consistency is achieved if the propositions and concepts are consistent with one another and with the assumptions of the model (Fitzpatrick & Whall, 1996). Newman's theory is internally consistent because the propositions for the relationships among movement, space, time, and consciousness are consistent within the conceptual framework, the theory, and later work by Newman. Newman's theory and conceptual framework are linked by the proposition that recognition of personal patterns, both physical and mental or emotional, facilitates the person's ability to move through the dimensions of time and space toward expanding consciousness, and the final state of unconditional love. The propositions, however, are in different publications, and not all stated together in one publication (Fawcett, 1993). The central concepts of the theory, health as expanding consciousness and pattern of the whole, and the propositions linking these concepts, are used in an internally consistent manner in her conceptual framework and theory.

Semantic consistency is achieved if the concepts or phenomena have the same names, definitions, and meaning throughout the theory (Dubin, 1978; Fawcett, 1995). Newman's integration of compatible theoretical, philosophical, and scientific sources facilitates semantic consistency. Three concepts of the conceptual framework (time, space, and consciousness) are used with semantic consistency within both the conceptual framework and the theory of health. The concept of movement is semantically inconsistent. Movement is described as different processes, including quantum movement of subatomic particles; physical movement over distance; movement pattern or personal tempo; distancing movement that creates personal space; movement from a given pattern to a higher pattern or progress; and movement in levels of consciousness. The multiple meanings of movement are logically consistent, however, within the context of Bohm's (1973, 1980) holographic universe, in which the totality of the whole is reflected in each part, and within the perspective of Sheldrake's (1981) theory of morphogenetic fields and Prigogine's (1976) theory of dissipative structures.

Analysis of Adequacy

A theory is evaluated for *logical adequacy,* validity of the theory's assumptions and concepts; *empirical adequacy,* testability of the theory (Hardy, 1974); and *pragmatic adequacy,* use of a theory in practice (Fawcett, 1999). Newman's theory of health is logically adequate because the assumptions and concepts are drawn from many diverse disciplines, ranging from theoretical physics to philosophy, all representing the unitary-transformative paradigm and addressing pattern of the whole. Newman's theory of health, however, has limited empirical adequacy. Current research methods (Schorr & Schroeder, 1989) and conceptual differences between the dominant particulate deterministic research paradigm and Newman's unitary-transformative paradigm limit empirical testing of health as expanding consciousness at this time. All grand theories, however, have limited empirical adequacy. The strength of grand theory lies in pragmatic adequacy—the ability to generate practical solutions to real world problems (Silva & Rothbart, 1984), rather than in empirical adequacy (Fawcett, 1999). Newman's theory has pragmatic adequacy because it focuses on the process of nursing assessment and the "practice wisdom" of nurses, which enables development of mid-range theories through praxis (Litchfield, 1999; Newman, 1990a). It also provides a practice approach that facilitates nurse-client partnership, elucidates healthcare needs from the client's perspective, and articulates client patterns that are important in their chronic illness experience.

Analysis of Significance

A theory is significant if it has wide scope and complexity (Ellis, 1968). A theory has theoretical and social significance if it addresses phenomena of interest to the discipline of nursing (Fawcett, 1999). A theory has wide scope if "it covers and relates a number of smaller generalizations or concepts and provides at least a potential framework for ordering observations [whereas a theory has complexity if it treats] multiple variables or relationships, or the complexity of a single variable" (Ellis, 1968, p. 219). Newman's theory is significant because it is both wide in scope and complex. The theory focuses on health as expanding consciousness using the interrelated concepts of movement, space, time, and consciousness, within the context of person-environment interaction and pattern of the whole. Newman's theory also has theoretical and social significance because it focuses on health, one of the nursing metaparadigm's concepts, and addresses phenomena relevant to nursing practice.

EXTERNAL ANALYSIS

The external theory analysis evaluates the use of Newman's theory in research, practice, education, and nursing classification systems. Early quantitative research using Newman's theory of health tested relationships among the four concepts of consciousness, movement, space, and time that were emphasized in Newman's (1979, 1986) two books. Over time, research and practice shifted to focus on health as expanding consciousness, recognition of pattern of the whole, and qualitative research as praxis methodology. The convergence of research- and practice-based scholarly activities reflects the evolution of knowledge derived from Newman's theory, and the change in focus of nurse scholars toward humanism and holism (Litchfield, 1999; Silva & Rothbart, 1984).

Relationship to Nursing Research

Three phases of research using Newman's theory can be identified: the quantitative theory description phase, the qualitative theory application and research as praxis phase, and the transcultural qualitative theory application and research as praxis phase. The first phase, quantitative description, focused on the description of the relationships among the concepts of consciousness, movement, space, and time, and their relationship to personality characteristics such as depression and to processes such as physical exertion. The theory description phase paralleled the initial development of the theory in Newman's (1979, 1986) two books, and the early studies were summarized by Engle (1989, 1996). Nurse researchers during the theory development phase included Newman (1971, 1972, 1976, 1982), Newman and Gaudiano (1984), Tompkins (1980), Engle (1983, 1985), Mentzer and Schorr (1986), Schorr and Schroeder (1989, 1991), and Schorr (Schorr, 1993; Schorr, Farnham, & Ervin, 1991). Quantitative studies by these nurse-researchers, however, were not able to adequately investigate the complexity of health as expanding consciousness and pattern of the whole.

The second phase, qualitative theory application and research as praxis, is congruent with elaboration and application of Newman's theory to research and practice, with emphasis on health as expanding consciousness, the process of pattern recognition, and research as praxis methodology. Nurse researchers during the second phase include Newman (Newman & Moch, 1991), Moch (1990), Fryback (1993), Smith (1995), Smith (1997a, 1997b), and Weingourt (1998).

Newman developed research as praxis methodology in parallel with her philosophical evolution. Newman changed from logical empiricism (Hempel, 1965; Nagel, 1961; Scheffler, 1963) to historicism (Lakatos, 1968; Lauden, 1977), and the use of qualitative research methodology (Bramwell, 1984; Parse, 1981; Patterson & Zderad, 1976; Watson, 1979). Newman (1979) searched for holistic methods of nursing inquiry and selected a phenomenological hermeneutic-dialectic process (Guba & Lincoln,

1989; Newman, 1994a) that emphasized the search for meaning, authentic involvement of the nurse-researcher, and process as content.

Newman developed her research as praxis methodology, "a process of inquiry characterized by negotiation, reciprocity, and empowerment" (Newman, 1990a, p. 38), based on the work of Lather (1986). Newman's research as praxis method identifies and describes the client's pattern of expanding consciousness by "a) establishing the mutuality of the process of inquiry, b) focusing on the most meaningful persons and events in the interviewee's life, c) organizing the data in narrative form and displaying it as sequential patterns over time, and d) sharing the interviewer's perception of the pattern with the interviewee and seeking revision or confirmation" (Newman, 1990a, p. 40). Newman (1997a) identifies the clients' stage of function using her adaptation of Young's (1976) model of human evolution, and movement in consciousness occurs in accord with Prigogine's (1976) theory of dissipative structures, as the client moves through and beyond the point of choice. The process of pattern recognition is the content and product of the research, and the research uses a priori theory (e.g., Newman's theory of health) to interpret this process (Lather, 1986; Newman, 1990a; Ray, 1990). Thus, science is "a process of knowing, a process of challenging, and a continuing revolution" (Newman, 1983c; Silva & Rothbart, 1983).

Research as praxis is communicated to the larger nursing community, whereas practice is not (Newman, 1991). Research as praxis is supported by Carter (1992), who suggests that scholarship derived from both practice and research should be communicated to the larger nursing community. Nurse-researchers using research as praxis include Newman (Newman & Moch, 1991), Moch (1990), Lamendola (Lamendola & Newman, 1994), and Weingourt (1998).

The third phase, transcultural qualitative theory application and research as praxis, focuses on the process of client assessment in Japan, New Zealand, and Iceland. Newman's theory was used as the conceptual framework, and research as praxis as the methodology because both are congruent for use with different cultures (Litchfield, 1999; Yamashita, 1998). Use of Newman's theory in different cultures strengthens its application to practice (Endo, 1998). Nurse researchers conducting transcultural theory application and research as praxis research include Connor (1998), Endo (1998), Jonsdottir (1998), Yamashita (1998), and Litchfield (1999).

Research as praxis methodology, however, may have limitations when critiqued from the perspective of logical empiricism. First, the research process itself may alter the process of pattern identification and the client's pattern (Batey, 1991). Second, client patterns rather than the nurse's process of pattern identification are studied. This prohibits identifying how skilled

nurses identify patterns, characteristics of expert nurses, how nurse characteristics influence client patterns (Silva, 1988), and how pattern identification can be taught to novice practitioners. Third, macroscopic patterns of
person-environment interaction are studied rather than microscopic patterns.
This precludes evaluation of physiological phenomena at the cellular and
system level. Fourth, the practice setting may prohibit adequate time for pattern identification and this may influence the quality of pattern recognition.
Fifth, research as praxis methodology may be more appropriate for study of
clients and nurses who are abstract thinkers, are verbally fluent, are cogni-
tively intact, use a linear time perspective, are highly motivated, and share a
common culture with the nurse. Last, research as praxis may be more appropriate for small-scale studies that may limit generalizability of results.

Newman, conversely, has stated that we need to "let go of the false dichotomy of investigator and subject, nurse and client. . . The concept of
'objective' is obsolete, but so also is the concept of 'subjective.' Validity is
a function of the relationship of two (or more) persons" (Newman, 1994a,
p. 85). Using a unitary-transformative paradigm, the ongoing interaction of
all phenomena precludes the possibility of the researcher's remaining separate from whatever phenomena are being studied. If nursing is to be viewed
as a human science (Meleis, 1992), nursing research must address the meanings and values of the lived experience of the people to whom care is extended (Leininger, 1995; Mitchell & Cody, 1992; Newman, 1994b; Parse,
1981; Upton, 1999). Qualitative methods such as hermeneutic phenomenology (Lincoln & Guba, 1985; Newman, 1994a), from which Newman's
research as praxis method is drawn, are appropriate because of their emphasis on clients' perspectives of phenomena of concern in their everyday
lives (Holstein & Gubrium, 1994; Young et al., 2001). In phenomenology,
the researcher and the informant interact by reflecting on the experience being studied such that the researcher becomes part of the nurse-client experience (Boyd, 1993). Thus, the logical empiricist principle of detachment
from the condition under study violates an important tenet of phenomenology and is inappropriate for consideration within a phenomenological research design. Thus, research as praxis methodology is more appropriate
than quantitative research methods for use with Newman's theory.

Newman previously espoused a metaparadigmatic disciplinary focus
that subsumed and transcended disparate paradigmatic perspectives
(Newman et al., 1991). She now states that the discipline of nursing is at a
choice point and needs to "break with a paradigm of health that focuses on
power, manipulation, and control and move on to one of reflective, compassionate consciousness," one that embraces wholeness and pattern (Newman,
1997b, p. 37). She implies that there should be only one paradigm and only
one research method. This is in contrast, however, to the assumption that dif-

ferent theories and research methods are better suited to answer different types of nursing questions (Chinn & Kramer, 1999; Fawcett, Watson, Neuman, Walker, & Fitzpatrick, 2001; Munhall, 1993; Oiler; 1982; Pribram, 1986).

Relationship to Nursing Practice

Principles from Newman's theory of health have been applied to practice at the individual practitioner level and at the healthcare organization level. In general, nurses use a process model to evaluate client patterns over time, looking for client learning and insight as evidence of movement in consciousness. Nurses have used Newman's principles to assess family patterns (Connor, 1998; Litchfield, 1999); to organize North American Nursing Diagnosis Association (NANDA) nursing diagnoses in parish nursing (Gustafson, 1990); to facilitate knowledge of personal patterns among students with juvenile diabetes (Schlotzhauer & Farnham, 1997); to understand the experience of primary family caregivers with a schizophrenic relative (Yamashita, 1998); to generate a model of bereavement (Solari-Twadell, Bunkers, Wang, & Snyder, 1995); and to facilitate clinical management of preterm labor in women's high-risk pregnancy (Kalb, 1990). Although Newman's theory of health does not include interventions per se, use of the theory by individual practitioners may be appropriate for energy-based interventions that promote repatterning of the client's energy field (Engle, 1996), such as light (Ference, 1988), music (Schorr, 1993), or therapeutic touch (Engle & Graney, 2000; Yamashita, Jensen, & Tall, 1998).

Application of Newman's theory to case management in community nursing organizations in Arizona (Ethridge, 1991, 1997; Newman, Lamb, & Michaels, 1992; Schraeder, Lamb, Shelton, & Britt, 1997) and in New Zealand (Connor, 1998) has been described. Case managers' practice is described as "a) the nurse coming together with clients at critical choice points in their lives and participating with them in the process of expanding consciousness, b) rhythmicity and timing in the relationship, c) letting go of the need to direct the relationship, d) pattern identification as an essential element in the process, and e) personal transformation" (Newman et al., 1992, p. 408). The process of nursing assessment and delivering quality, cost-effective care is emphasized. Ethridge (1991, 1997) reports nurse and client satisfaction, decreased client healthcare utilization and expenditures, and increased client participation in health promotion activities.

Newman (1990c) describes a model of differentiated nursing practice with three levels of practice based on educational preparation. Nurses with advanced practice skills, such as clinical nurse specialists and nurse practitioners, should have postbaccalaureate preparation in a unitary-transformative paradigm. Team leaders and "charge" nurses should have baccalaureate preparation, and staff nurses should have a diploma or associate's degree preparation. Newman does not, however, address how nurses with different levels of practice would use her theory, what nursing assessment process skills they would need, or what are quality indicators for the nursing assessment process.

Relationship to Nursing Education

Newman (personal communication, November 9, 1993) previously stated that nursing students should be exposed to many nursing theories. As her theory has developed, she now supports use of one paradigm (Newman, 1997b). It is a challenge for undergraduate nursing education programs to use Newman's theory as the basis for their curricula. The theory does not articulate with the six American Nurses Association (ANA) nursing classification systems, licensure examinations, or the allopathic healthcare system, because it emphasizes the process of nursing assessment as an intervention, rather than interventions and outcomes. Newman's theory has been used to foster creativity in undergraduate students (Jacono & Jacono, 1996) and to provide a practice framework for undergraduate students in nursing homes (Weingourt, 1998). Newman's theory may be more appropriate for use with graduate nursing education programs and would be consonant with graduate curricula in holistic nursing. The University of Akron has incorporated aspects of Newman's theory into the philosophical and conceptual framework of their master's program (Hensley, Keffer, Kilgore-Keever, Langfitt, & Peterson, 1989).

Relation to Nursing Classification Systems

Newman (1983a, 1984) initially used the NANDA Nurse Theorist Group's framework to classify identified client patterns because the framework's dimensions of person-environment interaction were conceptually consistent with her unitary-transformative paradigm. However, the NANDA framework addresses patterns at a single point in space-time and is therefore *temporally* inconsistent with Newman's theory of health. Newman views pattern as constantly evolving at each point in space-time, with nursing assessment of a series of client patterns (Newman, 1994a). Rather than using the NANDA framework, Newman now diagrams a sequence of patterns over the client's lifetime, with a concentration on present patterns (Newman, 1989a).

Newman likewise does not use individual NANDA nursing diagnoses because they are conceptually inconsistent with her theory (Newman, personal communication, November 9, 1993). The NANDA diagnostic categories were derived from clinicians' observations, removed from the context of the environment that gave meaning to the observation (Newman, 1984), and placed within the context of the particulate deterministic paradigm prevalent in current nursing practice and education. Because the six ANA-approved nursing classification systems were developed using the particulate deterministic paradigm, none of the classification systems are applicable for use with Newman's theory. Thus, nurses using Newman's theory of health must be able to switch back and forth between the particulate deterministic paradigm and unitary-transformative paradigm (Newman, 1990b) or find a paradigm broad enough to incorporate differing perspectives and methods because a "paradigm that integrates different levels of reality would be consistent with the content of nursing practice" (Newman, 1990b, p. 234).

Relation to Theory-Driven, Evidence-Based Practice

Evidence-based clinical practice literature using the medical model emphasizes empirical results from quantitative research using the gold standard of the randomized clinical trial (Fawcett et al., 2001). This emphasis, however, devalues theory-based nursing practice (Fawcett et al., 2001; Ingersoll, 2000; Mitchell, 1999) and removes clinical research results from the context of the environment. Because nursing's metaparadigm recognizes and addresses individual needs (Ingersoll, 2000; Meleis, 1992; Mitchell, 1999), the definition of evidence-based nursing practice should be different from the definition used in the medical literature (Ingersoll, 2000, p. 152): "Evidence based nursing practice is the conscientious, explicit and judicious use of theory-derived, research-based information in making decisions about care delivery to individuals or groups of patients in consideration of individual needs and preferences." Fawcett et al. (2001) contend that a more comprehensive approach to evidence-based practice should use Carper's (1978) patterns of knowing in nursing (empirics, ethics, person, aesthetics) as separate types of nursing *theory,* which have equal weight (Stein, Corte, Colling, & Whall, 1998), contain content identified through different processes (Chinn & Kramer, 1999), and are supported through different types of evidence. Application of Newman's theory of health to the different patterns of knowing follows.

Empirics. The pattern of empirical knowing is grounded in quantitative research methods emphasizing use of aggregate data. Newman's theory has limited usefulness for the verification of empirical questions because reality is seen as a dynamic, relational *process* that is a unitary manifestation of an implicate order at any given moment (Newman, 1997b). Reality includes the see-touch, behavioral, and inner experience realms. The inner experience realm in which expanding consciousness occurs cannot be studied using reductionistic quantitative research methods that require division of the whole. Newman (1997b, p. 38) has stated directly, "We need to study the meaning of the whole. The nature of wholeness is such that it cannot be addressed by the scientific method as currently conceived."

Ethics. The pattern of ethical knowing focuses on the moral component of nursing knowledge, matters of obligation or what ought to be done by nurses (Carper, 1978). Newman's theory does not address ethics per se. Rather, it is her discussion of the use of her theory in practice that addresses nursing's beliefs and values. Newman emphasizes identification and support of an individual's values as a nursing value. This emphasis on individual self-determination may include supporting client values in opposition to the medical system's values or the nurse's values (Bramlett, Gueldner, & Sowell, 1990; Newman, 1990c). Use of Newman's theory to guide inquiry into nursing's values shifts the emphasis from inquiry about groups of nurses' values to an individual client's values, and thus provides a broader focus for ethical inquiry. Her theory is therefore particularly relevant for a cross-cultural and lifespan approach to knowledge development for theory-guided, evidence-based nursing practice.

Personal. The pattern of personal knowing is concerned both with the quality of interpersonal interactions, relationships, and transactions between the nurse and client, and with the nurse's and the client's knowing and encountering of self (Carper, 1978). This is the most difficult pattern of knowing to master and teach, and yet the most essential to understanding the meaning of health (Carper, 1978). Of the four patterns of knowing, Newman's theory of health and use of her theory in practice have the greatest relevance for advancing knowledge about personal knowing. Newman focuses on the *process* of nursing assessment during which the nurse seeks to be fully present with the client, learns what is meaningful in the client's life, conceptualizes the patterns of client stories of important moments, and reflects these patterns to the client (Newman, 1997a). During the assessment process, both the client and nurse are transformed as they learn about themselves and each other, and in doing so, identify knowledge for use in clinical practice.

Aesthetics. The pattern of aesthetic knowing is related to the art of nursing: integrating scattered details into an experienced whole, identifying significant needs expressed in a client's behavior, and seeing the unity of nursing actions and results (Carper, 1978). Carper (1978) identifies empathy, knowledge of another's unique felt experience, as an important mode for aesthetic knowing. Use of Newman's theory in practice with its emphasis on pattern, rhythm, attunement, partnership, and presence provides the foundation for aesthetic knowing. This knowledge enables the nurse to perceive what is right and comforting for the client and to provide that in a skillful way.

SUMMARY

Newman's theory of health is a grand theory that focuses on health as expanding consciousness, using the interrelated concepts of movement, space, time, and consciousness within the context of person-environment interaction and pattern of the whole. Nursing practice focuses on the process of mutual pattern recognition, involving the client as co-participant and evaluated using research as praxis methodology. Although current nursing classification systems are not applicable for use with Newman's theory, principles from the theory may be particularly useful for guiding graduate nursing curricula, especially holistic nursing. Newman's theory has external, internal, and semantic consistency. The theory's unitary-transformative paradigm has logical and pragmatic adequacy, yet limited empirical adequacy, with the greatest relevance for personal knowing. Newman's theory of health as expanding consciousness is visionary, proposing a relational paradigm for nursing practice that reflects the changing focus of nurse scholars toward humanism and wholeness.

REFERENCES

Bateson, G. (1979). *Mind and nature: A necessary unity.* Toronto: Bantam.

Batey, M. (1991). The research-practice relationship: Commentary and response. *Nursing Science Quarterly, 4,* 100–103.

Bentov, I. (1977). *Stalking the wild pendulum.* New York: Sutton.

Bohm, D. (1973). Quantum theory as an indication of a new order in physics. B. Implicate and explicate order in physical law. *Foundations of Physics, 3,* 139–168.

Bohm, D. (1980). *Wholeness and the implicate order.* London: Routledge & Kegan Paul.

Boyd, C. O. (1993). Phenomenology: The method. In P. Munhall & C. Boyd (Eds.), *Nursing research: A qualitative perspective.* New York: National League for Nursing Press.

Bramlett, M., Gueldner, S., & Sowell, R. (1990). *Nursing Science Quarterly, 3,* 156–161.

Bramwell, L. (1984). Use of the life history in pattern identification and health promotion. *Advances in Nursing Science, 7,* 37–44.

Capra, F. (1982). *The turning point.* New York: Simon & Schuster.

Carper, B. (1978). Fundamental ways of knowing in nursing. *Advances in Nursing Science, 1,* 13–23.

Carter, M. (1992, Fall). *The meaning of scholarship in nursing: Practice and scholarship.* Presented at the American Association of Colleges of Nursing Fall Semi-Annual Meeting, Washington, DC.

Chinn, P., & Kramer, M. (1999). *Theory and nursing: Integrated knowledge development* (5th ed.). St. Louis: Mosby.

Connor, M. (1998). Expanding the dialogue on praxis in nursing research and practice. *Nursing Science Quarterly, 11,* 51–58.

de Chardin, T. (1959) *The phenomenon of man.* New York: Harper & Brothers.

Dubin, R. (1978). *Theory building.* New York: Free Press.

Ellis, R. (1968). Characteristics of significant theories. *Nursing Research 17,* 217–222.

Endo, E. (1998). Pattern recognition as a nursing intervention with Japanese women with ovarian cancer. *Advances in Nursing Science, 20,* 49–61.

Engle, V. F. (1983). Newman's model of health. In J. J. Fitzpatrick & A. L. Whall (Eds.), *Conceptual models of nursing.* Norwalk, CT: Appleton & Lange.

Engle, V. F. (1985). The relationship of movement and time to older adults' functional health. *Research in Nursing and Health, 9,* 123–129.

Engle, V.F. (1989). Newman's model of health. In J. J. Fitzpatrick & A. L. Whall (Eds.), *Conceptual models of nursing* (2nd ed.). Norwalk, CT: Appleton & Lange.

Engle, V. F. (1996). Newman's theory of health. In J. Fitzpatrick & A. Whall (Eds.), *Conceptual models of nursing: Analysis and application* (3rd ed.). Stamford, CT: Appleton & Lange.

Engle, V. F., & Graney, M. J. (2000). Bio-behavioral effects of therapeutic touch. *IMAGE: Journal of Nursing Scholarship, 32,* 287–293.

Ethridge, P. (1991). A nursing HMO: Carondelet St. Mary's experience. *Nursing Management, 22,* 22–27.

Ethridge, P. (1997). Historical perspective: The Carondelet experience. *Nursing Management, 28,* 26–27.

Fawcett, J. (1993). *Analysis and evaluation of nursing theories.* Philadelphia: F. A. Davis.

Fawcett, J. (1995). *Analysis and evaluation of conceptual models in nursing* (3rd ed.). Philadelphia: F. A. Davis.

Fawcett, J. (1999). *The relationship of theory and research* (3rd ed.). Philadelphia: F. A. Davis.

Fawcett, J., Watson, J., Neuman, B., Walker, P., & Fitzpatrick, J. (2001). On nursing theories and evidence. *Journal of Nursing Scholarship, 33,* 115–119.

Ference, H. M. (1988). *The theory of motion.* Nursing Science Institutes Monograph. Carmel, CA: Nightingale Society.

Fitzpatrick, J. (1983). A life perspective rhythm model. In J. Fitzpatrick & A. Whall (Eds.), *Conceptual models of nursing: Analysis and application.* Bowie, MD: Robert J. Brady.

Fitzpatrick, J., & Whall, A. (1996). *Conceptual models of nursing: Analysis and application* (3rd ed.). Stamford, CT: Appleton & Lange.

Fryback, P. (1993). Health for people with a terminal diagnosis. *Nursing Science Quarterly, 6,* 147–159.

Guba, E., & Lincoln, Y. (1989). *Fourth generation evaluation.* Newbury Park, CA: Sage.

Gustafson, W. (1990). In M. E. Parker (Ed.), *Nursing Theories in Practice.* New York: National League for Nursing.

Hardy, M. (1974). Theories: Components, development, evaluation. *Nursing Research 23,* 100–107.

Hempel, C. (1965). *Aspects of scientific explanation and other essays in the philosophy of science.* New York: Free Press.

Hensley, D., Keffer, M., Kilgore-Keever, K., Langfitt, J., & Peterson, L. (1989). Margaret A. Newman model of health. In A. Marriner-Tomey (Ed.). *Nursing theorists and their work* (2nd ed.). St. Louis: Mosby.

Holstein, J., & Gubrium, J. (1994). Phenomenology, ethnomethodology, and interpretative practice. In E. Denizen & S. Lincoln (Eds.). *Handbook of qualitative research.* Thousand Oaks, CA: Sage.

Ingersoll, G. (2000). Evidence-based nursing: What it is and what it isn't. *Nursing Outlook, 48,* 151–152.

Jacono, B, & Jacono, J. (1996). The benefits of Newman and Parse in helping nurse teachers determine methods to enhance student creativity. *Nurse Education Today, 16,* 356–362.

Jonsdottir, H. (1998). Life patterns of people with chronic obstructive pulmonary disease: Isolation and being closed in. *Nursing Science Quarterly, 11,* 160–166.

Kalb, K. (1990). The gift: Applying Newman's theory of health in nursing practice. In M. E. Parker (Ed.), *Nursing theories in practice*. New York: National League for Nursing.

Krieger, D. (1979). *The therapeutic touch: How to use your hands to help or heal*. Englewood Cliffs, NJ: Prentice-Hall.

Lakatos, I. (1968). Changes in the problem of inductive logic. In I. Lakatos (Ed.), *The problem of inductive logic*. Amsterdam: North-Holland Publishing Co.

Lamendola, F., & Newman, M. (1994). The paradox of HIV/AIDS as expanding consciousness. *Advances in Nursing Science, 16,* 13–21.

Lather, P. (1986). Research as praxis. *Harvard Educational Review, 56,* 257–277.

Lauden, L. (1977). *Progress and its problems: Towards a theory of scientific growth*. Berkeley, CA: University of California Press.

Leininger, M. (1985). *Qualitative research methods in nursing*. Orlando, FL: Grune & Stratton.

Leininger, M. (1995). *Transcultural nursing concepts, theories, and practices* (2nd ed.). New York: McGraw-Hill.

Lincoln, Y. S., & Guba, E. G. (1985). *Naturalistic inquiry*. Beverly Hills, CA: Sage.

Litchfield, M. (1999). Practice wisdom. *Advances in Nursing Science, 22,* 62–73.

Meleis, A. (1992) Directions for nursing theory development in the 21st century. *Nursing Science Quarterly, 5,* 3.

Mentzer, C., & Schorr, J. A. (1986). Perceived situational control and perceived duration of time: Expressions of life patterns. *Advances in Nursing Science, 9,* 12–20.

Mitchell, G. (1999). Evidence-based practice: Critique and alternative view. *Nursing Science Quarterly, 12,* 30–35.

Mitchell, G., & Cody, W. (1992). Nursing knowledge and human science. Ontological and epistemological considerations. *Nursing Science Quarterly, 5,* 54–61.

Moch, S. D. (1990). Health within the experience of breast cancer. *Journal of Advanced Nursing, 15,* 1426–1428.

Moss, R. (1981). *The I that is we*. Millbrae, CA: Celestial Arts.

Munhall, P. (1993). Epistemology in nursing. In P. Munhall & C. Boyd (Eds.), *Nursing research: A qualitative perspective*. New York: National League for Nursing Press.

Nagel, E. (1961). *The structure of science: Problems in the logic of scientific explanation*. New York: Harcourt Brace & World.

Newman, M. (1971). *An investigation of the relationship between gait tempo and time perception*. Unpublished doctoral dissertation, New York University, New York.

Newman, M. (1972). Time estimation in relation to gait tempo. *Perceptual and Motor Skills, 34,* 359–366.

Newman, M. (1976). Movement tempo and the experience of time. *Nursing Research, 25,* 273–279.

Newman, M. (1979). *Theory development in nursing*. Philadelphia: F. A. Davis.

Newman, M. (1982). Time as an index of expanding consciousness with age. *Nursing Research, 31,* 290–293.

Newman, M. (1983a). Editorial. *Advances in Nursing Science, 5,* x–xi.

Newman, M. (1983b). Newman's health theory. In I. Clements & F. Roberts (Eds.), *Family health: A theoretical approach to nursing care*. New York: Wiley.

Newman, M. (1983c). The continuing revolution: A history of nursing science. In N. L. Chaska (Ed.), *The nursing profession: A time to speak* (pp. 385–393). New York: McGraw-Hill.

Newman, M. (1984). Looking at the whole. *American Journal of Nursing, 84,* 1496–1499.

Newman, M. (1986). *Health as expanding consciousness*. St. Louis: Mosby.

Newman, M. (1987). Aging as increasing complexity. *Journal of Gerontological Nursing, 13,* 16–18.

Newman, M. (1989a). Nursing's emerging paradigm: The recognition of pattern. In A. M. McLane (Ed.), *Classification of nursing diagnoses*. St. Louis: Mosby.

Newman, M. (1989b). The spirit of nursing. *Holistic Nursing Practice, 3,* 1–6.

Newman, M. (1990a). Newman's theory of health as praxis. *Nursing Science Quarterly, 3,* 37–41.

Newman, M. (1990b). Nursing paradigms and realities. In N. L Chaska (Ed.), *The nursing profession: Turning points*. St. Louis: Mosby.

Newman, M. (1990c). Shifting to a higher consciousness. In M. E. Parker (Ed.), *Nursing theories in practice*. New York: National League for Nursing.

Newman, M. (1991). The research-practice relationship: Commentary and response. *Nursing Science Quarterly, 4,* 100–103.

Newman, M. (1992). Prevailing paradigms in nursing. *Nursing Outlook, 40,* 10–14.

Newman, M. (1994a). *Health as expanding consciousness* (2nd ed.). New York: National League for Nursing Press.

Newman, M. (1994b, Winter). Theory for nursing practice. *Nursing Science Quarterly, 7,* 153–157.

Newman, M. (1997a). Evolution of the theory of health as expanding consciousness. *Nursing Science Quarterly, 10,* 22–25.

Newman, M. (1997b). Experiencing the whole. *Advances in Nursing Science, 20,* 34–39.

Newman, M. (2000). *Health as expanding consciousness*. Sudbury, MA: Jones and Bartlett.

Newman, M., & Gaudiano, J. (1984). Depression as an explanation for decreased subjective time in the elderly. *Nursing Research, 33,* 137–139.

Newman, M., Lamb, G., & Michaels, C. (1992). Nursing case management: The coming together of theory and practice. *Nursing and Health Care, 12,* 404–408.

Newman, M., & Moch, S. (1991). Life patterns of persons with coronary heart disease. *Nursing Science Quarterly, 4,* 161–167.

Newman, M., Sime, A. M., & Corcoran-Perry, S. A. (1991). The focus of the discipline of nursing. *Advances in Nursing Science, 4,* 1–6.

Nollan, R. (2000). *Margaret A. Newman Collection: Database and inventory*. University of Tennessee Health Sciences Library and Biocommunications Center Historical Collections. Retrieved from http://library.utmem.edu/HSLBC/history/Displays/Newman/man_exhib.htm. Accessed 2/28/04.

Oiler, C. (1982). The phenomenological approach in nursing research. *Nursing Research, 31,* 178–181.

Parse, R. (1981). *Man-living-health: A theory of nursing*. New York: Wiley.

Parse, R. (1998). *The human becoming school of thought*. Thousand Oaks, CA: Sage.

Patterson, J., & Zderad, L. (1976). *Humanistic Nursing*. New York: Wiley.

Patterson, J., & Zderad, L. (1988). *Humanistic nursing*. New York: National League for Nursing.

Pressler, J. (1996). Fitzpatrick's rhythm model. In. J. J. Fitzpatrick & A. L. Whall (Eds.), *Conceptual models of nursing: Analysis and application* (3rd ed.). Stamford, CT: Appleton & Lange.

Pribram, K. (1976). Problems concerning the structure of consciousness. In G. Globus, B. Maxwell, & I. Savodnik (Eds.), *Consciousness and the brain: A scientific and philosophic inquiry*. New York: Plenum Press.

Pribram, K. (1986). The cognitive revolution and mind/brain issues. *American Psychologist, 41,* 507–520.

Prigogine, I. (1976). Order through fluctuation: Self-organization and social system. In E. Jantsch & C. H. Waddington (Eds.), *Evolution and consciousness*. Reading, MA: Addison Wesley.

Prigogine, I., Allen, P. M., & Herman, R. (1977). Long-term trends in the evolution of complexity. In E. Laszlo & J. Bierman (Eds.), *Goals in a global community: The original background papers for goals for mankind* (Vol. 1). New York: Pergamon.

Ray, M. (1990). Critical reflective analysis of Parse's and Newman's research methodologies. *Nursing Science Quarterly, 3,* 44–46.

Rogers, M. (1970). *An introduction to the theoretical basis of nursing.* Philadelphia: F. A. Davis.

Rogers, M. (1990). Nursing: Science of unitary, irreducible human beings: Update 1990. National League for Nursing NY, NY Pub. No. 15-2285.

Sarter, B. (1988). Philosophical sources of nursing theory. *Nursing Science Quarterly, 1,* 52–59.

Scheffler, I. (1963). *The anatomy of inquiry: Philosophical studies in the theory of science.* New York: Alfred A. Knopf.

Schlotzhauer, M., & Farnham, R. (1997). Newman's theory and insulin dependent diabetes mellitus in adolescence. *Journal of School Nursing, 13,* 20–23.

Schorr, J. A. (1993). Music and pattern change in chronic pain. *Advances in Nursing Science, 15,* 27–36.

Schorr, J. A., Farnham, R. C., & Ervin, S. M. (1991). Health patterns in aging women as expanding consciousness. *Advances in Nursing Science, 13,* 52–63.

Schorr, J. A., & Schroeder, C. A. (1989). Consciousness as a dissipative structure: An extension of the Newman model. *Nursing Science Quarterly, 2,* 183–193.

Schorr, J. A., & Schroeder, C. A. (1991). Movement and time: Exertion and perceived duration. *Nursing Science Quarterly, 4,* 104–112.

Schraeder, C., Lamb, G., Shelton, P., & Britt, P. (1997). Community nursing organizations: A new frontier. *American Journal of Nursing 91,* 63–65.

Sheldrake, R. (1981). *A new science of life: The hypothesis of formative causation.* Los Angeles: Tarcher.

Silva, M. (1988). Health as expanding consciousness: Silva's analysis. *Nursing Science Quarterly, 1,* 136–138.

Silva, M., & Rothbart, D. (1984). An analysis of changing trends in philosophies of science on nursing theory development and testing. *Advances in Nursing Science, 6,* 1–13.

Smith, C. (1995). The lived experience of staying healthy in rural African-American families. *Nursing Science Quarterly, 8,* 17–21.

Smith, S. (1997a). Women's experience of victimizing sexualization, part I: Responses related to abuse and home and family environment. *Issues in Mental Health Nursing, 18,* 395–416.

Smith, S. (1997b). Women's experience of victimizing sexualization, part II: Community and longer term personal impacts. *Issues in Mental Health Nursing, 18,* 417–432.

Solari-Twadell, P., Bunkers, S., Wang, C., & Snyder, D. (1995). The pinwheel model of bereavement. *IMAGE: Journal of Nursing Scholarship, 27,* 323–326.

Sperry, R. (1969). A modified concept of consciousness. *Psychological Review, 76,* 532–536.

Stein, K., Corte, C., Colling, K., & Whall, A. (1998). A theoretical analysis of Carper's ways of knowing using a model of social cognition. *Scholarly Inquiry for Nursing Practice, 12,* 43–60.

Tompkins, E. (1980). Effect of restricted mobility and dominance on perceived duration. *Nursing Research, 29,* 333–338.

Upton, D. (1999). How can we achieve evidence-based practice if we have a theory-practice gap in nursing today? *Journal of Advanced Nursing, 29,* 549–555.

Walker, L., & Avant, K. (1988). *Strategies for theory construction in nursing* (2nd ed.). Norwalk, CT: Appleton & Lange.

Watson, J. (1979). *Nursing: The philosophy of science and caring.* Boston: Little Brown.

Weingourt, R. (1998). Using Margaret A. Newman's theory of health with elderly nursing home residents. *Perspectives in Psychiatric Care, 34,* 25–30.

Yamashita, M. (1998). Newman's theory of health as expanding consciousness: Research on family caregiving in mental illness in Japan. *Nursing Science Quarterly, 11,* 110–115.

Yamashita, M., Jensen, E., & Tall, F. (1998). Therapeutic touch: Applying Newman's theoretic approach. *Nursing Science Quarterly, 11,* 49–50.

Yamashita, M., & Tall, F. (1998). A commentary on Newman's theory of health as expanding consciousness. *Advances in Nursing Science, 21,* 65–75.

Young, A. M. (1976). *The reflexive universe: Evolution of consciousness.* San Francisco: Robert Briggs.

Young, A., Taylor, S., & McLaughlin-Renpenning, K. (2001). *Connections: Nursing research, theory, and practice.* St. Louis: Mosby.

14

Watson's Model of Caring

Ann C. Glasgow and Diana Lynn Morris

Jean Watson's leadership as a scholar in human caring theory, human science, and caring science has been clearly established. With the publication of the postmodern transpersonal caring-healing paradigm, Watson (1999b) has transformed the original caring model into one that is useful to practitioners from nursing and other disciplines to guide clinical practice. By moving from the prevailing cure-disease paradigm to a caring model, the practitioner and client are empowered to be active participants in a caring-healing sacred moment by experiencing the quantum energy fields conducive to healing from a spiritual, mystical environment. In revisiting Nightingale's fundamental understandings of nursing, Watson gives credence to the integration of many of Nightingale's core principles to formulate an evolving transpersonal caring-healing paradigm supported by unitary caring science theory.

The theory of human caring, influenced by studies in nursing and social psychology, was developed in the late 1970s while Watson was a faculty member at the School of Nursing, University of Colorado. Watson earned a nursing diploma from Lewis Gale Hospital in Roanoke, VA; a bachelor's of science in nursing from the University of Colorado; a master's of science in psychiatric-mental health nursing from the University of Colorado; and a doctorate in Educational Psychology and Counseling from the University of Colorado. Dr. Watson is currently Distinguished Professor of Nursing and former Dean of the School of Nursing at the University of Colorado, and founder of the Center for Human Caring in Colorado.

Jean Watson is the recipient of honors from universities throughout the United States and many foreign countries. While Director of the Center for Human Caring, she established international affiliations with colleagues in the United Kingdom, Canada, New Zealand, Australia, Scandinavia, Brazil, Thailand, and Korea. Watson is a member of the American Academy of Nursing and has served as president of the National League for Nursing. In 1993, she received the National League for Nursing Martha E. Rogers Award, which recognized her as a nurse scholar who has made significant contributions to nursing knowledge to advance the science of caring in nursing and health sciences.

A plethora of publications can be credited to Watson. In 1979, Dr. Watson published *Nursing: The Philosophy and Science of Caring.* Continuing work on caring theory led to the publication of *Nursing: Human Science and Human Care* in 1985, with re-release in 1988 and 1999. Working with Bevis, Watson published *Toward a Caring Curriculum* in 1989, with a more recent reprinting in 2000, in which integration of caring science into the nursing curricula is described. In 1990, Leininger and Watson published *The Caring Imperative in Education.* Changes in Watson's theory are apparent in the 1999 book, entitled *Postmodern Nursing and Beyond* (Watson, 1999b), and the 2002 article, Caring Science and the Science of Unitary Human Beings: A Trans-Theoretical Discourse for Nursing Knowledge Development (Watson & Smith, 2002) which includes discussion of caring-healing for advanced practice in nurse. In 2002, Watson published *Assessing and Measuring Caring in Nursing and Health Science* (Watson, 2002a). Throughout her writings, Watson encourages all practitioners to focus on an integral caring-healing paradigm that emphasizes the spiritual aesthetics linked to caring, intentionality, and energy of the practitioner's power in healing and caring.

BASIC ELEMENTS

The main theme of Watson's theory has been based on her experiences and philosophical foundation in phenomenological-existential-spiritual dimensions of humanness. In the later writings she developed an intellectual blueprint that was transdisciplinary in nature and, thus, relevant to all health care professionals (Watson, 1999b). Accordingly, Boyd and Mast (1989) emphasized the globalization of Watson's model and its relevance as a broad conceptual model that guides human care concepts in the development of theories.

Boykin and Schoenhofer (1993) identified three caring knowledge categories as ontological, anthropological, and ethical caring. Subsequently, Swanson (1999) and Sherwood (1997) emphasized the ethical aspects and outcomes of caring in nursing. With more emphasis on caring knowledge, Watson and Smith (2002) acknowledged caring knowledge and ways of being effective in both personal and professional practices for patients and nurses. Watson considers caring as an ethical, ontological, and epistemological development requiring consistent exploration and expansion, as exemplified in her latest publications (Watson, 1999a & b, 2002a & b).

Definition of Nursing

According to Watson (1999a), nursing as a profession is undergoing de-construction from unreal loyalties and masculine principles prevailing within the medical paradigm. This reconstructed nursing understanding in-cludes new definitions and themes. These are unity of mind, body, and spirit; inner human potential and inner healing processes; healing environ-ments; expanding consciousness and human-environment-nature-universe field and energy source; and spirituality and soul care that interconnects feminine principles with the sacred universe.

In Watson's (1979) earlier writings, "nursing is concerned with pro-moting health, preventing illness, caring for the sick, and restoring health" (p. 7). From this view, she saw nursing focusing on *prevention, promotion,* and *rehabilitation.* Later, nursing science is defined as "a human science of persons and human health-illness-healing experiences that are mediated by professional, scientific, esthetic, and ethical human care transactions" (Watson, 1989, p. 221). Thus, the interaction between nurse and patient is fundamental. It is through this interaction that the nurse's goal was to as-sist the person in exploring the meaning of their health-illness experiences and assist the nurse and person in obtaining a higher degree of harmony within self to produce self-knowledge, self-reverence, self-healing, and self-care (Watson, 1989; George, 2001).

The transformation of the caring model for nursing with new defin-ing principles emerged in Watson's more recent publications. The follow-ing structure emerged from the feminine principles manifested in the developing caring-healing paradigm: "the result: nursing, both manifest-ing and simultaneously transcending its caring-healing paradigm; the par-adox: nursing is no longer nursing, as we have know it within the modern era; it has become something else, more nursing, not less" (Watson, 1999b, p. 84). These principles embraced the philosophical and moral foundation of professional models of caring-healing practices that include:

> . . . honoring deeper, subjective meanings and feelings about life, liv-
> ing the natural inner processes and choices; considering the relational,
> intuitive and receptive rather than the separatist and disconnected ways

of knowing and being; honoring art, beauty and aesthetics together with science and technology; living, researching and practicing from a call motivated by love: a love of life, humans, nature and all living things; discovering ourselves through the forms of inquiry rather than a desire to control or know an isolated event which stands outside ourselves; incorporating intersubjectivity, feelings, unknowns, transcendence, mystery and even chaos into our life, work, and play; seeking nurturing, cooperation, multiplicity, relatedness, and harmony in our relations with self, others, nature and the planet; following an inner and outer vision of wholeness and healing.

(Watson, 1999b, p. 85)

Watson was critical of nursing being defined as "the way of doing caring" (Watson, 1999b, p. 131), forcing nursing to become an integral component of the technological aspects of health care. In the shift to a postmodern understanding, caring becomes an evolving ontology with a caring practitioner developing a caring consciousness that is central to the healing process. In reconsidering Nightingale's model, Watson found that the unique focus of nursing embedded in Nightingale's work is congruent with the redefined caring-healing principles of nursing. Watson proposes that "nurses will need to play a critical role in creating healing space, facilitating, if not creating and directing, ontological design projects whereby professionals, employees, patients, friends, family, volunteers, visitors, community members and any members of the public who enter the space will experience a transforming, regenerating, healing environment" (1999b, p. 257). Therefore, the postmodern nurse is challenged with ontological, ethical, and epistemological premises that embrace *coordination, mediation,* and *collaboration* with a broader range of practitioners. The nurse in essence becomes a "sacred architect" who is critical to the healing process.

Definition of Person

An emerging definition of person in a caring-healing paradigm has its foundation in the earlier developments of Watson's caring model. In 1985, Watson defined person as the *"locus of human existence,"* which is "dormant until touched and activated by a rising spiritual power" (Watson, 1999b, p. 162). A person is a *"being-in-the-world"* having the capacity for experiencing and perceiving (Watson, 1989). Watson focused on the spiritual essence of the human being that transcends time and space. In recent work, Watson (1999a; 1999b) describes the transformation of the person from the body-physical to a metaphysical level based on Campbell's "kundalini," Myss's "chakra system," and Grey's art in "Sacred Mirrors" (Watson, 1999a; 1999b). Within a postmodern paradigm, a person begins with centering on self to reach a level in which the body connects with the soul. As Watson (1999b) stated, "eventually, mind, body and soul are embodied in one moment of being which is the goal of life and practice within the transpersonal paradigm. One then becomes more aware of the need for on-going spiritual, ontological development" (p. 175).

Definition of Health

Watson's (1979) original definition of health was founded on the World Health Organization's definition of health as: "The positive state of phys-ical, mental and social well-being with the inclusion of three elements:

1. A high level of overall physical, mental, and social functioning.
2. A general adaptive-maintenance level of daily functioning.
3. The absence of illness (or the presence of efforts that lead to its absence)"

(p. 220).

As her thinking evolved, Watson conceived of health as an experience of the whole person that included physical, esthetic, and moral domains (Watson, 1989). Disharmony represented an imbalance within the mind, body, and soul, and was equivalent to illness. Health then reflected as the unity and harmony between self and others, and self and nature (Watson, 1989).

Accordingly, Rafael (2000) acknowledged "the centrality of empow-erment to health promotion as clear in the WHO definition as it is in Watson's assertion that caring involves helping a person gain more self-knowledge, self-control, and readiness for self-healing" (p. 35). Based on Nightingale's foundations of health informed by postmodern thought, Watson viewed health residing in different frameworks than those of con-ventional medical treatment models (Watson, 1999b). For example Watson notes that Rogers proposed that more drugs, more technology, and more hospitals would not provide answers for health (1999a & b). Postmodern recognition of different theoretical models suggests that health is more than unity and harmony. In fact, health emerges from transformational ex-periences that give new meaning to self-actualization as a journey of dis-covery in search of peace within the spiritual realm.

Definition of Environment

In 1979, Watson stated, "Caring has existed in every society. Every soci-ety has had some people who have cared for others. A caring attitude is not transmitted from generation to generation through human genes. It is trans-mitted by the culture of the profession as a unique way of coping with its environment" (p. 8). She connected caring to the promotion of a "support-ive, protective, and/or corrective mental, physical, societal, and spiritual environment" (Watson, 1985, p. 75).

Watson has reconsidered her earlier conceptualization of environ-ment based on the foundations of nursing established by Nightingale, who gave special attention to the significant relationship between the environ-ment and healing (Watson, 1999a & b). Environment becomes more than the sterile environment that prevailed in conventional medicine and the-oretical foundations. The postmodern environment is a "caring-healing architecture" that is transformative and "resonates within the human soul and transcends whole being across time and conditions" (Watson, 1999b, p. 254). Within the context of the caring-healing paradigm, nurses are in-tegral to creation of transformative environments, and make explicit in consciousness the intentionality through which caring arts can potentiate wholeness. Influenced by Zukav's (1990) light and energy thesis, Watson viewed the nurse as the key to controlling the environment to promote higher energy fields conducive to healing. The environment then takes on an "ontological design framework for healing, wholeness, authenticity, relationship, consciousness and intentionality" (Watson, 1979, p. 255).

INTERNAL ANALYSIS AND EVALUATION

Metatheoretical Assumptions

Metatheoretical assumptions are premises and prepositional statements that conceptualize the foundation of the caring-healing paradigm. In 1979, Watson (pp. 8–9) proposed seven assumptions about the science of caring to form the framework of her human caring model:

- Caring can be effectively demonstrated and practiced only inter-personally.
- Caring consists of carative factors that result in the satisfaction of certain human needs.
- Effective caring promotes health and individual or family growth.
- Caring responses accept a person not only as he or she is now but as what he or she may become.
- A caring environment is one that offers the development of poten-tial while allowing the person to choose the best action for him or her at a given point in time.
- Caring is more "healthogenic" than is curing. The practice of car-ing integrates biophysical knowledge with knowledge of human behavior to generate or promote health and to provide ministrations

to those who are ill. A science of caring is therefore complementary to the science of curing.

- The practice of caring is central to nursing.

Watson (1985) described the basic concepts within the theory of human caring:

- Human caring is the moral ideal, the ethic of nursing; the intersubject human-to-human contact becomes a way of knowing self and other for both nurse and patient.
- Self is the process that synthesizes experiences and transforms what is perceived into knowledge as one is in the world.
- Transpersonal caring relationship is a specific type of professional, human-to-human contact having the goal of restoring the patient's experience of inner harmony with the release of feelings and thought transmitted and reflected in energy fields that potentiates transcendence.
- Phenomenal field is a subjective experience of the person, which represents the totality of human experience, of one's being in the world. A phenomenal field is created when nurse and person choose to engage in a transpersonal relationship.
- Caring occasion is a specific event such as engaging in a transpersonal caring relationship with its own unique phenomenal field.
- Carative factors are intervention processes or modalities used in a transpersonal caring relationship

(Watson, 1985).

Watson (1985) viewed caring as the most valuable attribute nursing has to offer to humanity. She contended that caring can assist the person to gain control, become knowledgeable, and promote health changes (George, 2001). Watson (1985) emphasized a humanistic value system as the foundation of the philosophy of caring and the transpersonal caring relationship:

- Having deep respect for the wonders and mysteries of life.
- Recognizing the power of humans to grow and change.
- Acknowledging a spiritual dimension of life.
- Acknowledging the internal power of the human care process.
- Having high regard and reverence for the spiritual-subjective sense of the person.
- Placing high values on how the person (patient and nurse) is perceived and experiencing health-illness conditions.
- Holding nonpaternalistic values that recognize human autonomy and freedom of choice.

- Emphasizing helping a person gain more self-knowledge, self-control, and readiness for self-healing regardless of the present health-illness condition.
- Placing high value on the relationship between the nurse and the person.
- Recognizing the nurse as a coparticipant in the human care process (pp. 34–35).

Watson made the following 11 assumptions about the human care model:

- Care and love are the most universal and the most mysterious of cosmic forces which comprise primal and universal psychic energy.
- Often the need for love and care is overlooked; or we know that people need each other in loving and caring ways, but often do not behave well toward each other. If we are to sustain our humanity, however, we need to become more caring and loving, to nourish our humanity and evolve as a civilization.
- Because nursing is a caring profession, its ability to sustain its caring ideal and ideology in practice will affect the development of civilization and determine nursing's contribution to society.
- We first have to impose our will to care and love upon ourselves. We have to treat ourselves with gentleness and dignity before we can respect and care for others with gentleness and dignity.
- Nursing has always held a human care and caring stance in regard to people with health-illness concerns.
- Caring is the essence of nursing and the most central and unifying focus of nursing practice.
- Human care, at the individual and group levels, is receiving less and less emphasis in the healthcare delivery system.
- The quality of caring has been devalued; therefore, sustaining human care ideals and a caring ideology in nursing practice and in society is critical. The human care role is threatened by increasingly sophisticated medical technology and bureaucratic-managerial institutional constraints. At the same time, radical treatment techniques have proliferated, often without regard to costs.
- Preservation and advancement of human care as both an epistemic and a clinical endeavor is a significant issue for nursing today and in the future.
- Human care can be effectively demonstrated and practiced only interpersonally. The Intersubjective human process keeps alive a common sense of humanity; it teaches us how to be human by identifying ourselves with others, whereby the humanity of one is reflected in the other.

- Nursing's social, moral, and scientific contributions to humankind lie in its commitment to human care ideals in theory, practice, and research (1985, pp. 32–33).

In addition to these assumptions, Watson delineated seven basic premises of the human care model:

- A person's mind and emotions are windows to the soul. Nursing care can be and is physical, procedural, objective, and factual, but at the highest level of nursing the nurse's human care responses, the human care transactions, and the nurse's presence in the relationship transcend the physical and material world, bound in time and space, and made contact with the person's emotional and subjective world as the route to the inner self and the higher sense of self.
- A person's body is confined in time and space, but the mind and soul are not confined to the physical universe. One's higher sense of mind and soul transcends time and space and helps to account for such notions as the collective unconscious, causal past, mystical experiences, parapsychological phenomena, and a higher sense of power, and may be an indicator of spiritual evolution.
- A nurse may have access to a person's mind, emotions, and inner self indirectly through any sphere—mind, body, or soul—provided the physical body is not perceived or treated as separate from the mind and emotions and the higher sense of self (soul).
- The spirit, inner self, or soul (geist) of a person exists in and for itself. The spiritual essence of the person is related to the human ability to be free, which is an evolving process in human development. The ability to develop and experience one's essence freely is limited by the extent of others' ability to "be." The destiny of one's being is to develop the spiritual essence of self, to become more Godlike. However, each person has to question his or her own essence and moral behavior toward others, because if people are dehumanized at a basic level such as a human care level, that dehumanizing process is not capable of reflecting humanity.
- People need the care and love of others. Love and caring are the two universal givens. We need to become more loving, caring, and moral to nourish our humanity, advance civilization, and live together. We need to love, respect, and care for ourselves and treat ourselves with dignity before we can respect, love, and care for others and treat them with dignity.
- A person may have an illness that is "completely hidden from our eyes." To find solutions it is necessary to find meanings. A person's

human predicament may not be related to the external world as much as to the person's inner world as he or she experiences it.

- The totality of experience at any given moment constitutes a phenomenal field. The phenomenal field is the individual's frame of reference and comprises the subjective internal relations and the meanings of objects and subjects, past, present, and future, as perceived and experienced (1985, p. 50–51).

With the emergence of the reconstructed postmodern and beyond nursing (or medicine) model, Watson's (1999a) transpersonal caring-healing era III/paradigm III model was born based on the following major assumptions:

- Caring is based on an ontology and ethic of relationship and connectedness, and of relationship and consciousness.
- Caring consciousness, in relation, becomes primary.
- Caring can be most effectively demonstrated and practiced interpersonally and transpersonally.
- Caring consists of "caritas" consciousness, values, and motives. It is guided by carative components founded in earlier assumptions.
- A caring relationship and a caring environment attend to "soul care": the spiritual growth of both the one caring and the one being cared for.
- A caring relationship and a caring environment preserve human dignity, wholeness, and integrity; they offer an authentic presenting and choice.
- Caring promotes self-growth, self-knowledge, self-control, and self-healing processes and possibilities.
- Caring accepts and holds safe space (sacred space) for people to seek their own wholeness of being and becoming, not only now but also in the future, evolving toward wholeness, greater complexity and connectedness with the deep self, the soul, and the higher self.
- Each caring act seeks to hold an intentional consciousness of caring. This energetic, focused consciousness of caring and authentic presenting has the potential to change the field of caring, thereby potentiating healing and wholeness.
- Caring, as ontology and consciousness, calls for ontological authenticity and advanced ontological competencies and skills. These, in turn, can be translated into professional ontologically based caring-healing modalities.
- The practice of transpersonal caring-healing requires an expanding epistemology and transformative science and art model for further advancement. This practice integrates all ways of knowing. The art and science of a postmodern model of transpersonal caring-healing

is complementary to the science of medical curing, modern nursing, and medical practices (pp. 102–103).

Within the postmodern, transpersonal, caring-healing era III/paradigm III framework, Watson (1999a) makes these basic premises explicit:

- There is an expanded view of the person and what it means to be human—fully embodied, but more than body physical; an embodied spirit; a transpersonal, transcendent, evolving consciousness; unity of mind-body-spirit; person-nature-universe as oneness, connected.
- Acknowledgment of the human-environment energy field-life energy field and universal field of consciousness; universal mind.
- Positing of consciousness as energy; caring-healing consciousness becomes primary to the caring-healing practitioner.
- Caring potentiates healing, wholeness.
- Caring-healing modalities (sacred feminine archetype of nursing) have been excluded from nursing and health systems; their development and reintroduction are essential for postmodern, transpersonal, caring-healing models and transformation.
- Caring-healing processes and relationships are considered sacred.
- Unitary consciousness as the worldview and cosmology, such as viewing the connectedness of all.
- Caring as a moral imperative to human and planetary survival.
- Caring as a converging global agenda for nursing and society alike (pp. 129–130).

By 2002, caring knowledge was described by Watson and Smith as increasingly transdisciplinary. This led to further emergence and expansion of assumptions for caring science:

- Developing knowledge of caring cannot be assumed; it is a philosophical-ethical-epistemic endeavor that requires on-going explication and development of theory, philosophy, and ethics, along with diverse methods of caring inquiry that inform caring-healing practices.
- Caring science is grounded in a relational ontology of unity within the universe (in contrast to a separatist ontology that guides conventional science models); this relational ontology of caring establishes the ethical-moral relational foundation for care science (and for nursing) and informs the epistemology, methodology, pedagogy, and praxis of caring in nursing and related fields.
- Caring science embraces epistemological pluralism, seeking the underdeveloped intersection between arts and humanities and clinical sciences, that accommodates diverse ways of knowing, being-becoming,

evolving; it encompasses ethical, intuitive, personal, empirical, aesthetic, and even spiritual/metaphysical ways of knowing and being.

- Caring science inquiry encompasses methodological pluralism whereby the method flows from the phenomenon of concern, not the other way around; the diverse forms of caring inquiry seek to unify ontological, philosophical, ethical, and theoretical views, while incorporating empirics and technology (Watson & Smith, p. 6).

As a result of Watson's (Watson & Smith, 2002) efforts to embrace a model of knowledge development that encompasses spirit and healing and caring within a unitary paradigm, a unitary caring science has emerged that transcends a specific disciplinary perspective.

Central Components

The major conceptual elements of the original and emergent theory are the carative factors or the clinical caritas processes, the transpersonal caring relationship, and the caring moment or caring occasion. Watson (2002b) viewed the emerging model of transpersonal caring as evolving from carative to caritas processes that transcend conventional models of nursing, while simultaneously evoking both the past and the future. For example, the future of nursing is grounded in Nightingale's sense of "calling" guided by a deep sense of commitment and an ethic of human service so that members of the discipline cherish our phenomena, our subject matter, and those we serve. Thus, it is when we include caring and love in our work and our life that we discover and affirm that nursing, like teaching, is more than just a job, but a life-giving and life-receiving career for a lifetime of growth and learning. Maturation of the discipline that includes integration of past, present, and future leads to transformation of self, those we serve, and our institutions, including the profession.

As we more publicly and professionally assert these positions for our theories, our ethics, and our practices, even our science, we also locate ourselves and our profession and discipline within a new, emerging cosmology. Such thinking calls for a sense of reverence and sacredness with regard to life and all living things. It incorporates both art and science, as they are redefined, acknowledging a convergence between art, science, and spirituality. As we enter into the transpersonal caring theory and philosophy, we simultaneously are challenged to relocate ourselves in emerging ideas and question how caring-healing theory speaks to us. We are invited into a new relationship with self and beliefs about life, nursing, and theory. Thus, to engage in unitary caring science, the nurse clinician, nurse educator, and nurse scientist embraces a philosophy and way of life that is not limited to one's professional role. To live a healing-caring framework one is asked, if not enticed, to examine and explore the critical intersection between the personal and the professional; to translate one's unique talents, interests, and gifts into human service of caring and healing, concentric circles of caring—from individual, to others, to community, to world, to Planet Earth, to the universe" (p. 1).

For the postmodern paradigm, the 10 original carative factors are transformed into the following clinical caritas processes:

1. Formation of humanistic-altruistic system of values, becomes: "Practice of loving-kindness and equanimity within context of caring consciousness";
2. Instillation of faith-hope, becomes: "Being authentically present, and enabling and sustaining the deep belief system and subjective life world of self and one-being-cared-for";
3. Cultivation of sensitivity to one's self and to others, becomes: "Cultivation of one's own spiritual practices and transpersonal self, going beyond ego self";
4. Development of a helping-trusting, human caring relationship, becomes: "Developing and sustaining a helping-trusting, authentic caring relationship";
5. Promotion and acceptance of the expression of positive and negative feelings, becomes: "Being present to, and supportive of, the expression of positive and negative feelings as a connection with deeper spirit of self and the one-being-cared-for";
6. Systematic use of a creative problem-solving caring process, becomes: "Creative use of self and all ways of knowing as part of the caring process; to engage in artistry of caring-healing practices";
7. Promotion of transpersonal teaching-learning, becomes: "Engaging in genuine teaching-learning experience that attends to unity of being and meaning, attempting to stay within other's frame of reference";
8. Provision for a supportive, protective, and/or corrective mental, physical, societal, and spiritual environment, becomes: "creating healing environment at all levels, physical as well as non-physical, subtle environment of energy and consciousness, whereby wholeness, beauty, comfort, dignity, and peace are potentiated";
9. Assistance with gratification of human needs, becomes: "assisting with basic needs, with an intentional caring consciousness, administering 'human care essentials', which potentiate alignment of mind-body-spirit, wholeness, and unity of being in all aspects of care"; tending to both embodied spirit and evolving spiritual emergence;

10. Allowance for existential-phenomenological-spiritual forces, becomes: "opening and attending to spiritual-mysterious and existential dimensions of one's own life-death; soul care for self and the one-being-care-for"

(Watson, 2002b, p. 2).

Watson proposes that the clinical caritas framework is a transformation of the original caring model which emphasizes the merging of spirituality, an evocation of love and caring to provide new paradigm for the millennium. "This work posits a value's explicit moral foundation and takes a specific position with respect to the centrality of human caring, "caritas" and love as now an ethic and ontology, as well as a critical starting point for nursing's existence, broad societal mission, and the basis for further advancement for caring-healing practices found to be congruent with recent reports on health care and health professional educational reform, which call for 'centrality of caring-healing relationships' as the foundation for all health professional education and practice reform" (Watson, 2002b, pp. 1–2).

A transpersonal caring relationship is foundational to the caring-healing paradigm. According to Watson (2002b):

- The transpersonal caring relationship moves beyond ego-self and radiates to spiritual, even cosmic concerns and connections that tap into healing possibilities and potentials. Transpersonal caring seeks to connect with, embrace the spirit or soul of the other, through the processes of caring and healing and being in authentic relation, in the moment. Such a transpersonal relation is influenced by the caring consciousness and intentionality of the nurse as she or he enters into the life space or phenomenal field of another person, and is able to detect the other person's condition of being (at the soul, spirit level). It implies a focus on the uniqueness of self and other, and the uniqueness of the moment, wherein the coming together is mutual and reciprocal, each fully embodied in the moment, while paradoxically capable of transcending the moment, open to new possibilities.
- Transpersonal caring calls for an authenticity of being and becoming, an ability to be present to self and other in a reflective frame; the transpersonal nurse has the ability to center consciousness and intentionality on caring, healing, and wholeness, rather than on disease, illness, and pathology. Transpersonal caring competencies are related to ontological development of the nurse's human competencies and ways of being and becoming; thus

"ontological caring competencies" become as critical in this model as "technological curing competencies" were in the conventional modern, Western nursing-medicine model, now coming to an end.

- Within the model of transpersonal caring, clinical caritas consciousness is engaged at a foundational ethical level for entry into this framework. The nurse attempts to enter into and stay within the other's frame of reference for connecting with the inner life world of meaning and spirit of the other; together they join in a mutual search for meaning and wholeness of being and becoming, to potentiate comfort measures, pain control, a sense of well-being, wholeness, or even spiritual transcendence of suffering. The person is viewed as whole and complete, regardless of illness or disease (Watson, 1996, 2002, pp. 5–6).

- "A caring occasion occurs whenever the nurse and another come together with their unique life histories and phenomenal fields in a human-to-human transaction. The coming together in a given moment becomes a focal point in space and time. It becomes transcendent whereby experience and perception take place, but the actual caring occasion has a greater field of its own, in a given moment. The process goes beyond itself, yet arises from aspects of it that become part of the life history of each person, as well as part of some larger, more complex pattern of life. A caring moment involves an action and choice by both the nurse and other. The moment of coming together presents them with the opportunity to decide how to be in the moment, in the relationship—what to do with and in the moment. If the caring moment is transpersonal, each feels a connection with the other at the spirit level, thus it transcends time and space, opening up new possibilities for healing and human connection at a deeper level than physical interaction."

(Watson, 1985, pp. 59–60; 1996, p. 157)

The fundamental key to understanding human caring, transpersonal relationship and caring occasion is the spiritual nature of human beings. It is the spirit or soul of the person that strives for inner harmony. Harmony is experienced as health and human "becoming," as the inner strength and power of the human spirit are engaged and transcendent healing experiences occur. Transcendent healing results from a phenomenal field that goes beyond the event of an actual caring occasion. It is manifest in a field of consciousness. The transpersonal dimensions of a caring moment are affected by the nurse's consciousness in the caring moment, which in turn affects the field of the whole. The role of consciousness with respect to a holographic view of science includes these points:

- "The whole caring-healing-loving consciousness is contained within a single caring moment.
- The one caring and the one being cared for are interconnected; the caring-healing process is connected with the other human(s) and the higher energy of the universe.
- The caring-healing-loving consciousness of the practitioner or nurse is communicated to the one being cared for.
- Caring-healing-loving consciousness exists through and transcends time and space and can be dominant over physical dimensions." (Watson, 1999b, p. 111)

It is the caring-healing consciousness, "held as an intentionality and moral ideal during the transpersonal caring moment that directs practitioners and nurses toward new ontologies and epistemologies in developing postmodern theory and postmodern nursing science" (Watson, 1999b, p. 114). Furthermore, Watson connects intentionality with the concepts of consciousness, energy, and light prevalent in Zukav's metaphysical concepts, thus focusing on the power of the caring-healing consciousness and its relationship to energy, transcendence, and the postmodern caring-healing paradigm.

SUMMARY OF RELATIONSHIPS OF COMPONENTS

Watson's humanistic, existential, and metaphysical conceptualization of human beings informs her understanding of health and illness (Rafael, 2000). Human beings have been described by Watson as beings-in-the-world composed of mind-body-soul. More recently, Watson has embraced a unitary prospective of caring-healing that suggests an understanding of human beings as unitary phenomena rather than additive wholes. Health is harmony, while conversely, illness results from conscious or subconscious disharmony that may lead to disease. Inherent in Watson's conceptualization of human beings is the metaphysical potential for self-healing and transcendence to higher levels of consciousness. The person is an active agent of change responsible for allowing healing to occur. External agents, such as the nurse, may on occasion coparticipate in healing change (Rafael, 2000).

Watson notes that the soul or spirit is the essence and highest sense of the human being. Furthermore, actualization of spirit is the most basic human need (Rafael, 2000). Actualization of spirit expands one's consciousness and empowers the person to self-healing that can include intuitive and mystic experiences. For a transpersonal caring relationship to occur, the spirit of the person-patient and the spirit of the person-nurse are present to each other and mutually engage in the caring occasion moment using caritas processes. The caring occasion is an intra- and intersubjective experience that requires the nurse to be fully present and conscious, or awake to the other (person-patient) and the caring occasion. Thus the intentional evocation of love and caring by the nurse empowers the caritas processes and the actual caring occasion as the person-patient transcends to higher levels of consciousness and actualizes spirit self.

The clinical caritas processes are the core of nursing actions and facilitate therapeutic healing processes and the transpersonal relationship (Rafael, 2000). Both the nurse and person-patient are affected by the caritas processes. To use Watson's caring-healing paradigm, the nurse must explore and embrace the values and principles represented in the caritas processes. This requires self-exploration and self-knowledge and openness to living the paradigm both personally and professionally. Thus, the nurse seeks actualization of one's own spirit through evolving consciousness and self-healing in preparation for caring for others. Human caring based on human values such as kindness, concern, and love of self and others (Watson, 1985, 1989).

Human caring values are described in the caritas processes. Three are fundamental to the nurse's preparation: humanistic-altruistic systems of values, faith and hope, and sensitivity to others. For example, the humanistic-altruistic value system begins early in life and is influenced through interactions with others, including nurse-educators, and can be developed through consciousness raising and introspection (Rafael, 2000). In this sense, altruism is not self-sacrifice but expresses the fullness of being that allows the nurse to be authentically present with person-patients. Furthermore, the process of faith-hope interacts with humanistic altruism to enhance caring-healing.

Influenced by Carl Rogers, Watson asserted that a balanced sensitivity to one's self is necessary to empathetic knowing of the other (Rafael, 2000). Self-exploration and knowing is a life-long process that includes value clarification, self-reflection, self-acceptance and love, and spiritual actualization. Such self-knowing is the foundation for loving and accepting the human experience of others. As one's consciousness is raised and one recognizes a unitary ontology, the nurse, or person, becomes aware of the interconnectedness of all beings and experiences, thus transforming the nurse's practice and vision of what is possible.

Four caritas processes are reflected in the transpersonal caring relationship. These processes focus on interpersonal communication between nurse and the person-patient that is the basis of what is known as the therapeutic relationship (Rafael, 2000). Again Watson's thinking has been informed by Carl Rogers' discussion of the helping relationship that emphasizes the necessity for the care provider to be congruent, empathetic, and warm or caring. According to Watson, the transpersonal caring relationship is a helping-trusting, human care relationship based on intentionality and consciousness so that one is fully present and focused on the person's actualization of spirit.

The last five caritas processes describe assessment of the person-patient's health goals and evaluation effectiveness of the caritas processes on the transformative healing that evolves from the actual caring occasion (Rafael, 2000). The person-patient and nurse mutually engage in the processes that establish goals, identify needs, select actions, determine the role of the person-patient and nurse, and evaluate outcomes.

Rafael (2000) has proposed that each caritas process can be used for reflective, creative problem solving (e.g., the nursing process) to plan, direct, and evaluate care in clinical practice. The nurse provides professional expertise and guidance while facilitating the person-patient's active engagement, self-determination, and self-healing. The person-patient, not the nurse, is responsible and empowered through the transpersonal, therapeutic relationship for transformative self-healing. The nurse is a genuinely present, empathetic facilitator-guide.

In early work, Watson addressed mental, physical, social, and spiritual environments. Internal and external environments were described in particularistic terms that had characteristic factors such as comfort, privacy, safety, and clean aesthetic surroundings (Rafael, 2000). More recently, Watson revisited Nightingale's writings and reflected on the importance of creating an environment that facilitates health. Thus, in the explication of postmodern nursing, environment was conceptualized as the context for transformative healing to occur. In fact, Watson challenges nurses to create a healing environment that nurtures the caritas process during the actual caring occasion. Thus, Watson has developed a spiritual, healing environment. Drawing on sources such as Eastern philosophy, Hildegard von Bingen, and Alex Gray, Watson describes the body with spirit within a consciousness that is integral to all consciousness (Rafael, 2000). Through intentionality and evocation of love, the nurse is a unitary healing environment mutually cocreating self-healing with the person-patient coparticipant. Within a unitary paradigm, all consciousness is, and is connected, so as Watson suggests, the intentional awakening to and sharing of consciousness can create a context for healing potential.

Watson initially drew on the work of Maslow as she described a systematic way of attending to an individual's symptom management, comfort, and well-being. Watson categorized human needs in terms of biophysical; psychophysical needs, (e.g., sexuality); psychosocial needs; and intrapersonal-interpersonal needs. This framework for human needs, along with a systematic review of internal and external environments and consideration of existential-phenomenological-spiritual forces, provided a schema for organizing an assessment (Rafael, 2000). More recent work on Watson's caring theory reflects the evolution of her thinking influence by Eastern and mystical writings as well as feminist thought. Watson has continued to work on clarification of model assumptions and values as well as conceptual and theoretical clarification of the model of caring as it has evolved to a caring-healing paradigm embedded in a unitary caring science. Watson's caring-healing paradigm focuses on the relationships between the human being's quest for spirit actualization through transformative self-healing that is informed and guided by the caritas processes. Healing can be facilitated by the mutual transpersonal caring relationship between the nurse and person that is entered into intentionally with love in the context of a healing environment. The nurse who is fully present facilitates the person-patient's "exploration of the meaning of an experience, the means by which the person transcends life's predicaments, the meaning of life and death, and belief systems through the person-patient finds a sense of purpose" (Rafael, 2000, p. 7).

Analysis of Consistency

Reflections on theory contribute to understanding how it relates to practice, research, and education. Chinn and Kramer (1999) established these questions for critical reflection: "How clear is this theory? How simple is this theory? How general is this theory? How accessible is this theory? How important is this theory?" (p. 100).

Fawcett (1993) connected internal consistency with congruency of the philosophical claims and elements with the conceptual model. Watson's theoretical conceptualization of the human caring model has been criticized for the incongruent use of abstract terminology in defining the components and relationships within the original human caring theory and the postmodern transpersonal caring-healing paradigm (Mitchell & Cody, 1992; Paley, 2001).

Accordingly, Chinn and Kramer (1999) reflected the clarity of a theory by focusing on semantic clarity, semantic consistency, structural clarity, and structural consistency. Semantic clarity and consistency refer to the understandability of theoretical meaning as it relates to concepts and connectedness between concepts within the theory. Watson has taken the original components and progressively transformed them into transdisciplinary concepts. Because of the complexity of her conceptualizations through borrowing concepts from the philosophical, phenomenological, existential, and spiritual realms, clarity has become obscure. Clarity is affected by excessive narration and verbiage found within Watson's publication on postmodern nursing.

Fawcett (1993) suggested that Watson (1992) attempted to address the criticisms from Mitchell and Cody (1992) by using the term "human mind-body-spirit" to describe her understanding of person. Semantic consistency reflects consistent use of meanings explicitly stated with those implied within the theory (Chinn & Kramer, 1999). The earlier conceptual inconsistencies in the human care model have lead to the progressive transformation into the transpersonal caring-healing paradigm that is transdisciplinary. In the ontological shift, the nurse was viewed as an active participant in healing. The inconsistencies may in fact be the complexity of the explication of human care concepts limited by language. Paley (2001) was decidedly critical of such inconsistencies in conceptual terminology. Paley (2001) was highly critical of Watson's theoretical and conceptual origins and of interchangeable use of metaphysical terminology. Watson and Smith (2002), in an attempt to address the criticisms, further expanded on the science of caring by describing caring-healing as a unitary caring science.

Structural clarity and consistency refers to how understandable the connections of the components are and how consistent their use is throughout the theory (Chinn & Kramer, 1999). These structural components should convey a simple conceptual map that enhances the clarity of the concepts and associated relationships as seen in the original concept on human caring. With the emergence of the postmodern transpersonal caring-healing paradigm, analysis of these components are difficult because of Watson's integrated beliefs and premises from several philosophical and epistemic perspectives such as seen in Zukav's concepts on the relationship among consciousness, energy and light, and Myss's work on charkas as energy centers that depict sacred, ancient imagery related to the human. Once again the complexity of the current paradigm has lead to what is viewed as inconsistencies. For those without a metaphysical-phenomenological-epistemological-philosophical-spiritual   background, the complexity of the paradigm would be difficult to comprehend and would be viewed with much criticism.

On the surface, Watson's conceptual foundation reflects highly complex philosophical and epistemic perspectives. Within the main structure there are three key components around which all the basic concepts revolve, so it is conceptually simple in structure. Although it has a few structural components, the concepts account for a broad range of empiric experiences, which lends to generality (Chinn & Kramer, 1999). Theories with a high degree of generality are useful in organizing and generating ideas and hypotheses. A plethora of publications have been generated based on caring from Watson's human caring theory.

According to Chinn and Kramer (1999), "accessibility addresses the extent to which empiric indicators can be identified for concept with the theory and how attainable the projected outcomes of the theory are. If a theory is to be used for explaining some aspect of the practice world, its theoretic concepts must be linked to empiric indicators available in practice" (p. 106). In Watson's (2002) publication on assessing and measuring caring, a variety of tools are available to operationalize indicators of caring to determine outcomes in a practice. To avoid conceptual inconsistencies with the context of theories, clearly defined components of each tool are given. Empirical accessibility is important if a theory is to be used to guide research and shape nursing practice (Chinn & Kramer, 1999). Watson's caring model has been used in research (Rafael, 2000; Maeve & Vaughn, 2001; Lagana, 2000; Dorsey, Phillips, & Williams, 2001; Updike, Cleaveland, & Nyberg, 2000; Touhy, 2001; Griffith, 1999; Mullaney, 2000) and in shaping nursing practice found in the daily practices at the Center for Human Caring in Colorado and through the Nursing Doctorate curriculum at the University of Colorado.

Analysis of Adequacy

In assessing the adequacy of a theory, Walker and Avant (1995) consider: "Is there a system whereby predictions can be made from the theory independent of its content? Can scientists in the discipline in which the theory is developed agree on those predictions? Does the actual content make sense? And are there obvious logical fallacies?" (p. 141). Hardy (1974) bases the adequacy of a theory on two criteria: meaning and logical adequacy, and operational and empirical adequacy.

Accordingly, Watson (1985) presented an extensive, well-organized argument for the philosophical assumptions and premises for the human caring model. With the transformation and reconstructing of the postmodern model into the transpersonal caring-healing paradigm, Watson (1999b) expanded her assumptions and premises to embrace an ontological shift and to broaden the scope of the model to one that is a multidisciplinary in nature. The content is complex and eludes the knowledge of those lacking a background grounded in the sciences and philosophies, as well as the mystical and spiritual realms. The realm of the transpersonal relationship and actual caring occasion, no longer exclusive to nursing, was expanded to include other disciplines and practitioners. The nurse becomes a practitioner of caring-healing processes within a unitary caring science. The person is empowered to become an active participant in the healing force. The environment is a sacred realm of spiritual, mystical energetic fields in which caring-healing processes occur.

Concerns continue to be expressed about the extant and emerging caring conceptualizations within the discipline regarding the various caring concepts and philosophical perspectives, including the utility of caring theory in the context of practice. Specifically, George (2001) has questioned the pragmatic value of Watson's theory in the current health system with high acuity levels, short stays, and technology. It is suggested that quality care in a cost-benefit ratio environment may not be the goal of bureaucratic care provider structures focused on task completion that rewards the "trim" and not the "core" of nursing, placing the nurse in an untenable position. The pragmatics of the economic and political pressures surrounding health care and nursing practice are important to consider. However, the caring-healing paradigm that Watson proposes can provide a philosophical foundation for understanding the human experience and guiding a nurse's approach to practice in any health care environment. Furthermore, within the expanded focus on multiple ways of knowing and theory development in nursing, such as proposed by Fawcett, Watson, Neuman, Walker, and Fitzpatrick, (2001), Watson's conceptualization has great relevance. Furthermore, the nurse is challenged to understand the environment of care in a way that challenges the practitioner to promote the therapeutic or healing potential of the environment in which a caring-healing encounter takes place.

A conceptual model, because of its level of abstraction, usually cannot meet the criteria of operational and empirical adequacy. Watson's specific constructs and concepts were not operationally defined for the purposes of empirical observations. From the original theory, an instrument was developed for measuring the caring dimensions (Watson, 2002a). Many other researchers have developed caring instruments based on Watson's theory of human caring and the 10 carative factors, thus lending empirical validation of the theory (Watson, 2002a). In her writings about a postmodern paradigm, Watson has continued to redefine concepts and relationships as her thinking has evolved.

EXTERNAL ANALYSIS

Nursing Research

The Center for Human Caring at the University of Colorado School of Nursing has emphasized the development of knowledge in human caring and healing across the life span. Research activities at the Center include the development and testing of practice modalities to facilitate and promote human integrity and health. The human care model also has been used to guide studies by nurse-scientists who are not connected to the Center for Human Care, and by students in the master's and doctoral programs within and outside the United States. In addition, the Center for Human

Care offers a summer visiting fellowship program for academics who want to be mentored in caring-healing theory and research methods.

It is important to note that Watson (1985) thinks that traditional research methods are not adequate for knowledge development in the human care model. Given the focus on knowledge of caring-healing for the human spirit, human phenomenal fields, and meanings related to health-illness experiences, Watson suggests qualitative-naturalistic-phenomenological methods. Descriptive phenomenological approaches are proposed as the best methods for understanding the human predicament and the meaning attached to health-illness given current knowledge of scientific methods. It also may be appropriate to consider the usefulness of feminist theory and constructivism, which engage the "subject/stakeholder" as a coparticipant in the research process.

Nursing Education

Watson has suggested that the nursing discipline needs to develop new paradigms for educational preparation (Watson & Phillips, 1992). To this end the human care model has been used as the basis for curricula in the nursing doctoral (ND) program at the University of Colorado and other nursing education programs in the United States and Canada. An advanced postgraduate program of study is available through the Center for Human Care that includes mentored study of caring-healing for educators.

An educational process based on the human care model requires knowledge of the humanities, art, basic sciences, ethics, and discipline-specific caring-healing (Watson & Phillips, 1992). An academic program guided by the philosophy and ethics of the human care model has the potential to develop a nursing professional who is self-aware and spiritually aware. As noted by Boyd and Mast (1989), "the emphasis on art, discovery, esthetics, wholeness, and spirituality offers a refreshing alternative" for academic preparation in nursing.

Nursing Practice

The human care model and the postmodern transpersonal caring-healing paradigm are being used as clinical practice models in the United States and Canada in acute, community, and long-term care settings. Dissemination and implementation of a human care practice model is supported by direct consultation with Watson and colleagues at the Center for Human Care and indirectly through videotapes and electronic bulletin boards. Clinicians also can study caring praxis at the Center and obtain a certificate in caring skills.

The moral ideal and transpersonal care process delineated by Watson in the human care model provide a welcome frame of reference for contemporary nursing practice. At a time when the disease-cure-for-profit healthcare system seems to be more dehumanizing and nihilistic, a return to the philosophical roots of modern nursing is evident within the postmodern paradigm as a guide to clinical practices. The postmodern nurse emerges as a healing practitioner with increased emphasis on an intention to care and recognition of the healing potential of the human spirit of both practitioner and patient within the context of a caring-healing environment. At the same time, Watson asks those in the discipline and profession of nursing to reconnect with the roots of nursing and values first articulated by Nightingale, who spoke of a "calling" and "service" to others. Concurrently, Watson proposes that the transpersonal caring-healing paradigm is transdisciplinary and is useful to multiple disciplines that choose to engage in a caring-healing relationship and caring moment that is required for a sacred healing moment to occur. Herein lies a dilemma for many who will struggle with a caring-healing paradigm that has its foundation in Nightingale's work but has been transformed into a caring-healing paradigm meaningful to multiple disciplines. It challenges the nurse scholar and practitioner to re-examine basic philosophical positions about the nature, focus, and uniqueness of the discipline called nursing.

Relationship to Nursing Classification System

England (1989) discussed two definitions of the nursing diagnosis. Nursing diagnosis has been defined as a response to actual or potential health problems that nurses are legally responsible and accountable to treat (Moritz, 1982). This reflects a problem-oriented, disease-model frame of reference. England (1989) suggested that the definition of nursing diagnosis derived from a view of humans as unitary beings is most useful to nursing. The latter perspective emphasized phrases that describe empirical indicators illustrating patterns of unitary beings (Roy, 1982). Adam (1989) cautioned that the data interpretation (nursing diagnosis) and data collection processes upon which interpretations are based are concrete operations. Furthermore, she notes that a conceptual framework that is substantially more abstract should guide data collections.

Watson does not believe that the extant nursing diagnosis taxonomy is philosophically or conceptually congruent with the human care model. She acknowledges, however, that some nurses who are implementing the model may use a particular nursing diagnosis label. For instance, the pattern of valuing addresses one diagnostic category, "spiritual distress," referred to as distress of the human spirit. Within the context of the Watson's original caring model, it seemed more appropriate to derive conclusions about human care needs based on the human care model than the current taxonomy of the North American Nursing Diagnosis Association (NANDA). The proposed caring-healing paradigm, or unitary caring science, is not congruent with the NANDA taxonomy.

Within the context of the human care model, diagnostic conclusions would be based on the intersubjective experience of the nurse and patient during an actual caring moment. The nurse's knowledge of the caritas processes and their potential usefulness in a given transpersonal caring relationship would also inform the naming of the phenomenal experience of the nurse-patient sacred healing field. With the development of the transpersonal caring-healing paradigm applicable to multiple disciplines, questions remain about the use of such taxonomy in those practices not familiar with nursing. Watson (2002b) considers her work more a philosophical, ethical, intellectual blueprint for nursing's evolving disciplinary/professional matrix, rather than a specific theory.

SUMMARY

The transpersonal caring-healing paradigm is considered a philosophical and moral/ethical foundation for professional nursing and part of the central focus for practitioners in multidisciplinary levels. Watson (2002a) believes that

> A model of caring includes a call for both art and science; it offers a framework that embraces and intersects with art, science, humanities, spirituality, and new dimensions of mind-body-spirit medicine and nursing evolving openly as central to human phenomena of nursing practice. This work posits a value's explicit moral foundation and takes a specific position with respect to the centrality of human caring, "caritas" and love as now an ethic and ontology, as well as a critical starting point for nursing's existence, broad societal mission, and the basis for further advancement for caring-healing practices. The ideas as originally developed, as well as in the current evolving phase provide a chance to assess, critique and see where or how, or if, one may locate self within the framework or the emerging ideas in relation to their own "theories and philosophies of professional nursing and/or caring practice." (p. 8)

Watson's work, in both its original and evolving forms, seeks to develop caring as an ontological and theoretical-philosophical-ethical framework for the profession and discipline of nursing, and clarify its mature relationship and distinct intersection with other health sciences.

Activities based on the nursing caring theory have become guides to practice, education and research, and have developed throughout the United States and other parts of the world. Watson's work is consistently one of the theories of caring used by nurse educators, practitioners, and researchers.

Watson's (1999a) conception of nursing is transformed in the ontological shift found in her transpersonal caring-healing paradigm. Nursing became a transcendent synthesis of metaphysics, spirituality, and existential phenomenology. This model is significant in its transforming, healing power of the human spirit of both practitioner and patient in a sacred phenomenon occurring at a special moment between two energy fields within a spiritual, mystic environment. In essence, the artistry of caring has been transformed to "soul-to-soul" as the paramount focus of nursing (Schmidt, Bunkers, Mitchell, & Northrup, 1999). The complexity of such a theory is supported by Watson's fluidity of expression at a higher intellectual level.

REFERENCES

Adam, E. (1989, October). *Levels of abstraction in nursing content development*. Paper presented at the Second Annual Rosemary Ellis Scholars' Retreat. Frances Payne Bolton School of Nursing, Case Western Reserve University, Cleveland, OH.

Bevis, E. O., & Watson, J. (1989). *Toward a caring curriculum: a new pedagogy for nursing*. New York: National League for Nursing.

Boyd, C., & Mast, D. (1989). Watson's model of human care. In J. J. Fitzpatrick and A. Whall (Eds.), *Conceptual models of nursing: Analysis and application* (2nd ed., pp. 371–383). Norwalk, CT: Appleton & Lange.

Boykin, A., & Schoenhofer, S. (1993). *Nursing as caring*. New York: National League of Nursing.

Chinn, P., & Kramer, M. (1999). *Theory and nursing: Integrated knowledge development* (5th ed.). St. Louis: Mosby.

Dorsey, C., Phillips, K. D., & Williams, C. (2001). Adult sickle cell patients' perceptions of nurses' caring behaviors. *American Black Nurses Association Journal, 12*(5), 95–103.

England, M. (1989). Nursing diagnosis: A conceptual framework. In J. J. Fitzpatrick & A. L. Whall (Eds.). *Conceptual models of nursing: Analysis and application* (2nd ed). Norwalk, CT: Appleton & Lange.

Fawcett, J. (1993). *Analysis and evaluation of nursing theories*. Philadelphia: F. A. Davis.

Fawcett, J., Watson, J., Neuman, B., Walker, P., & Fitzpatrick, J. (2001). On nursing theories and evidence. *Journal of Nursing Scholarship, 33*(2), 115–120.

George, L. (2001). *Nursing theories: The base for professional nursing practice* (5th ed.). St. Louis: Mosby.

Griffith, K. (1999). Holism in the care of the allogeneic bone marrow transplant population: Role of the nurse practitioner. *Holistic Nursing Practice, 13*(2), 20–27.

Hardy, M. (1974). Theories: Components, development, evaluation. *Nursing Research, 23*, 100–107.

Lagana, K. (2000). The "right" to a caring relationship: The law and ethic of care. *Journal of Perinatal & Neonatal Nursing, 14*(2), 12–24.

Leininger, M., & Watson, J. (Eds.). (1990). *The caring imperative in education.* New York: National League for Nursing.

Maeve, M., & Vaughn, M. (2001). Nursing with prisoner: The practice of caring, forensic nursing or penal harm nursing? *Advances in Nursing Science, 24*(2), 47–64.

Mitchell, G. J., & Cody, W. K. (1992). Nursing knowledge and human science: Ontological and epistemological considerations. *Nursing Science Quarterly, 5,* 24–30.

Moritz, D. A. (1982). Nursing diagnosis in relation to the nursing process. In M. J. Kim & D. A. Moritz (Eds.), *Classification of nursing diagnoses: Proceedings of the third and fourth national conferences* (pp. 53–57). New York: McGraw-Hill.

Mullaney, J. (2000). The lived experience of using Watson's actual caring occasion to treat depressed women. *Journal of Holistic Nursing, 18*(2), 129–142.

Paley, J. (2001). An archaeology of caring knowledge. *Journal of Advanced Nursing, 36*(2), 188–198.

Rafael, A. (2000). Watson's philosophy, science, and theory of human caring as a conceptual framework for guiding community health nursing practice. *Advances of Nursing Science, 23*(2), 34–49.

Roy, C. (1982). Theoretical framework for classification of nursing diagnoses. In M. J. Kim & D. A. Moritz (Eds.), *Classification of nursing diagnoses: Proceedings of the third and fourth national conferences* (pp. 215–221). New York: McGraw-Hill.

Schmidt, S., Bunkers, G., Mitchell, J., & Northrup, D. (1999). Reconstructing nursing: Beyond art and science. *Nursing Science Quarterly, 12*(4), 348–355.

Sherwood, G. (1997). Metasynthesis of qualitative analysis of caring. *Advances in Nursing Science, 3,* 32–42.

Swanson, K. (1999). What is known about caring in nursing science? In A. Hinshaw, S. Feetham, & J. Shaver (Eds.). *Handbook of clinical nursing research* (pp. 31–60). Thousand Oaks, CA: Sage Publications.

Touhy, T. (2001). Nurturing hope and spirituality in the nursing home. *Holistic Nursing Practice, 15*(4), 45–56.

Updike, P., Cleaveland, M., & Nyberg, J. (2000). Complementary caring-healing practices of nurses caring for children with life-challenging illnesses and their families: A pilot project with case reports. *Alternative Therapies in Health and Medicine, 6*(4), 112–119.

Walker, L., & Avant, K. (1995). *Strategies for theory construction in nursing* (3rd ed.). Englewood Cliffs: Prentice Hall.

Watson, J. (1979). *Nursing: The philosophy and science of caring.* Boston: Little Brown.

Watson, J. (1985). *Nursing: Human science and human care: A theory of nursing.* Norwalk, CT: Appleton-Century-Crofts.

Watson, J. (1989). Watson's philosophy and theory of human caring in nursing. In J. Riehl-Sisca (Ed.), *Conceptual models for nursing practice* (pp. 219–236). Norwalk, CT: Appleton & Lange.

Watson, J. (1992). Window on theory of human caring. In M. O'Toole (Ed.). *Miller—Keane encyclopedia and dictionary of medicine, nursing, and allied health* (5th ed., p. 1481). Philadelphia: Saunders.

Watson, J. (1999a). *Nursing: Human science and human care.* Sudbury, MA: Jones and Bartlett.

Watson, J. (1999b). *Postmodern nursing and beyond.* London: Churchill Livingstone.

Watson, J. (2002a). *Assessing and measuring caring in nursing and health science.* New York: Springer Publishing Company.

Watson, J. (2002b). *Theory of human caring.* Retrieved July 7, 2002, from http://www.2.uchsc.edu/son/caring.

Watson, J., & Smith, M. C. (2002). Caring science and the science of unitary human beings: A trans-theoretical discourse for nursing knowledge development. *Journal of Advanced Nursing, 37*(5), 452–461.

Watson, J., & Phillips, S. (1992). A call for educational reform: Colorado nursing doctorate model as exemplar. *Nursing Outlook, 40,* 20–26.

Watson, M. J. (1996). Watson's theory of transpersonal caring. In P. Hinton Walker & B. Neuman (Eds.). *Blueprint for use in nursing models.* (pp. 141–184). New York: NLN Press.

Zukav, G. (1990). *The seat of the soul.* New York: Fireside Books.

15

Fitzpatrick's Life Perspective Rhythm Model

Original Chapter by Jana L. Pressler
Updated by Kristen S. Montgomery

As pointed out in the 1989 critique of Fitzpatrick's rhythm model (Pressler, 1989), Fitzpatrick's scholarly endeavors have changed since her first description of the life perspective rhythm model in 1983 (Fitzpatrick, 1983a), and today are continuing to evolve. Consistent with one of Fitzpatrick's theoretical premises regarding the evolutionary development of person and environment (Fitzpatrick, 1983a, 1989), her own work and that of others reflect open systems of pattern and organization congruent with her idea of rhythmicity along a life perspective.

This chapter examines changes or derivations emanating from Fitzpatrick's model pertinent to advancing nursing knowledge. An analysis of the model is presented along with comments concerning areas in which the model has the potential for better serving the needs and goals of the nursing discipline. The main ideas addressed include how a consideration of rhythmic methodologies might develop nursing knowledge pertaining to nursing classification systems and theory-driven, evidence-based practice.

The major focus of Fitzpatrick's scholarly activities continues to be the development of a community of nurse-scholars and the development of nursing within a broader scope of inquiry. Although she still serves as the chairperson for doctoral dissertations, her primary scholarly activities include advancing nursing science and development at a broader level.

BASIC CONSIDERATIONS OF THE MODEL

According to Fitzpatrick (1986), interactions of the community of scholars and the field of inquiry are necessary to develop nursing knowledge. For such nursing knowledge to be useful, it must undergo differentiation, organization, and hierarchical ordering to become fully developed as a distinct body of knowledge (Fitzpatrick, 1986). Although Fitzpatrick recommends that interaction take place between scholars and the field of inquiry, she has not been working recently to further develop her rhythm model in this regard. The major elements of her rhythm model, and their relationships with each other, remain much as they were originally conceptualized.

Fitzpatrick presented her rhythm model as the field of inquiry for nursing. Person, environment, health, and nursing are distinctively defined and related in the model. All of these elements have been linked with the idea that meaning is essential to life. Fitzpatrick (1983a, 1989) has asserted that meaning is the most crucial piece of human experience. She (Fitzpatrick, 1979, 1980, 1983a, 1989) sees meaning as necessary to enhance and maintain life. Fitzpatrick has incorporated Rogers' (1979, 1983) postulated correlates of human development as a basis from which to differentiate, organize, and order life's reality.

Correlates of Human Development

Rogers' (1979, 1983) correlates of shorter, higher-frequency waves that manifest shorter rhythms and approach a seemingly continuous patterning serve as Fitzpatrick's foci for hypothesizing the existence of *rhythmic patterns*. Rogers' position that the human life span approximates transformation with human development aimed toward transcendence has been incorporated within Fitzpatrick's quantitative and qualitative descriptions of life perspective. The developmental correlate whereby time seems timeless represents a beginning of Fitzpatrick's theorizing regarding *temporal patterns*. *Motion patterns* have been similarly derived from Rogers' proposal of motion seeming to be continuous as development proceeds. *Consciousness patterns* are closely aligned with Rogers' idea that one progresses from sleeping to waking and from there to a pattern that is beyond waking. The correlates of "visibility" become more ethereal in nature, and "heaviness" approaching a more weightless phase serves as the basis for Fitzpatrick's *perceptual patterns*.

Definitions of Person and Environment

Fitzpatrick's definitions of person and environment result from her interpretation of Rogers' (1979, 1983) developmental correlates and definitions of person and environment (Rogers, 1980). Envisioned as patterns within a pattern, or rhythms within a life rhythm (Fitzpatrick, 1983a, 1989), Fitzpatrick's rhythm patterns are explicit operational modes that specify the pattern of person and environment explicated by Rogers (1980, 1983). Occurring within the context of rhythmic person-environment interaction, Fitzpatrick identifies indices of holistic human functioning as temporal, motion, consciousness, and perceptual patterns (Fitzpatrick, 1979, 1980, 1982a, 1983a, 1989). Overall, Fitzpatrick's writings are consistent with the Rogerian position regarding person and environment being open systems in continuous interaction.

Fitzpatrick (1983a, 1989) has asserted that the four indices of human functioning identified above are intricately related to health patterns throughout the life span. She also has proposed that these indices can be described as rhythmic in nature. In a projection of Rogers' (1979, 1980, 1983) principle regarding the continuous interaction of persons and their environments, Fitzpatrick (1982a) postulated the dynamic concepts of *congruency, consistency,* and *integrity* as complementary with rhythmic patterns. The nonlinear character of patterns by Rogers has supported Fitzpatrick's incorporation of Rogers' (1980, 1983) specifications regarding four-dimensionality.

Definition of Health

Two distinct interpretations of Smith's (1981) clinical and eudemonistic models of health/illness are contained in Fitzpatrick's explanation of health. According to Fitzpatrick (1983a), health shares the health interpretations of Smith (1981), that is, absence of disease (clinical interpretation), and quality of life and maximum wellness (eudemonistic interpretation). Conceptualizing about health further, Fitzpatrick (1981a, 1989) stated that health is a basic human dimension undergoing continuous development. She has offered a heightened awareness of the *meaningfulness of life* as an example of a more fully developed phase of human health (Fitzpatrick, 1989).

Definition of Nursing

The ontogenetic and phylogenetic interactions among person and health have been looked upon as the essence of nursing (Fitzpatrick, 1983a). Fitzpatrick has not only attended to relationships within or between these juxtaposed elements, but also has included latent relationships "outside" of person and health proper. Having the salient concern of these relationships as the meaning attached to life, nursing has been understood to be a discipline worthy of professional status (Fitzpatrick, 1982c, 1985a). Nursing interventions have been interpreted as facilitating the developmental process toward health. As stated by Fitzpatrick (1989), "Nursing interventions can be focused on enhancing the developmental process toward health so that individuals may be led to develop their potential as human beings" (p. 406).

An important clarification should be made regarding Fitzpatrick's usage of *perspective* in characterizing her life perspective rhythm model for nursing. More limited in scope than a *worldview,* the concept of perspective described by Fitzpatrick might be interchanged with the term *paradigm* or *paradigmatic view.* As defined by Kuhn (1970), a paradigm represents a unique description of phenomena yet lacks a dramatically new worldview. Paradigms usually have obvious associations with existing worldviews and share like orientations. Fitzpatrick's reliance on Rogers' (1970) five basic assumptions and homeodynamic principles (Rogers, 1970, 1980, 1983) substantiates a bond with an established worldview for nursing.

Relationship Among Concepts

Person, environment, health, and nursing have been addressed in Fitzpatrick's model. Because person and environment have been considered integral with one another and as having no real boundaries, one might assume that environment is implied when the term *person* is used. Although Fitzpatrick (1983a, 1989) has not gone into great detail in outlining her perception of environment, her publications consistently mirror a basic Rogerian (1980, 1983) definition of environmental field. The human element is treated as an open, holistic rhythmic system that can best be described by temporal, motion, consciousness, and perceptual patterns. Her fourfold entity of person is enhanced by awareness of the meaningfulness of life, or health. The meaningfulness of life is thought to be enhanced after a crisis experience (Fitzpatrick, 1989).

INTERNAL ANALYSIS

Basic Assumptions of the Model

Emanating from the time when Rogers served as a mentor for Fitzpatrick when she was a doctoral student at New York University, Fitzpatrick (1983a, 1989) has constructed her model primarily with the conceptual underpinnings of Rogers (1970, 1980, 1983). Rogers' (1970) five explicit assumptions about man as a unified whole, man and environment as open systems, the life process evolving irreversibly along space time, pattern and organization identifying man, and man as a sentient being, capable of abstraction, language, and thought, have provided a framework for Fitzpatrick's basic considerations about person, environment, health, and nursing. Energy fields, openness, pattern, and organization and four-dimensionality (Rogers, 1980), along with Rogers' (1979) 10 postulated correlates of human development, have further assisted Fitzpatrick in proposing rhythmic patterns of holistic human functioning. Rogers' (1970, 1980, 1983) homeodynamic principles of helicy, resonancy, and integrality, and also helicy, resonancy and complementarity (Rogers, 1980), have reflected Fitzpatrick's basic beliefs regarding the evolutionary development of person and environment.

Several implicit assumptions pertinent to an understanding of Fitzpatrick's model have been identified through an examination of early writings. These include the following:

1. Differences in behavioral manifestations are more easily identified during the peaks of wave patterns (Fitzpatrick, 1980, p. 153);
2. Identified by congruency, consistency, and integrity of rhythmic patterns, health is the manifestation of symphonic interaction of persons and their environments (Fitzpatrick, 1982a, p. 33).
3. Emphasized through selected research on temporality, the meaning attached to life is a central concern of nursing (Fitzpatrick, 1981c); and
4. Nursing is a philosophy, a science, and an art

(Fitzpatrick, 1982c, p. 5).

The fourth assumption is emphasized and reinforced when Fitzpatrick (Fitzpatrick & Carnegie, 1991) proposed that Florence Nightingale might concur with her that nursing is an important scientific endeavor as well as being the finest of arts.

The central components of Fitzpatrick's model for nursing are distinguishable through the above assumptions. *Person, environment, rhythmic patterns,* the *meaning attached to life,* health, and nursing all are viewed essential in the *life perspective rhythm model.* Because the meaning attached to life has been regarded by Fitzpatrick as "the basic understanding of human existence" (Fitzpatrick, 1989, p. 406), it appears that this particular dimension of one's health is of utmost concern.

According to Hardy (1974), a first step in evaluating a theoretical premise is an appraisal of the validity of the assumptions, the validity of meanings attributed to the concepts, and the logic of the theoretical system. This kind of analytical sector allows for an overall assessment of meaning and logical adequacy.

The explicit Rogerian (1970) assumptions (regarding the essence of man and environment) postulated by Fitzpatrick are representative of a synthesis of a number of areas of knowledge. Clearly, Fitzpatrick's (1980) first implicit assumption about peaks of wave patterns was primarily derived from biologic rhythm theory (Haus, 1964; Luce, 1970) and Caplan's (cited in Fitzpatrick, 1982a) interpretation of crisis theory. Fitzpatrick's (1982a, 1989) reformulation of the crisis perspective in relation to Rogers' (1970, 1980, 1983) conceptualizations was related to Rogers' second assumption concerning health. Similar to Rogers' (1970, 1980, 1983) approach, the concept of health continues to remain somewhat abstract. Health research that supports the existence of congruency, consistency, and integrity per se within Fitzpatrick's rhythmic patterns (described as peaks and troughs) of human functioning has yet to be documented.

Fitzpatrick has not laid claim directly to any of the implicit assumptions identified in this or an earlier critique (Pressler, 1983). Therefore, it is understandable that Fitzpatrick's conceptualization of health might be characterized somewhat differently in her model. However, the third assumption is supported by her past extensive work with temporality (Donovan, Fitzpatrick, & Johnston, 1980, 1981; Fitzpatrick, 1975, 1977, 1980, 1981d, 1982a; Fitzpatrick & Donovan, 1978a, 1978b; Fitzpatrick, Donovan, & Johnston, 1979; Fitzpatrick, Johnston, & Donovan, 1980b; Johnston, Fitzpatrick, & Donovan, 1981). In addition, Rogers' (1970) view of nursing is again visible within the final implicit assumption. As articulated by Fitzpatrick (1981b, 1981c, 1983b), the broader dimensions of the discipline of nursing can be characterized as philosophical, scientific, and artistic. These complementary types of nursing inquiry have constituted an evolving theme in Fitzpatrick's work.

All of the explicit and implicit assumptions, except those of congruency, consistency, and integrity of human rhythmic patterns, seem clearly and logically defined within the model. Fitzpatrick (1989) does allude to congruency, in that one has patterns (temporal, motion, consciousness, and perceptual) within a pattern, or rhythms within a rhythm; consistency, in that one's overall life rhythm pattern may continue an infinite number of times, and also that consistencies between environmental rhythms such as light, dark, and the human rhythms of sleep, wake, emotions and moods, pain, and level of consciousness or mental alertness exist; and integrity, in that basic human rhythms describe holistic human functioning. However, if congruency, consistency, and integrity were explicated more fully using specific scientific findings, these ideas would seem more useful in describing phenomena of concern.

Phenomena of Concern

An internal analysis of a model attempts to determine the overall soundness and strength of the model as the foundation for nursing inquiry. In addition to establishing the validity and adequacy of the underlying assumptions, the model should provide an explicit guide to phenomena of concern within the field of study.

Currently, the nature of the phenomena of concern associated with the life perspective model could be classified as being more implicit than explicit. Brief theoretical descriptions for the elements of person, environment, health, nursing, and nursing activity have been stated in Fitzpatrick's (1983a) beginning sketch of the model. Of these five terms, the major discussion rests with person and health.

Rogerian explanations have been used as Fitzpatrick's foundation for identifying person and environmental phenomena, even though Rogers' (1980, 1983) definitions of human field and environmental field were not presented in the model. According to Fitzpatrick (1983a, 1989), human phenomena can be further characterized by basic rhythms in the form of *temporal patterns, motion patterns, consciousness patterns,* and *perceptual patterns,* and *life's crisis experiences* have been thought to represent the rhythmic peaks in the human developmental process (Fitzpatrick, 1989). As stated earlier, ideas for the patterns noted were synthesized from Rogers' (1979, 1983) correlates of human development. All of the proposed patterns have been presented as being equal in importance. However, perceptual patterns appear to be subsidiary to and/or dependent upon consciousness patterns. The notion of "visibility" and "heaviness" contained in perceptual patterns would logically fit within or overlap with one's dimension of consciousness. Similarly, the notion of the perceptual rhythms of emotions and moods (Fitzpatrick, 1989) would seem to be driven by patterns of consciousness.

Fitzpatrick (1983a) has contended that the phenomena related to health are closely affiliated with the meaning attached to life: "It seems as if the meaning attached to life is intimately linked to health, no matter whether health is defined as absence of disease, quality of life or maximum wellness" (Fitzpatrick, 1983a, p. 295). However, the words "no matter" made this statement a little confusing in determining how health phenomena were actually being conceptualized. One interpretation might have been that the meaning attached to life was intimately linked to health, with a notion of health including aspects of absence of disease, quality of life, or maximum wellness. Because she specifically gave three commonly used descriptions of health, one might deductively have selected the latter meaning of health.

In a revised presentation of her model, Fitzpatrick (1989) deleted the words "no matter" (p. 401) from this statement and it became even more apparent that she did not intend that health be defined as maximum wellness. In that discussion, Fitzpatrick (1989) stated that ". . . health is viewed as a continuously developing characteristic of humans with the full life potential that may characterize the process of dying—the heightened awareness of the meaningfulness of life—representing a more fully developed dimension of health" (pp. 405–406). Here it seems that the meaningfulness of life is the key determinant of one's health, and that it is a developmental phenomenon.

In addition, as a continuously developing characteristic of humans, or a basic human dimension, Fitzpatrick (1983a) has implied that health is in a perceptual phase of flux or rhythm. She contended that the development of health could be related to the full life potential, the process of dying, heightened awareness of the meaningfulness of life, and more fully developed humanness. It is clear from these descriptions that Fitzpatrick relates to health phenomena and that her consideration of health continues to evolve.

Fitzpatrick (1983a, 1983b, 1989) has presented two different definitions for nursing. Nursing, as a noun, has been described as a developing discipline with a central concern for the meaning attached to life (Fitzpatrick, 1989). As a verb, nursing, or nursing activity, has focused on enhancing the developmental process toward health so that individuals might develop their potential as human beings (Fitzpatrick, 1983a, 1983b, 1989).

The way in which nursing as a philosophy fits in with such explanations of nursing as a noun or verb was unclear from the 1983 publication (Fitzpatrick, 1983a). Yet nursing as a philosophy was identified as a type of nursing inquiry in a Distinguished Scholar Lecture later that same year (Fitzpatrick, 1983b). Fitzpatrick supported the inclusion of philosophical ways of knowing in the development of nursing as a discipline as early as 1981. She wrote: "Have we, in our quest for scientific and academic legitimacy and autonomous practice, lost sight of the philosophical basis for nursing?" (Fitzpatrick, 1981b, p. 1).

Fitzpatrick has been careful in specifying the aim of nursing inquiry. She stated that nursing inquiry is knowledge generation: knowledge that is applied in professional practice rather than a "practice theory" approach to nursing inquiry (Fitzpatrick, 1982a). She has pointed out that because knowledge and practice were complementary rather than similar, attempts to study the practice of nursing would fall short.

Syntax for Knowledge Development

Finally, a model should include syntax. Syntax is the logic for generating governing principles, and the resultant governing principles of such logic, for the discovery and validation of a field of study. More specifically, syntax is used as the procedural basis for conducting inquiry (for example, empirical inquiry, esthetic inquiry, philosophical inquiry, and historical inquiry) and also as the procedural basis for interpreting the meaning(s) of study findings.

Fitzpatrick has not discussed the specific principles that govern empirical, esthetic, philosophical, or historical inquiry, nor has she discussed the logic upon which such principles would be derived. However, her model has provided rudimentary assumptions from which syntax might be developed. Her explicit and implicit assumptions connect the essential nursing concepts of person, environment, health, and nursing into a unified whole with the meaning of life (refer to the prior discussion (page 327) regarding the implicit assumption that looks at health). In addition, there has been a consistent internal flow of ideas beginning with the assumptions and proceeding to the derived nursing interventions suggested. Nonetheless, without the logic and governing principles for conducting inquiry and establishing meaning(s), it is difficult to proceed to the subsequent step of organizing meanings into a coherent whole.

EXTERNAL ANALYSIS

Evaluating a model's external validity demonstrates its overall potential usefulness to the discipline in transmitting current knowledge and in generating new knowledge. According to Ellis (1968), the essential criticism of theoretical usefulness is use in practice along with a careful observation of the results. Hardy (1978) continues by reporting that theoretical ideas cannot be empirically valid if they are logically inadequate. She also contends that empirical validity is perhaps the single most important criterion for evaluating a theoretical tradition intended for subsequent application in a practice setting. Theoretical postulations must be rigorously tested by research studies before they can be accepted and actually utilized in nursing practice. One can identify how Fitzpatrick developed specific conceptualizations by examining previous research related to rhythmic phenomena.

Holistic Approach

A holistic approach to inquiry consists of the identification of patterns that are reflective of the whole (Newman, 1979). Newman (1979) asserts that this type of research method is not to be confused with a complex, multivariate approach, nor the summing of many factors to make a whole.

To include patterns of holistic human functioning in a model, it is necessary to determine scientific ways for measuring behaviors characteristic of the patterns, and the relationships among them. Because this is a challenging undertaking, no direct testing of the basic relationships posited has been completed. Because, as a whole, the model is not operationally defined in measurable terms, certainly the empirical adequacy of the perspective cannot be analyzed in any straightforward manner. What follows is an overview of the nursing research that exists for including particular components in the model's theoretical claims.

Nursing Research on the Model

Various kinds of support are suggested for the human rhythmic patterns of temporality, motion, consciousness, and perception from data gathered during student research projects. Fitzpatrick's conceptualizations have been investigated by graduate students in nursing both at the master's and doctoral levels. Studies looking at temporality in combination with adult and elderly populations (Smokvina, 1976; Brausell, 1977; Jones, 1977; Bouwman, 1979; Johnston, 1980; Kotal, 1980; Engle, 1981; Moore, 1981; Ramin, 1982; Schorr, 1982), temporality in association with psychiatric clients (Grider, 1977; Nalinnes, 1977; Mack, 1978; Chaffer, 1979; Alford, 1981), temporality in relation to terminally ill individuals (Hartline, 1978), and temporality in terms of planned adolescent pregnancy (Montgomery, 2000) provide a workable base from which to establish the existence of temporal patterns. From a holistic perspective of life span, however, the rhythm model continues to lack nursing research focused on infants' and children's notions of temporality, and knowledge development regarding adolescents' temporality needs to be expanded.

Both younger and elderly groups have been addressed in investigating motion (Smokvina, 1976; Goldberg & Fitzpatrick, 1980; Roberts & Fitzpatrick, 1983; Sipols-Lenss, 1982). Nevertheless, patterns of consciousness have again been exclusively examined in older age group contexts (Flaherty & Fitzpatrick, 1978; Jablonski, 1978; Pacini & Fitzpatrick, 1982; Roslaniec & Fitzpatrick, 1979; Floyd, 1982b; Horowitz, Fitzpatrick, & Flaherty, 1984).

Other types of perceptual patterns (i.e., perception of color [Fromme, 1979; McDonald, 1981] and music [Ludwig-Bonney, 1981]) have been investigated. Because one's perception would seem to be dependent on a present sense of consciousness, these studies would relate to the patterns of consciousness. In a sense, Shiao (1993) has investigated very low birth weight (VLBW) infants' perceptual patterns, such as perception of interference with breathing, oxygen saturation, and sucking with simultaneous nasal gastric tube feedings. However, Shiao refers to sucking and breathing as distinct biologic rhythms having temporal and perceptual characteristics, rather than as some type of temporal, motion, consciousness, or perceptual rhythm per se. Primarily, Shiao has used Fitzpatrick's rhythm model as the perspective for her study; that is, that human development is characterized by rhythm and that an individual infant's rhythms exist within his or her overall life rhythm.

Yarcheski and Mahon (1995) conducted a study to examine the four manifestations of human-environmental field patterning, including human field motion, human field rhythms, creativity, and sentience. They examined these patterns in relation to perceived health status in adolescents. The authors note that although Fitzpatrick (1983a) identified that the life perspective rhythm model provided a framework for research with human rhythms and health, the relationship between human field rhythms and health had not been previously studied (Yarcheski & Mahon, 1995). The authors found that human field rhythms were associated with health during late adolescence (age 18–21 years), but not during early (age 12–14 years) or middle adolescence (age 15–17 years). The authors note that these findings are consistent with Fitzpatrick's conceptualization that rhythms and health are basic processes of human development that advance and mature simultaneously over time (Yarcheski & Mahon, 1995).

Recognizing that her investigative efforts have been primarily centered on temporal patterns, Fitzpatrick (1983a, 1989) has summarized some of the results that lend support to the theoretical model. Furthermore, she points out that in order to examine the meaning attached to life, it is critical for phenomena to be explored using a multidimensional approach.

Most recently, nursing has witnessed an expansion and greater acceptance of qualitative research methods, which has resulted in a cadre of new literature support for the life perspective rhythm model. This expansion of research has been particularly evident in the areas of phenomenology, which as a method has the goal of discovering the "lived experience" and the meaning the experience has for the individual. The philosophical underpinnings for the phenomenological methods are consistent with Fitzpatrick's ideas regarding life meaning. Thus, many phenomenological researchers compare and contrast their findings with Fitzpatrick's life perspective rhythm model.

Montgomery (2000) conducted a phenomenological investigation of young adolescent girls' experiences planning a pregnancy. Several participants indirectly addressed the meaning the pregnancy or baby had on their lives (Montgomery, 2001). Increased responsibility, adulthood, being able to care for the baby, and personal growth were identified as meaningful in their lives. As part of their descriptions about the lived experience of planning a pregnancy as an adolescent, several participants made reference to situations that could be perceived as crisis experiences. Two individuals in this study talked about their pregnancies in terms of a self-chosen way to end the crisis in their lives and to move their lives forward. For example, one participant talked about her life being in disarray and that she needed something to work toward to pull herself together (Montgomery, 2001). After the pregnancy was achieved, her description of her life indicated she had gained meaning through the pregnancy.

Criddle (1993) conducted a phenomenological study of patient's experiences of healing following surgery. Participants in her study were in good health and all were expected to have a full recovery following the procedure with no loss of function. Criddle found that the meaningfulness of the participant's life was enhanced following their illness episode that prompted the surgical intervention. She notes that this finding is consistent with Fitzpatrick's ideas as health developing on a continuum and that increased life meaningfulness can be found following crisis experiences (Criddle, 1993). Many individuals consider major surgical procedures (and illness) crisis experiences (Gray, Fitch, Phillips, Labrecque, & Klotz, 1999; Perry, 1990; Isaacs, 1989).

Moore (1997) conducted a phenomenological study of the meaning of life in older suicidal adults. Eleven participants between the age of 64 and 92 years were interviewed at an acute care psychiatric facility. The life descriptions provided by these participants indicated that they felt their lives were no longer meaningful and thus they did not want to live. These findings are consistent with Fitzpatrick's belief that the meaning attached to life is essential to health and that "those who have no meaning do not continue to live" (Fitzpatrick, 1983a, p. 295).

Several other nurse-researchers have examined the meaning of life within other contexts, including breast cancer (Chiu, 1999; Cowan, 1995), menopause (Pasquali, 1999), and teaching spiritual care (Ross, 1996). Chiu (1999) examined women's experiences searching for meaning during treatment for breast cancer. She found that participants described searching for meaning as a "spiritual journey" that included gaining meaning through creativity, relationships, and experiencing situations. These explanations are consistent with Fitzpatrick's notion of gaining meaning through a crisis experience and these women's descriptions support Fitzpatrick's notion that the meaningfulness of life is a developmental process.

Cowan (1995) conducted a pilot study to examine the use of holistic nursing interventions for the treatment of breast cancer and how life meaning was influenced by such treatments. Pasquali (1999) conducted an ethnographic study of women who experienced premature menopause. The focus of her research was the women's concept of self and how this change influenced their lives. Women in this study experienced their situations of premature menopause as a stressful time, but once they were able to move beyond the crisis situation they were able to move their lives forward. These results are consistent with Fitzpatrick's ideas regarding crisis experiences resulting in growth for an individual (1989).

Empirical support for the existence of nonlinear temporal patterns emerged from a number of research endeavors (Fitzpatrick, 1989). Results from Fitzpatrick's 1975 study helped to identify the need for generating questions about ways to measure the experience of time. The prevalence of temporal directions on the basis of differences in development was apparent in subsequent studies (Fitzpatrick & Donovan, 1978a; Johnston et al., 1981). A sense of timelessness was described as being characteristic of behaviors identified among death-involved individuals (Fitzpatrick, 1980; Fitzpatrick et al., 1980a, 1980b). Descriptions of temporal rhythm patterns throughout the developmental process and during different crisis experiences have been stated as necessary subsequent research targets. As an investigator, Fitzpatrick has yet to embark upon equally robust research foundations for motion patterns, consciousness patterns, and perceptual patterns.

Pressler, Wells, and Hepworth (1993) investigated methodologic issues relevant to VLBW, very preterm (VP) infant outcomes based on the idea of the existence of microrhythms within some larger rhythmic pattern. By applying time series techniques and fuzzy subsets to the analysis of massive amounts of longitudinal data collected in the neonatal intensive care unit (NICU) environment, this study examined single-subject results for generalizations across individuals. In general terms, what is presently known about the sequelae and risks associated with the NICU per se for VLBW (i.e., < 1,500 g) and VP (i.e., < 30 weeks) gestation neonates is that information processing deficits and attention deficit-hyperactivity disorders are not uncommon during the preschool (Klein, Hack, Gallaher, & Fanaroff, 1985) and school-age years (McCormick, 1989). It is speculated that these types of problems might reflect these infants' earlier inabilities to attend to and cope with stresses and/or care received while hospitalized in the NICU environment. Although researchers are continuing to investigate potential regulatory mechanisms within infants coping with extrauterine life (for example, the roles of primitive newborn reflexes [Allen & Capute, 1990], the autonomic nervous system [Als, 1982; Porges, 1986, 1991, 1992; Porges & Byrne, 1992; Porges, Matthews, & Pauls, 1992], and self-stimulating behaviors [Guess & Carr, 1991]), such investigations are either system specific or completed over a short span of time, or have failed to adequately account for the interactive complexity of infants' dynamic functioning.

According to Pressler et al. (1993), the problem of addressing the complexity of infants' neurologic functioning is potentiated by the fact that infant assessment itself is a very complex process. It is thought that conducting thorough infant assessments will help develop understandings of change over time within infants, so that caregivers can meet an infant's proximate goals for the diagnosis of health problems, establish significant positive and negative baseline parameters essential for identifying the infant's needs, and meet the infant's ultimate goals for well-being and health.

Nonetheless, as suggested by Zadeh (1990) and his construct of fuzzy logic, because complexity and fuzziness are positively correlated, approximations rather than precise assessments might be needed to understand the complex and uncertain situations surrounding the NICU care of VLBW and VP infants. Such approximations might be achieved using time series and spectral analyses of longitudinal infant and environmental data. For example, when one considers the types of developmental disabilities experienced by VLBW and VP infants (e.g., dyslexia, attentional deficits), it seems possible that if one tracked the development of the disabilities across time, some might be explained by asynchronous rhythmic functioning in response to the environment. It has been hypothesized that asynchronous rhythmic functioning might develop during early infancy in response to overly stressful or incomprehensible stimuli that are part of being cared for in the NICU.

What is clear from prior infant outcome studies is that current methods have had limitations that must be dealt with in order to prevent inaccurate assessments and unwise decision making with respect to interventions for individual infants while in NICUs. Second, there is a complexity inherent in describing the behavioral patterns of VLBW and VP infants that has not been addressed adequately. The use of an ecotechnologic approach (Waller, 1989) to study preterm infant outcomes, in interaction with the theoretical idea of the existence of microrhythms within a larger overall rhythm, might be one valid way of adequately addressing their biobehavioral complexity and dynamic functioning. Given that crucial aspects of term infants' behavior have been shown to be ordered and organized at the level of microrhythms (i.e., high-frequency cycles lasting fractions of seconds (Beebe, Stern, & Jaffe, 1979), with social interactive regulation specifically occurring at a microlevel (Stern, 1971), and that circadian rhythms have not been found in infants less than 30 weeks gestation (Mirmiran, Kok, Boer, & Wolf, 1992), it seems appropriate that preterm infants' microlevel biobehavioral rhythmic interactions be investigated using a different approach if caregivers are to understand their health and functional status.

The analytic phase of the above research will consist of quantitative, qualitative, and fuzzy analyses toward the establishment of categorical structures for individual infant differences in biologic functioning, behavior, the environment as related to neonatal outcomes, family member visits, and the cost of care. Fitzpatrick's (1983a, 1989) ideas of temporal, motion, consciousness, and perceptual rhythms will be examined using the biobehavioral data and fuzzy logic.

In summary, the major focus on Fitzpatrick's scholarly activities continues to be the development of nursing within a broader scope of inquiry. Although Fitzpatrick still serves as the chairperson for doctoral dissertations, her primary scholarly activities surround her broader involvement with advancing the nursing discipline.

Other Types of Inquiry and Support

At present, empirical inquiry is the only type of nursing research that has been used to investigate phenomena relevant within Fitzpatrick's model. Esthetic and philosophical modes have not been explored. If the discipline of nursing is, indeed, more than empirics (science), then it is crucial that investigations necessitating other types of inquiry be completed. Otherwise, the development of nursing knowledge and its corresponding practice subsequently will be limited to nursing science.

Knowledge Transmission

Knowledge is transmitted through both the community of scholars and the field of inquiry with the express purpose of education, practice, and further inquiry. Fitzpatrick's involvement in graduate nursing education is related to the development of her theoretical views. Her teaching of graduate level nursing theory and nursing research courses has influenced her own and her students' conceptualizations of nursing inquiry and knowledge. Ashworth's (1980), Laffrey's (1982), Loveland-Cherry's (1982), and Reed's (1982) studies were related to health, life perspective, and/or well-being. Doctoral students attending Fitzpatrick's research-based seminars on rhythmic phenomena have used topics related to rhythmic phenomena for dissertations (Floyd, 1982b; Quillin, 1983; Shiao, 1993). Fitzpatrick's interests in suicidology and gerontologic nursing have also played a part in students' selection of research topics.

Nursing interventions have been derived from results stemming from the investigations on rhythmic patterns (Fitzpatrick, 1982b). For example, specific indications for reality orientation, rocking, reminiscence, music therapy, and rhythm profiles have been suggested based on certain research findings. With respect to temporal dimensions, identified nursing activities are believed to enhance the meaningfulness of life.

Fitzpatrick's overall model continues in its development and, therefore, has yet to have an observable impact on nursing education. In upcoming years, her ideas about human rhythm patterns and health could fit readily into nursing curricula.

NURSING CLASSIFICATION SYSTEMS AND THE MODEL

The North American Nursing Diagnosis Association (NANDA), Nursing Intervention Classification (NIC), Nursing Outcomes Classification (NOC), Home Health Care Classification, Ozbolt Patient Care Data Set, and the Omaha system represent the current nursing classifications that are in use or under development in the United States. Each of these classification systems shares a similar goal of uniting nursing practice through a common language. The development of such classification systems emerged from the need for nurses to have a common language with which to communicate, bill for services, and measure outcomes.

With further development and clarification of terminology, the life perspective rhythm model could provide the theoretical base and organization for any of these classification systems. One such benefit of using a conceptual model as an organizing framework for any of these classification systems is that the model would provide structure and represent nursing functions in a way that captures what nurses do. Capturing what nurses do and how nurses influence patient outcomes are key to nursing's value to the health care system and to billing for nursing services.

THEORY-DRIVEN, EVIDENCE-BASED PRACTICE AND THE MODEL

The life perspective rhythm model certainly has components that are applicable to the practice setting; however, at present much more support needs to be provided for the essential elements of the model before implementation into practice can occur. The life perspective rhythm model is particularly suited for use with patient populations who are undergoing major life-changing events, which may be perceived as positive (childbirth, marriage, graduation) or negative (e.g., divorce, death of a loved one, major surgery) crisis experiences. Nurses in a variety of roles can assist such individuals to cope with these and other stressful life-changing events so as to successfully adapt and hence, add meaning to their lives. Further research into the central elements of the life perspective rhythm model may provide support for nursing interventions to assist individuals to cope with crisis experiences and promote health to the fullest extent possible.

SUMMARY OF THE MODEL CRITIQUE

A perspective is thought to lead to a knowledge system (Ellis, 1982). Ellis' (1968) characteristics of significant theories are applied to Fitzpatrick's (1983a) ideas and allow conclusions to be drawn about the relevance of the model for nursing. More specification is needed regarding syntax before formal conclusions can be made about testability and usefulness. As illustrated in the upcoming discussion, broadness in scope, complexity, implicit values, and information generated are potentially accounted for in this developing model.

Fitzpatrick's understanding of interactions between person and health continue to permit a broad application and interpretation of nursing phenomena. Conceptual relationships proposed in the model illustrate the potential scope for future investigations in nursing. Fitzpatrick's descriptions of person, environment, the indices of holistic human functioning, the meaning attached to life, the domain of health, the manner of deriving meaningful nursing activities, and the essence of nursing are undoubtedly complex. Even though Fitzpatrick and others have tested fragments of the model, some of the basic relationships have not been examined. As shown in the interventions emanating in gerontologic counseling (Fitzpatrick, 1982b), Fitzpatrick's model has usefulness in guiding the nature and direction of nursing practice through nursing classification systems. Through its close linkage with the meaning attached to life, Fitzpatrick's model highlights the value of health by means of investigations of suicide and temporal dimensions related to the elderly, the terminally ill, and hospitalized individuals. In addition, as doctoral students, Floyd (1982a) found support for Fitzpatrick's rhythm research interests in the reformulation of rhythm theories to a psychiatric-mental health nursing application, and Shiao (1993) found support for Fitzpatrick's model in developing an approach to study biologic rhythms in VLBW infants. Persisting weaknesses of the model at this time include a lack of parsimony in terminology and that the notion of health implicitly overlaps with a connotation of life perspective. Likewise, perceptual patterns might realistically be embodied within patterns of consciousness.

SIGNIFICANCE OF THE MODEL FOR THE DISCIPLINE

Donaldson and Crowley (1977) have isolated two major factors that are necessary for the continued growth, significance, and utility of the discipline of nursing. First, theories must be viewed in terms of the more basic structural conceptualizations of the discipline. Second, researchers must place their research within the context of the discipline.

Fitzpatrick has pointed out ways in which a community of scholars can be developed. She has articulated and continues to support means through which individual scholarship can be increased. She has discussed specific measures to enhance individual scholars' transmission of knowledge. Finally, Fitzpatrick has identified ways through which scholars might become increasingly organized as a group. If temporal, motion, consciousness, and perceptual patterns were used to guide the nursing classification efforts, theory-driven, evidenced-based practice could be realized. What is currently needed, however, is direct and concentrated attention to the development of the field of inquiry. What are the underlying mechanisms for how the field of inquiry can be organized into a recognizable and coherent whole? Although admittedly a difficult assignment, answers to these questions might be pursued through the development of syntax. The manner in which the community of scholars becomes hierarchically ordered cannot be addressed until some probable and/or tentative answers to the preceding questions are made available. In conclusion, progress is being made concerning the development of a field of inquiry, and the significance of Fitzpatrick's model for the ongoing development of a distinct discipline seems forthcoming.

SUMMARY

Fitzpatrick's Life Perspective Rhythm Model was developed as a field of inquiry for nursing and includes the metaparadigm concepts of person, environment, health, and nursing. One of the main ideas of the model is that meaning is essential to human life and a critical element of the human experience. Meaning is viewed as necessary to enhance and maintain life. The model is based on the work of Rogers' Science of Unitary Human Beings and Crisis Theory.

REFERENCES

Alford, P. A. (1981). *Temporal experience of individuals in a suicidal crisis.* Unpublished master's research project, Wayne State University, Detroit.

Allen, M. C., & Capute, A. J. (1990). Tone and reflex development before term. *Pediatrics, 85,* 393–399.

Als, H. (1982). Toward a synactive theory of development: Promise for assessment and support of infant individuality. *Infant Mental Health Journal, 3,* 229–243.

Ashworth, P. E. (1980). *Health status perception in middlescence I and middlescence II.* Unpublished master's research project, Wayne State University, Detroit.

Beebe, B., Stern, D., & Jaffe, J. (1979). The kinesic rhythm of mother-infant interactions. In A. W. Siegman & S. Feldstein (Eds.), *Of speech and time: Temporal patterns in interpersonal contexts* (pp. 110–132). Hillsdale, NJ: Erlbaum.

Bouwman, D. W. (1979). *Temporal perspective in middlescence I, middlescence II, and late adulthood.* Unpublished master's research project, Wayne State University, Detroit.

Brausell, J. M. (1977). *A comparison of psychological changes produced in aged persons as a result of passage of time, empathetic-clarifying counseling and response-outcome dependence counseling.* Unpublished master's research project, Wayne State University, Detroit.

Chaffer, N. R. (1979). *Temporal experiences of individuals in a suicidal crisis.* Unpublished master's research project, Wayne State University, Detroit.

Chiu, L. (1999). A phenomenological study on searching for meaning-in-life in women living with breast cancer [Abstract]. *Nursing Research (China), 7,* 119–128.

Cowan, C. (1995). The use of holistic nursing interventions in the treatment of breast cancer: A pilot study [Abstract]. *New Zealand Practice Nurse, 80,* 82–82.

Criddle, L. (1993). Healing from surgery: A phenomenological study. *IMAGE: Journal of Nursing Scholarship, 25,* 208–213.

Donaldson, S. K., & Crowley, D. M. (1977). Discipline of nursing: Structure and relationship to practice. *Communicating Nursing Research, 10,* 1–22.

Donovan, M. J., Fitzpatrick, J. J., & Johnston, R. L. (1980, September). *Temporal experiences related to the developmental process of aging.* Paper presented at the American Psychological Association Convention, Montreal, Canada.

Donovan, M. J., Fitzpatrick, J. J., & Johnston, R. L. (1981, August). *Aging, time and health.* Paper presented at the American Psychological Association Annual Convention, Los Angeles, CA.

Ellis, R. (1968). Characteristics of significant theories. *Nursing Research, 17,* 218–222.

Ellis, R. (1982). Conceptual issues in nursing. *Nursing Outlook, 30,* 406–410.

Engle, V. F. (1981). *A study of the relationship between self-assessment of health, function, personal tempo and time perception in elderly women.* Unpublished doctoral dissertation, Wayne State University, Detroit.

Fitzpatrick, J. J. (1975). *An investigation of the relationship between temporal orientation, temporal extension, and time perception.* Unpublished doctoral dissertation, New York University, New York.

Fitzpatrick, J. J. (1977, November). *Time and motion: Behavioral correlates among the aged.* Paper presented at Wayne State University, College of Nursing Research Reports, Detroit.

Fitzpatrick, J. J. (1979, June 13). Possible new variables for assessment and intervention. Paper presented at Indiana University, School of Nursing, Seminar in Nursing Futurology, Indianapolis, IN.

Fitzpatrick, J. J. (1980). Patients' perceptions of time: Current research. *International Nursing Review, 27,* 148–153.

Fitzpatrick, J. J. (1981a). Is nursing the science of health? *Center for Health Research NEWS,* Wayne State University, 2(2), Detroit.

Fitzpatrick, J. J. (1981b, April). *The essence of nursing.* Paper presented at the Lambda Chapter, Sigma Theta Tau Induction Ceremony, Detroit.

Fitzpatrick, J. J. (1981c, May). *The path of nursing: The path of science?* Paper presented at the Fourth Annual Nursing Research Symposium, Sigma Theta Tau Nursing Research Consortium, Detroit.

Fitzpatrick, J. J. (1981d, May 15). *Suicide and temporality: Programmatic research.* Paper presented at the University of Iowa, College of Nursing, Iowa City, IA.

Fitzpatrick, J. J. (1982a). The crisis perspective: Relationship to nursing. In J. J. Fitzpatrick, A. L. Whall, R. L. Johnston, & J. A. Floyd, *Nursing models and their psychiatric mental health applications* (pp. 19–36). Bowie, MD: R. J. Brady.

Fitzpatrick, J. J. (1982b). *Gerontological counseling.* In S. Lego (Ed.), *Lippincott manual of psychiatric nursing* (pp. 357–363). Philadelphia: J. B. Lippincott.

Fitzpatrick, J. J. (1982c, May 8). *Visions of nursing.* Paper presented at the Doctoral Homecoming, Wayne State University, College of Nursing, Detroit.

Fitzpatrick, J. J. (1983a). A life perspective rhythm model. In J. J. Fitzpatrick & A. L. Whall (Eds.), *Conceptual models of nursing: Analysis and applications* (pp. 295–302). Bowie, MD: R. J. Brady.

Fitzpatrick, J. J. (1983b, September 27). *Nursing science today and beyond.* Paper presented as a Distinguished Scholar Lecture, The Ohio State University, College of Nursing, Columbus, OH.

Fitzpatrick, J. J. (1985a, March 25). *Demystifying the research process.* Paper presented as part of the Yingling Scholars Series, Medical College of Virginia, Richmond, VA.

Fitzpatrick, J. J. (1986). Endowed chairs in nursing: State of the art. *Journal of Professional Nursing, 2,* 261–262.

Fitzpatrick, J. J. (1989). A life perspective rhythm model. In J. J. Fitzpatrick & A. L. Whall (Eds.), *Conceptual models of nursing: Analysis and application* (2nd ed., pp. 401–407). Norwalk, CT: Appleton-Century-Crofts.

Fitzpatrick, J. J., & Carnegie, M. E. (1991). Endowed chairs in nursing. *Nursing Outlook, 5,* 218–221.

Fitzpatrick, J. J., & Donovan, M. J. (1978a, May 13). *Temporal experiences among hospitalized individuals: A pilot study.* Paper presented at the First Sigma Theta Tau Nursing Research Symposium, Wayne State University, Detroit.

Fitzpatrick, J. J., & Donovan, M. J. (1978b). Temporal experience and motor behavior among the aging. *Research in Nursing and Health, 1,* 60–68.

Fitzpatrick, J. J., Donovan, M. J., & Johnston, R. L. (1979, May 5). *Temporal experiences among terminally ill cancer patients: An exploratory study.* Paper presented at the Second Annual Nursing Research Symposium, Sigma Theta Tau Nursing Consortium, Ann Arbor, MI.

Fitzpatrick, J. J., Donovan, M. J., & Johnston, R. L. (1980a). Experience of time during the crisis of cancer. *Cancer Nursing, 3,* 191–194.

Fitzpatrick, J. J., Johnston, R. L., & Donovan, M. J. (1980b, May 2). *Hospitalization as a crisis: Relation to temporal experiences.* Paper presented at the 13th Annual Conference of the Western Society for Research in Nursing, Los Angeles.

Flaherty, G. G., & Fitzpatrick, J. J. (1978). Relaxation technique to increase comfort level of postoperative patients: A preliminary study. *Nursing Research, 27,* 352–355.

Floyd, J. A. (1982a). Rhythm theory: Relationship to nursing conceptual models. In J. J. Fitzpatrick, A. L. Whall, R. L. Johnston, & J. A. Floyd (Eds.). (1983). *Nursing models and their psychiatric mental health applications* (pp. 95–116). Bowie, MD: R. J. Brady.

Floyd, J. A. (1982b). *Hospitalization, sleep-wake patterns and circadian type of psychiatric patients.* Unpublished doctoral dissertation, Wayne State University, Detroit.

Fromme, S. G. (1979). *The relationship between stated color preference and the vital signs of temperature, pulse rate, and respiratory rate.* Unpublished master's research project, Wayne State University, Detroit.

Goldberg, W. G., & Fitzpatrick, J. J. (1980). Movement therapy with the aged. *Nursing Research, 29,* 339–346.

Gray, R. E., Fitch, M. I., Phillips, C., Labrecque, M., & Klotz, L. (1999). Presurgery experiences of prostate cancer patients and their spouses. *Cancer Practice, 7,* 130–135.

Grider, J. A. (1977). *A descriptive study of time perception among hospitalized psychiatric patients.* Unpublished master's research project, Wayne State University, Detroit.

Guess, D., & Carr, E. (1991). Emergence and maintenance of stereotypy and self-injury. *American Journal of Mental Retardation, 96,* 299–319.

Hardy, M. E. (1974). Theories: Components, development, evaluation. *Nursing Research, 23,* 100–107.

Hardy, M. E. (1978). Perspectives on nursing theory. *Advances in Nursing Science, 1,* 37–48.

Hartline, C. A. (1978). *Temporal perspectives among terminally ill individuals.* Unpublished master's research project, Wayne State University, Detroit.

Haus, E. (1964). Periodicity in response to susceptibility to environmental stimuli. *Annals of the New York Academic Sciences, 107,* 361–373.

Horowitz, B. F., Fitzpatrick, J. J., & Flaherty, G. G. (1984). Relaxation techniques for pain relief after open heart surgery. *Dimensions in Critical Care Nursing, 3,* 364–371.

Isaacs, P. J. (1989). Crisis prevention in an outpatient surgery center. *MCN: The American Journal of Maternal Child Nursing, 14,* 352–354.

Jablonski, A. (1978). *Environmental effects of hospitalization on the mental status of elderly individuals.* Unpublished master's research project, Wayne State University, Detroit.

Johnston, R. L. (1980). *Temporality as a measure of unidirectionality within the Rogerian conceptual framework of nursing science.* Unpublished doctoral dissertation, Wayne State University, Detroit.

Johnston, R. L., Fitzpatrick, J. J., & Donovan, M. J. (1981, September). *Developmental stage: Relationship to temporal dimensions.* Paper presented at the ANA Council of Nurse Researchers Annual Meeting, Washington, DC.

Jones, E. K. (1977). *A comparison of temporal orientation in elderly institutionalized individuals.* Unpublished master's research project, Wayne State University, Detroit.

Klein, N., Hack, M., Gallaher, J., & Fanaroff, A. A. (1985). Preschool performance of children with normal intelligence who were very low birth weight infants. *Pediatrics, 75,* 531–537.

Kotal, B. A. (1980). *Subjective speed of time passage among adults.* Unpublished master's research project, Wayne State University, Detroit.

Kuhn, T. (1970). *The structure of scientific revolutions* (2nd ed.). Chicago: University of Chicago Press.

Laffrey, S. (1982). *Health behavior choice as related to self-actualization, body weight and health conception.* Unpublished doctoral dissertation, Wayne State University, Detroit.

Loveland-Cherry, C. (1982). *Family system patterns of cohesiveness and autonomy: Relation to family members' health behavior.* Unpublished doctoral dissertation, Wayne State University, Detroit.

Luce, G. G. (1970). *Biological rhythms in psychiatry and medicine.* Washington, DC: National Institute of Mental Health, U.S. Department of Health, Education, and Welfare.

Ludwig-Bonney, G. L. (1981). *The effect of tape recorded music on the pain experience of burn patients.* Unpublished master's thesis, Wayne State University, Detroit.

Mack, H. (1978). *Temporal experiences among psychiatric patients.* Unpublished master's research project, Wayne State University, Detroit.

McCormick, M. (1989). Long term follow-up of infants discharged from neonatal intensive care units. *JAMA, 261,* 1767–1772.

McDonald, S. (1981). *A study of the relationship between visible lightwaves and the experience of pain.* Unpublished doctoral dissertation, Wayne State University, Detroit.

Mirmiran, M., Kok, J. H., Boer, K., & Wolf, H. (1992). Perinatal development of human circadian rhythms: Role of the foetal biological clock. *Neuroscience and Biobehavioral Reviews, 16,* 371–378.

Montgomery, K. S. (2000). *Creating consistency and control out of chaos: The lived experience of planning a pregnancy as an adolescent.* Unpublished doctoral dissertation, Case Western Reserve University, Cleveland, OH.

Montgomery, K. S. (2001). Planned adolescent pregnancy: What they needed. *Issues in Comprehensive Pediatric Nursing, 24*(3), 19–29.

Moore, G. (1981). *Perceptual complexity, memory and human duration experience.* Unpublished doctoral dissertation, Wayne State University, Detroit.

Moore, S. L. (1997). A phenomenological study of meaning in life in suicidal older adults. *Archives of Psychiatric Nursing, 11,* 29–36.

Nalinnes, K. (1977). *Depression and temporal experience.* Unpublished master's research project, Wayne State University, Detroit.

Newman, M. A. (1979). *Theory development in nursing.* Philadelphia: F. A. Davis.

Pacini, C. M., & Fitzpatrick, J. J. (1982). Sleep patterns of hospitalized and non-hospitalized individuals. *Journal of Gerontological Nursing, 8,* 327–332.

Pasquali, E. A. (1999). The impact of premature menopause on women's experience of self [Abstract]. *Journal of Holistic Nursing, 17,* 346–364.

Perry, G. R. (1990). Loneliness and coping among tertiary-level adult cancer patients in the home. *Cancer Nursing, 13,* 293–302.

Porges, S. W. (1986). Respiratory sinus arrhythmia: Physiological basis, quantitative methods, and clinical implications. In P. Grossman, K. Jansen, & D. Vaitl (Eds.), *Cardiorespiratory and cardiosomatic psychophysiology* (pp. 206–211). New York: Plenum.

Porges, S. W. (1991). Vagal tone: An autonomic mediator of affect. In J. Garber & K. A. Dodge (Eds.), *The development of emotion regulation and dysregulation* (pp. 111–128). Cambridge: Cambridge University Press.

Porges, S. W. (1992). Vagal tone: A physiologic marker of stress vulnerability. *Pediatrics, 90,* 498–504.

Porges, S. W., & Byrne, E. A. (1992). Research methods for measurement of heart rate and respiration. *Biological Psychology, 34,* 93–130.

Porges, S. W., Matthews, K. A., & Pauls, D. L. (1992). The biobehavioral interface in behavioral pediatrics. *Pediatrics, 90,* 789–797.

Pressler, J. L. (1983). Fitzpatrick's rhythm model: Analysis for nursing science. In J. J. Fitzpatrick & A. L. Whall (Eds.), *Conceptual models of nursing: Analysis and application* (pp. 302–322). Bowie, MD: R. J. Brady.

Pressler, J. L. (1989). Fitzpatrick's rhythm model: A second look. In J. J. Fitzpatrick & A. L. Whall (Eds.), *Conceptual models of nursing: Analysis and application* (2nd ed., pp. 409–426). Norwalk, CT: Appleton-Century-Crofts.

Pressler, J. L., Wells, N., & Hepworth, J. T. (1993). *Methodological issues in preterm infant outcomes.* Research grant, NIH, NINR, 1 RO1 NR-03691, Vanderbilt University, Nashville, TN.

Quillin, S. M. (1983). *Growth and development of infant and mother and mother-infant synchrony.* Unpublished doctoral dissertation, Wayne State University, Detroit.

Ramin, C. J. (1982). *Reminiscence therapy: Changes in morale and self-esteem.* Unpublished master's thesis, Wayne State University, Detroit.

Reed, P. G. (1982). *Religious perspective, death perspective and well-being among death-involved and non-death involved individuals.* Unpublished doctoral dissertation, Wayne State University, Detroit.

Roberts, B. L., & Fitzpatrick, J. J. (1983). Improving balance: Therapy of movement. *Journal of Gerontological Nursing, 9,* 151–156.

Rogers, M. E. (1970). *An introduction to the theoretic basis of nursing.* Philadelphia: F. A. Davis.

Rogers, M. E. (1979). *Postulated correlates of unitary human development.* Unpublished course materials, New York University, Division of Nursing, New York, NY.

Rogers, M. E. (1980). Nursing: A science of unitary man. In J. P. Riehl & C. Roy (Eds.), *Conceptual models for nursing practice* (2nd ed., pp. 329–337). New York: Appleton-Century-Crofts.

Rogers, M. E. (1983). *Science of unitary human beings: A paradigm for nursing.* Unpublished manuscript, New York University, New York.

Roslaniec, A., Fitzpatrick, J. J. (1979). Changes in mental status in older adults with four days of hospitalization. *Research in Nursing and Health, 2,* 177–187.

Ross, L. A. (1996). Teaching spiritual care to nurses [Abstract]. *Nurse Education Today, 16,* 38–43.

Schorr, J. (1982). *Behavior patterns, temporal orientation and death anxiety.* Unpublished doctoral dissertation, Wayne State University, Detroit.

Shiao, S-Y. P. K. (1993). *Nasal gastric tube placement: Effect on sucking and breathing in very low birth weight infants.* Unpublished doctoral dissertation, Case Western Reserve University, Cleveland, OH.

Sipols-Lenss, M. (1982). *Vestibular stimulation: Effects on gross motor activity and weight of premature infants.* Unpublished master's thesis, Wayne State University, Detroit.

Smith, J. A. (1981). The idea of health: A philosophical inquiry. *Advances in Nursing Science, 3,* 43–50.

Smokvina, G. J. (1976). *Aging and institutionalization as determinants of temporal and motor phenomena: The data collection process and problems.* Unpublished master's research project, Wayne State University, Detroit.

Stern, D. (1971). A micro-analysis of mother-infant interaction. *Journal of the American Academy of Child Psychiatry, 10,* 501–517.

Waller, L. (1989). Fuzzy logic: It's comprehensible, it's practical—and it's commercial. *Electronics, 3,* 102–103.

Yarcheski, A., & Mahon, N. E. (1995). Rogers's pattern manifestations and health in adolescents. *Western Journal of Nursing Research, 17,* 383–397.

Zadeh, L. A. (1990, April 20). *Fuzzy logic: Approximate reasoning in solving complex problems.* Unpublished paper presented at Vanderbilt University, School of Nursing, Nashville, TN.

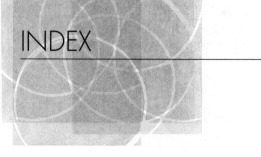

INDEX

Page numbers followed by "b" indicate boxed material
Page numbers followed by "f" indicate a figure
Page numbers followed by "t" indicate a table